HUMAN NUTRITION

Formerly **The Heinz Handbook of Nutrition**

EDITORIAL BOARD

HUMAN NUTRITION

Formerly **The Heinz Handbook of Nutrition**

THIRD EDITION

A Textbook of Nutrition in Health and Disease

Benjamin T. Burton, Ph.D.

National Institute of Arthritis, Metabolism, and
Digestive Diseases
National Institutes of Health

Published for **H. J. HEINZ COMPANY**
McGRAW-HILL BOOK COMPANY

A BLAKISTON PUBLICATION

New York   St. Louis   San Francisco   Auckland   Düsseldorf
Johannesburg   Kuala Lumpur   London   Mexico   Montreal   New Delhi
Panama   Paris   São Paulo   Singapore   Sydney   Tokyo   Toronto

Library of Congress Cataloging in Publication Data

Burton, Benjamin T
    Human nutrition.

    "A Blakiston publication."
    Includes index.
    1. Nutrition. 2. Diet in disease. I. Heinz (H. J.)
Company. II. Heinz (H. J.) Company. The Heinz handbook
of nutrition. III. Title. [DNLM: 1. Diet therapy.
2. Nutrition. 3. Nutrition disorders. QU145 B974h]
QP141.H4 1976   612'.3   75-4875
ISBN 0-07-009282-6
ISBN 0-07-009281-8 pbk.

HUMAN NUTRITION

5 6 7 8 9 0 K P K P 7832109

This book was set in Times Roman by Black Dot, Inc.
The editors were J. Dereck Jeffers and Michael LaBarbera;
the cover was designed by Pencils Portfolio, Inc.;
the production supervisor was Judi Frey.
The drawings were done by ECL Art Associates, Inc.
Kingsport Press, Inc., was printer and binder.

Contents

Part 3
NUTRITION IN HEALTH

Part 4
NUTRITION IN DISEASE

Part 5
ADDITIONAL ASPECTS OF HUMAN NUTRITION

Foreword

The first edition of this textbook of human nutrition in health and disease was published in 1959 under the title *The Heinz Handbook of Nutrition*. Since then it has seen two editions and worldwide distribution, including translation into Spanish and Arabic.

The change in the title to *Human Nutrition* is made in the belief that a title of broader connotation would better serve the classroom, the medical profession, and nutrition scientists. I feel justified in saying that we are proud that this book which we initiated is now in its third edition, that the author and distinguished editorial board have concurred in a continuous updating of the content during the last fifteen years.

The science of nutrition and its application are worldwide in scope. Solutions to problems of nutrition appear vital to long range improvement of public health, to the prevention of disease, and the advancement of human welfare. We sincerely hope that this textbook will continue to play a useful role in the achievement of these objectives.

H. J. HEINZ II

Preface

During the last two decades, the science of nutrition has grown progressively broader in scope. It has therefore become increasingly difficult to contain this multifaceted body of knowledge in one volume and still do justice to its various aspects. The subject matter of this book is organized as follows: The first part deals with the basic physiology and biochemistry of the human body as it relates to food intake and utilization. The second part presents the various nutrients, their sources, metabolism, physiology, and interrelationships. The third part encompasses human nutritional requirements and nutrition under varying conditions of health and in periods of physiologic stress. The fourth part is devoted to nutrition in disease—the relationship between nutrition and specific diseases and the practical therapeutic and preventive aspects of special diets. The fifth part presents miscellaneous, but essential, aspects of nutrition not directly related to the first four subdivisions.

A determined effort was made to have the material in this book represent the mainstream of accepted contemporary scientific and clinical opinion. Since a slight degree of empiricism is almost unavoidable in diet therapy, only the most convincing evidence was used for guidance in the presentation of special diets. Specific literature references were not cited since it was felt that the object of this book is to present concise, up-to-date and accepted information—not to serve as a key to the existing voluminous literature. Moreover, the knowledge of nutrition and its application in medicine is progressing so rapidly that the reader interested in a deep study of a specific topic must use current literature to keep abreast of all developments. In order to avoid needless duplication and to correlate better the subject matter, numerous cross references are made from chapter to chapter.

The last fifteen years have seen a heartening acceptance of this book, both in the United States and abroad. In 1961, it was published in Arabic translation in Cairo, Egypt. In 1966 it was translated into Spanish and published by the Pan American Health Organization for distribution in Latin America under the title "Nutricion Humana," followed by a second edition in 1969. It is hoped that in the years to come the present, considerably enlarged and revised, third edition will continue to further nutrition education at home and overseas.

The six members of the Editorial Board have been generous advisers in the editing of this edition, and their help is gratefully acknowledged. The death of one of them, Dr. Grace Goldsmith, just prior to publication, is a sorrow to all in the field of nutrition.

BENJAMIN T. BURTON

HUMAN NUTRITION

Formerly **The Heinz Handbook of Nutrition**

Part One

Utilization of Foods

Chapter 1

The Physiology of the Gastrointestinal Tract and Digestion

The term *food* embraces those substances which are taken into the body to support growth, maintain body functions, repair or replace tissues, and provide energy. As a rule we regard as foods only substances which enter the body through the alimentary tract, though, strictly speaking, oxygen fits into the definition.

The preliminary steps in the utilization of foods often involve profound physical and chemical changes which are essential to render the nutritive substances digestible and absorbable.

Mastication

In the mouth food undergoes repeated maceration through the grinding and crushing action of the teeth. Simultaneously, the food mass is being moistened and softened by saliva. Saliva acts as a lubricant and thus aids in swallowing; it also serves a chemical function since it contains ptyalin, a starch-splitting enzyme, which hydrolyzes starch into dextrins and maltose. This action depends on a neutral or alkaline pH and is inhibited by an acid environment; it starts in the mouth and is brought to partial completion in the stomach and small intestine since the masticated food does not remain in the mouth long enough, nor is it alkaline or neutral for very long in the stomach.

In the mouth the moistened and macerated food comes into intimate contact with the end organs for the sense of taste, located in the tongue and palate. If agreeable, the taste sensation (really the result of the combined action of taste and smell) serves as a psychic stimulus for continued food intake. It also serves the important purpose of stimulating the flow of gastric digestive juices. The mouth is instrumental in preservation of the body's water balance; the drying of the oral mucous membranes arouses the sensation of thirst, which serves as a protective mechanism against dehydration.

Also, while in the mouth and throat, masticated food comes in contact with a recently discovered fat-splitting enzyme—pharyngeal lipase—which facilitates the hydrolysis of triglyceride fats into free fatty acids and mono- and diglycerides. This lipolytic activity is initiated in the throat upon swallowing and continues during passage of the masticated food through the esophagus and stomach.

Deglutition

After mastication has been completed, the food bolus is placed far back upon the tongue, at which point reflex swallowing contractions force the food backward and downward through the pharynx, the common air and food passage, into the upper part of the esophagus. With the initiation of deglutition the individual loses voluntary control over the fate of the ingested food until he is ready to expel the unusable portion of the ingesta.

Once the food bolus has reached the upper region of the esophagus, a wave of contraction propels it toward the distal end, where the cardiac sphincter, a circular ring of muscle, guards the entrance to the stomach. This may open to permit immediate entrance to the food or may await the second peristaltic wave to admit food from both waves simultaneously.

The Stomach

Three main divisions of the stomach are recognized: the upper, cardiac portion; the large rounded pouchlike main body, the fundus; and the lower outlet, the pylorus. The fundus serves to store food and is the site where the major portion of gastric juice is secreted and the largest part of gastric digestion occurs. The muscular pyloric region and its sphincter provide the mechanism for manipulation and expulsion of the gastric contents at the proper time. The semisolid food aggregates which enter the stomach accumulate in a somewhat stratified mass. That which entered first spreads out toward the periphery, while that which was swallowed later remains in the center of the mass. This arrangement of the ingesta permits the center of the mass in the fundus to remain alkaline or neutral and to continue salivary digestion for 30 minutes or more. In the meanwhile, gastric digestion begins in the outer layers. The acid gastric juices are gradually worked into the mass by tonic contractions. Eventually, peristaltic waves which begin at about the middle of the stomach break up the food aggregates and sweep them toward the duodenum. These contractions vary in depth and strength; their tempo increases as digestion progresses.

The pyloric sphincter is a powerful ring of muscle located at the lower outlet of the stomach. Normally it is quiescent and relaxed, but it contracts strongly when a peristaltic wave approaches it. The sphincter opens after three or four peristaltic waves and permits the chyme, the thoroughly mixed and liquefied acid food mass, to be propelled into the duodenum. Subsequently the sphincter will remain shut until the chyme in the proximal part of the duodenum has changed from an acid to a neutral pH. In addition to resisting untimely gastric evacuation, the pyloric sphincter normally prevents any except minimal duodenal regurgitation.

Ordinarily, portions of the average mixed solid meal remain in the stomach 3 to $4^{1}/_{2}$ hours. In contrast to solid foods, liquids seem to take the path of least resistance and remain in the stomach for very brief periods only. Gastric peristaltic contracture is influenced by both the nature of the food and emotional mechanisms. Of the solids, fats display an inhibitory action on gastric motility and evacuation; they pass through the stomach at a slow rate. Proteins traverse the stomach somewhat more rapidly, and carbohydrates pass through it still faster. Hostility, anger, and resentment may result in contractile gastric hyperfunction; fear and depression, on the other hand, may result in gastric hypofunction and hypomotility.

Gastric Digestion

The gastric mucosa secretes hydrochloric acid, mucin, water, and a number of enzymes: (1) pepsin, which digests proteins, (2) rennin, which curdles milk, and (3) gastric lipase, which has a relatively weak lipolytic effect. Another proteolytic enzyme in gastric juice, *gastricsin*, has been described and characterized. It is said to account for about half the proteolytic activity of gastric juice. The normal gastric mucosa also elaborates a substance of protein or polypeptide nature, which facilitates the absorption of vitamin B_{12} (Chap. 11). The chief digestive action of the stomach is the splitting of proteins. This takes place in an acid medium only, at an optimum pH of 1.5, and is facilitated by the hydrochloric acid secreted by the parietal cells of the gastric mucosa. The proteolytic action of gastric pepsin is limited and does not go much beyond the formation of proteoses and peptones, relatively large intermediates in the breakdown of protein molecules to their component amino acids (Chap. 7). Rennin splits the principal milk protein casein into soluble paracasein, which forms an insoluble curd in the presence of calcium. In addition to these changes, the amylolytic action of the salivary enzyme ptyalin continues in the central parts of the food bolus which have not become acidified.

Gastric mucin serves as a mechanical lubricant and emollient and may protect the mucosa against the acid digestive juice through its local buffering effect.

The secretion of gastric juice is stimulated by psychic, nervous, chemical, and mechanical factors. Smelling or tasting food, as well as seeing or thinking about it, may initiate gastric secretion. Conversely, anger, fear, and excitement or repulsive sights and odors tend to inhibit the flow of gastric juice. A direct mechanical stimulation of gastric secretion is caused by the distention of the stomach musculature by the food. Chemical stimulation of the gastric mucosa has a much more pronounced effect; proteoses and peptones, meat extractives and broths evoke a copious secretion. The postulated mechanism for this excitation involves the formation of a hormone, gastrin, in the pyloric mucosa in the presence of food and particularly protein breakdown products; gastrin is then absorbed into the bloodstream and carried to the cells of the fundus, where it excites secretion of gastric juice.

The gastric glands are also subject to humoral control originating in the duodenum. The contact of food or protein-split products with the duodenal mucosa will excite an increased flow of gastric juice. Conversely, gastric secretion is decreased when ingested fats reach the small intestine.

A discussion of gastric physiology would be incomplete without mention of the protective action exerted by the highly acid gastric juice in destroying or inhibiting the many and varied microorganisms which accompany normal food intake. The bacteriocidal or bacteriostatic action of the stomach secretions probably constitutes the body's first and major defense against food-borne infection; it also aids in maintaining qualitative stability in the intestinal flora distal to the stomach.

The Small Intestine

The most important digestive processes take place in the small intestine, and most of the end products of digestion are absorbed into the bloodstream here. After passing into the intestine, the chyme is subject to a variety of muscular movements. Two types of peristaltic waves propel the chyme caudally: (1) sluggish contractions, moving slowly for short distances of the intestine, and (2) sweeping rush waves which carry the intestinal contents for longer distances. In addition, the chyme is mixed and brought into intimate contact with the intestinal mucosa by segmenting movements, rhythmic annular contractions which repeatedly divide and subdivide the food mass.

The digestive secretions in the small intestine come from three sources: the pancreas, the glands of the intestinal mucosa, and the liver.

Pancreatic Secretions

The pancreatic secretions contribute several enzymes:

1 Trypsin is a strongly proteolytic enzyme capable of splitting proteins into polypeptide fragments. Trypsin appears to attack only specific linkages in the interior of a native peptide chain, those next to arginine or lysine moieties. Trypsin is secreted by the pancreatic cells in the form of the inactive precursor trypsinogen, which is converted into the active enzyme trypsin in the presence of enterokinase of the intestinal juice.

2 Chymotrypsin is secreted as the inactive precursor chymotrypsinogen. Chymotrypsin, like trypsin, splits proteins into polypeptide fragments and attacks only specific linkages in the interior of a native peptide chain, those next to tyrosine, phenylalanine, tryptophan, or methionine.

3 Pancreatic carboxypeptidase hydrolyzes polypeptides into smaller peptides and amino acids. This enzyme specifically attacks peptide linkages next to a terminal amino acid (on a polypeptide chain) which possesses a free carboxy group, splitting off single amino acids from the chain.

4 Pancreatic amylase hydrolyzes starch to dextrins and maltose.

5 Pancreatic lipase is a fat-splitting enzyme which hydrolyzes fats to glycerol and fatty acids, probably through the stages of mono- and diglycerides.

Pancreatic secretion is under both nervous and humoral control. Nervous stimulation, conditioned by the cephalic sensations associated with food intake, is not extensive. The major stimulation for secretion of pancreatic juice is through secretin, a hormone liberated by the intestinal mucosa when it comes in contact with the acid chyme from the stomach. Secretin enters the bloodstream and is carried to the pancreatic cells, where it stimulates active secretion. Acid chyme also causes the mucosal cells of the duodenum and upper jejunum to release into the circulation the hormone pancreozymin-cholecystokinin, which stimulates the production of pancreatic enzymes.

Intestinal Secretions

The succus entericus, or intestinal juice, is secreted by the glands of the intestinal mucosa. Mechanical stimulation of the wall of the intestine promotes active secretion of the succus entericus. A hormonal stimulatory mechanism has also been demonstrated. The hormone enterocrinin is elaborated in the intestinal mucosa in the presence of the chyme and appears to activate the cells of the intestinal glands directly.

The intestinal juice is alkaline in reaction. It contributes the following digestive enzymes:

1 Peptidases, which hydrolyze polypeptides into smaller peptides and amino acids. In contrast to pancreatic carboxypeptidase, intestinal peptidases specifically attack peptide linkages next to a terminal amino acid which possesses a free amino group, splitting off single amino acids from the chain.

2 Phosphatases, which hydrolyze phosphorylated compounds like hexosephosphates, glycerophosphates, and nucleotides into inorganic phosphate and the organic component of the molecule.

3 Carbohydrases, which split disaccharides like maltose, lactose, and sucrose into their respective monosaccharide components, liberating glucose, galactose, and fructose.

4 Intestinal lipase, a fat-splitting enzyme of relatively little importance.

Bile

Bile is secreted by the hepatic cells and accumulates in the gallbladder during interdigestive periods. The gallbladder mucosa concentrates the dilute biliary secretion through selective reabsorption of water. Both hormonal and nervous mechanisms cause the gallbladder to empty; the latter pathway is apparently of less importance. The presence of certain food components, especially fats, in the small intestine initiates the elaboration of pancreozymin-cholecystokinin in the intestinal mucosa. When brought to the gallbladder by the bloodstream, this hormone specifically causes contraction of the storage organ and evacuation of the concentrated bile into the duodenum via the common duct.

Bile contains the bile salts sodium glycocholate and taurocholate, bile pigments, lecithin, and cholesterol. It does not contain digestive enzymes of importance, but is of extreme significance for proper digestion and absorption of fat by virtue of its efficient emulsifying action. The bile salts lower the surface tension of large fat globules and particles in the semiliquid intestinal contents and thus facilitate their subdivision into progressively smaller globules under the constant mechanical churning action of the small intestine. Consequently, the food fat is reduced into a fine emulsion which exposes an enormously increased surface of fine fat globules to the saponifying action of pancreatic lipase. The bile salts also facilitate the solution in the aqueous medium of the long-chain fatty acids which are liberated by the hydrolysis of fats to fatty acids and glycerol. In the absence of bile, neither partially hydrolyzed fat (mono- and diglycerides) nor fatty acids can traverse the mucosal barrier into the blood and lymph vessels of the intestine. The absorption of the fat-soluble vitamins and carotenes also depends on the presence of bile salts.

The bile pigments play no part in the digestive process. Bilirubin and biliverdin are hemoglobin breakdown products which are formed in cells of the reticuloendothelial system. The bile serves mainly as a pathway of excretion for these pigments, which lend their color to the feces.

Normally the liver converts significant amounts of cholesterol to bile salts, and this bile constitutes a major route of disposal of this substance. A relationship between the conversion of excessive amounts of cholesterol to bile salts and the maintenance of blood cholesterol levels is highly probable.

The Large Intestine

The large intestine serves as the terminal reservoir of the gastrointestinal tract. It absorbs the last remaining digested food constituents and actively reabsorbs any excess fluid from the semiliquid digested mass. Most of the water and dissolved electrolytes were secreted into the food mass by the more proximal parts of the gastrointestinal tract, and this function of the large intestine is essential for the body's water and electrolyte economy. A certain amount of active excretion of substances from the bloodstream into the visceral lumen may take place here as well. The large intestine also serves as an incubator which permits bacteria to degrade some materials which were resistant to the previous process of digestion.

The movements of the colon are sluggish in comparison with those of the small intestine. To a certain extent the contents of the large intestine move caudally because of the pressure exerted by the material expelled from the ileum. Weak peristalsis can be demonstrated throughout the length of the large intestine; however, antiperistaltic waves have also been observed in the proximal portions. The function of such waves would be to retard the passage of material which has been insufficiently dehydrated.

The Intestinal Flora

At birth, the gastrointestinal tract is sterile, but thereafter establishment of a microbial population proceeds rapidly. Until a more varied, solid diet is introduced, *Lactobacillus bifidus* predominates in the intestine of the breast-fed infant and *L. acidophilus* in infants fed cow's milk. Later, a more varied microflora becomes established. Among these organisms, *Escherichia coli*, other members of the coli-aerogenes group, *Bacillus subtilis*, yeasts, and molds have been recognized in the past. New studies indicate that the usually recognized forms normally represent a very small proportion of the intestinal flora. The bulk are anaerobic organisms belonging to the genera *Streptococcus, Lactobacillus,* and *Diploccus.*

The feeding of a predominantly carbohydrate diet leads to an increase in gram-positive, fermentative organisms, and, conversely, a high protein intake promotes a more gram-negative, putrefactive flora.

The microbial population of the large intestine and cecum plays a more important role than has been ascribed to it in the past. Experimental animals whose intestinal flora has been significantly altered or depressed with the aid of antibiotics have exhibited a wide spectrum of deficiency syndromes, attesting to the fact that they are normally dependent on synthesis of several essential nutritional factors by the normal microbial population which inhabits the large intestine. The synthesis of vitamin K, vitamin B_{12}, thiamin, biotin, folic acid, and perhaps niacin by the intestinal flora has been indirectly demonstrated in this fashion in laboratory animals.

The establishment of an intestinal flora in the human newborn alleviates its hypoprothrombinemia through the elaboration of vitamin K in the large intestine (which is absorbed and subsequently facilitates prothrombin synthesis in the liver). Part of the human vitamin B_{12} and thiamin requirements is probably satisfied in a similar fashion, as is the (still somewhat doubtful) requirement for biotin. The human need for many vitamins of the B complex varies with the nature of the ingested carbohydrates. In contrast to refined mono- and disaccharides, complex polysaccharides and sorbitol seemingly lower the B complex requirement by causing changes in the intestinal micro-flora which are inducive to increased absorption or bacterial vitamin synthesis. Conversely, the presence of thiamin-splitting bacteria in the intestinal tract will increase the thiamin requirement of the individual harboring such an organism. The thiamin blood level of patients suffering from "thiaminase disease" is significantly lower than that of normal persons; thiamin given orally to the patients is actually decomposed by a specific thiamin-splitting enzyme elabo-rated in the intestinal tract by such organisms.

The Feces

Up to one-third of the human feces is composed of bacteria originating in the large intestine. The rest is composed of cellular material desquamated into the lumen of the gastrointestinal tract, intestinal secretions and excretions, and to a smaller extent unabsorbed food residues. The residue of indigestible cellulose, hemicellulose, and lignin is greater when large amounts of fruits and vegetables are eaten. These indigestible residues of plant origin, commonly referred to as *roughage, fiber,* or *bulk*, contribute little or nothing of nutritional value per se to the body. However, it is desirable to have some indigestible residue left in the lower gastrointestinal level to maintain muscle tone of the colon and to keep it functioning normally. If the bulk of material in the lower intestine is too small, there is little stimulation for the intestinal musculature to move the residue along and produce evacuations frequently enough to make for intestinal well-being.

Chapter 2

Absorption, Cell Metabolism, and Excretion

Gastrointestinal digestion and absorption of nutrients in the human is extremely efficient. The fecal excretion of protein, carbohydrate, and fat constitutes only a very small percentage of the oral intake of these substances. The nitrogen content of the feces is practically independent of the quality of dietary protein; it is usually about 1.5 g per day and rarely exceeds 3 g daily in the healthy individual. (Pancreatic disease with concomitant impaired protein digestion or an excess of indigestible roughage in the diet will, however, result in higher fecal nitrogen figures.) Evidently, the fecal nitrogen is derived primarily from the bacterial residue and the secretions of the gastrointestinal tract.

Ordinarily, more than 95 percent of the dietary fat is absorbed, and only negligible quantities of carbohydrates are found in the feces, even when the carbohydrate intake is high.

Gastric Absorption

Absorption of nutrients from the stomach is practically nonexistent. Even water passes through this organ, to be absorbed subsequently in the intestine. Alcohol constitutes the main exception; it is absorbed to a large extent from the stomach.

Intestinal Absorption

Practically all the absorption of nutrients takes place in the intestine, most of this in the small intestine. Preliminary gastrointestinal digestion has broken down proteins, carbohydrates, and fats into more soluble, simple compounds of smaller molecular size which are capable of diffusion through the semipermeable mucosal barrier into the network of intestinal capillaries and lymphatics. Absorption is thus concerned with amino acids, fatty acids, glycerol, monosaccharides, minerals, and vitamins and their transportation across the cells of the intestinal mucosa into the circulation. This process is far from being a passive diffusion of solutes governed only by the physical factors involved. In a simple collodion membrane system the factors influencing diffusion from one compartment to the other are permeability of the membrane (which depends primarily on size of the pores), diffusibility of the solute (which depends primarily on the size of the molecule), concentration of the solute on both sides of the membrane, surface tension, temperature, and electrical membrane potentials. To a large extent these factors are also operative in the passive diffusion of soluble nutrients across the mucosal barrier. However, transit of nutrients from the intestinal lumen to the blood and lymph is also subject to the forces exerted by the living properties of the mucosa. In many instances absorption from the gut runs counter to the laws of simple diffusion because of the active participation of the epithelial cells in transportation of the nutrient across the mucosal barrier and chemical transformation of the nutrient in the mucosal cells before it passes into the circulation.

The absorption of individual nutrients is discussed in later chapters dealing with the various food constituents.

Transportation

Once the various nutrients have entered the bloodstream, they are carried to the liver by way of the portal vein and from there to the tissues. Fat which has passed into the lymphatics is carried into the thoracic duct, the main lymphatic channel draining the intestinal lymph vessels, and thence into the venous circulation at large. As the various nutrients are swept to the body tissues by the blood, an osmotic exchange takes place locally between the capillary blood, the extracellular interstitial fluid, and the cell which requires the nutrients. The nutrient, be it an amino acid, hexose sugar, or mineral salt, is present in the arterial capillary blood in a higher concentration than in the interstitial fluid or the cell proper. Following the existing concentration gradient, the food element diffuses through the endothelial cells which make up the capillary wall and dissolves in the extracellular fluid in which the local tissue cell is bathed. Following osmotic forces, it then diffuses into the cells, which exhibit a lower concentration of the particular nutrient. The transfer of oxygen (which should be considered another nutrient) from the arterial capillary blood to the cell level follows a similar course, though the mechanism involved is somewhat more complicated.

Cell Metabolism

Within the individual tissue cell occur the chemical transformations of nutrients which are lumped together under the term *metabolism*—oxidation and degradation, release of energy, interconversion and transformation, synthesis and storage. These chemical reactions are catalyzed by a host of specific enzymes which constitute the inherent armamentarium of each cell. The complement of enzymes which a cell possesses is specific for the particular tissue. For instance, liver cells, charged with the major chemical activity in the body, contain a much wider spectrum of enzymes (each one specific for a particular type of transformation) than the chemically relatively inert fat storage cells in the human subcutaneous adipose tissue.

The specific nature of the metabolism of each cell is determined by its inherent complement of enzymes, its native protoplasmic content and cellular structure, surface phenomena, and lesser factors. The rate at which cellular metabolic reactions proceed depends on the concentrations of the reacting compounds and availability of the enzyme; however, the rate is also under the control of hormones, chemical regulators secreted by the endocrine glands and carried by the bloodstream to the tissues on which they exert their regulatory action. Hormones are specific in their activity. They influence particular tissues only and regulate specific types of reactions; nevertheless, a hormone, although primarily concerned with one aspect of metabolism, indirectly influences others as well. Altogether, it is evident that the normal balance of cellular metabolism, or *metabolic homeostatis,* depends on an adequate supply of nutrients, on a normal synthesis of cellular enzymes which catalyze the cellular transformations, and an adequate secretion of hormones to regulate their rate. Abnormalities and deficiencies in any one of these factors upset the metabolic equilibrium of the body.

Individual enzymes, hormones, and metabolic reactions are discussed in later chapters.

Excretion

Just as the absorbed nutrients are transported to the cells by way of the extracellular fluids, the metabolic end products are swept from the cells to the excretory organs by the same fluids. Carbon dioxide and water, which are the ultimate end products of the complete degradation of carbohydrates (and to a major extent of proteins and fats as well), diffuse into the interstitial fluid surrounding the cell, and thence through the endothelial cells of the venous capillaries into the venous circulation. The carbon dioxide is subsequently eliminated from the venous blood by the lungs, and any excess of water in the extracellular fluids is eliminated by the kidney (and to a less extent by the lungs and skin). Urea, and to a much less extent ammonium salts, which are the other ultimate end products of amino acid catabolism, are also selectively eliminated by the kidney from the circulating blood. The kidney and lungs thus serve as the major excretory organs for metabolic end products. To a minor extent excretion of some substances takes place into the intestinal lumen, either directly or by way of the bile. This will be taken up whenever the specific food constituents are discussed.

Chapter 3

Fluid, Electrolyte, and Acid-Base Balance

The normal life processes of an organism depend on its ability to maintain a constant internal environment, a state of internal equilibrium, or homeostasis, which rules out physical and chemical extremes that are detrimental to its welfare. Some of the mechanisms with which the human body maintains its homeostasis are touched upon below.

External Fluid Balance

Water and electrolytes (ionizable salts) are essential dietary constituents for normal cell metabolism. The tissue cell is in positive balance with regard to water and electrolytes when it accumulates them and in negative balance when it loses them. In contrast to the nutritional balance of carbohydrates, fats, and proteins, the consequences of abnormal gain or loss of water and electrolytes are markedly acute. Water and electrolytes must be supplied to the individual regularly to compensate for the obligatory losses connected with the daily normal physiologic processes.

Water enters the body in the form of imbibed fluids and as a component of most solid foods. Some water is also formed within the body by the oxidation of the hydrogen which is a component of the solid nutrients. Most conventional solid foods contain between 65 and 90 percent water and thus account for a considerable portion of the daily water intake. Water is excreted from the body by the kidney in the form of urine and is lost through evaporation from the skin and lungs and as a component of the feces. The loss of water through the air expired in the lungs may be considerable in a dry climate even though the individual produces no visible sweat. Table 1 illustrates the daily water balance in the average individual in a temperate climate.

When fluid intake is restricted or ceases outright, obligatory losses of water through the kidney, skin, and lungs continue. The earliest sign of water depletion is thirst, which is felt when 2 percent of the body weight, or more, is lost through dehydration. Apparently two mechanisms actively allay thirst. One is the learned reflex of drinking whenever the mucous lining of the mouth feels dry. An unconscious stimulus to drinking is apparently mediated through special cells, located in the hypothalamic region of the brain, which respond to changes in the osmotic pressure of the blood serum (and extracellular fluids in general). When water deprivation occurs, the kidney attempts to compensate by excreting a more concentrated urine containing more solutes and less water. In more severe conditions of water depletion, the kidney excretes smaller quantities of solutes and a still smaller volume of urine in an effort to conserve body water.

Electrolyte depletion may occur under conditions of abnormal loss of body fluids when water alone is being replaced. This may be observed when an individual perspires excessively under conditions of hard physical labor in a very hot environment and drinks large quantities of water to allay his thirst. Under such circumstances, large quantities of sodium chloride are lost to the body through excessive perspiration. Other instances of pathologic electrolyte loss are represented by the acutely ill individual who vomits profusely, losing large quantities of chloride (from the gastric hydrochloric acid) with his stomach contents. Another example is the person with copious diarrhea who

Table 1 Typical Individual Water Balance

Intake	Volume, cc
Liquid foods	1,300–1,500
Moisture from solid foods	500–800
Water derived from oxidation of foods in the body	300–500
	2,100–2,800
Average	2,450
Output	
Urine	1,080–1,650
Feces	100–150
Evaporation from the skin (sweat)	550–600
Expired from the lungs as moist air	370–400
	2,100–2,800
Average	2,450

loses electrolytes and other secretions from the intestinal tract, or the patient who has a fistula with extensive fluid loss, or gastric and intestinal suction with loss of large volumes of secretions. Replacement of these body fluids with water or a parenteral water-dextrose infusion does not make up for the existing electrolyte loss. When water alone is replaced, the kidney will attempt to compensate by excreting a dilute urine, conserving the body's electrolytes but eliminating the water.

The Fluid Compartments and Osmotic Equilibrium

Capillary walls and cell membranes divide the water of the body into three major fluid compartments. The intracellular fluid compartment consists of the fluid inside all body cells, the bulk of the body water. The extracellular compartment, which contains the remainder, has been divided into the intravascular compartment, blood plasma, and the extravascular compartment, the interstitial fluid. The former accounts for about 5 percent of the body weight, and the latter for about 10 to 20 percent. The intracellular fluid compartment represents about 40 to 50 percent of the body weight and is comparatively stable. The extravascular compartment is quantitatively the most elastic; adjustments in its size permit the body to maintain the homeostasis of the intracellular and intravascular fluids in the face of a sometimes variable fluid intake from the intestine and fluid loss via the kidney, skin, and lungs.

The internal membranes of the body which separate the various fluid compartments permit water to traverse them without major restraint. If the membrane is freely permeable to a solute present in one compartment, this solute will migrate through it and distribute itself uniformly in the water of both compartments. In this case the solute has no influence on the distribution of water between the compartments. However, if the membrane is impermeable to a solute (or relatively so), the partition of water on both sides of the membrane is affected by the *osmotic pressure* (or water-retaining tendency) exerted by the solute, which is restricted, through selective permeability, to one side of the membrane.

The cell requires a surrounding fluid medium of relatively stable isoosmotic pressure and molecular composition. The osmotic pressure of the extracellular fluid is due to the dissolved solutes, of which ionized electrolytes are the most important. Na^+, Ca^{2+}, Cl^-, and HCO_3^- are found in greater concentration in the extracellular fluid, while K^+, Mg^{2+}, and organic phosphate are found in much greater concentration within the cell. Glycogen and nucleoproteins are exclusively intracellular; proteins, nucleotides, and enzymes are primarily intracellular and found in much lower concentration in the extracellular fluid. In any one compartment, the sum of cations must equal the sum of anions. The cations sodium and potassium do not readily diffuse across the cell membranes, and being the chief cations of the extra- and intracellular fluid compartments, respectively, they exert a profound osmotic influence. The shift of water from one compartment to the other serves to adjust differences in intra- and extracellular osmotic pressures.

In contrast to the relationship between intra- and extracellular solutes, there is a relatively free exchange of all solutes across the capillary walls between the blood and the extravascular fluid compartment. Any difference in osmotic pressure across the capillary wall is due to the osmotic effect exerted by the plasma proteins, which normally cannot diffuse across the capillary barrier. When the plasma protein concentration becomes very low, fluid moves from the blood to the interstitial spaces, resulting in swollen, waterlogged, soft tissues. This condition is termed *edema*. Normally the liver maintains sufficiently high plasma protein levels through constant synthesis. The osmotic effect exerted by the plasma proteins prevents the diffusion of intravascular fluid into the extravascular compartment and also any excessive elimination of water from the blood by the kidney.

Neutrality Regulation

The carbohydrates, fats, and amino acids are transported in the blood to the various tissues as neutral or nearly neutral substances. In addition to these nutrients, the blood also conveys oxygen to the cells. This oxygen provides the means by which the energy of the foodstuffs is liberated in the tissues by biologic combustion. In contrast to the neutral substances which are the raw materials for these biologic oxidations, the metabolic end products are mostly acids or bases and water. Most of the carbon contained in carbohydrates, fats, and amino acids is eventually oxidized to carbon dioxide, which exists in solution as carbonic acid; the sulfur contained in the amino acids cystine and methionine is oxidized to sulfate; much of the ingested phosphorus (in the form of phosphate esters) is metabolized chiefly to inorganic phosphate; and the sodium or potassium moiety of ingested organic or inorganic salts is liberated as cations of a strong base. These metabolic end products diffuse from the tissue cells into the surrounding extracellular fluid and would upset its hydrogen-ion concentration were it not for compensatory mechanisms.

In health, the hydrogen-ion concentration of the extracellular fluids is maintained between pH 7.35 and 7.45. A number of mechanisms exist to ensure a strict regulation of this pH range, which is essential for normal body metabolism and function. Probably the simplest available mechanism is dilution. When tissue cells produce an excess of CO_2, the concentration of dissolved HCO_3^- in the body fluids as a whole is not markedly affected, since the total body water is about 70 percent of the lean body mass. The second mechanism for the maintenance of optimal pH range is the ability of the body fluids to buffer excesses of cations and anions. The blood has several efficient buffer systems which permit the transport of acidic and basic metabolites from the site of formation, the cells, to the excretory organs, the lungs and kidneys, with minimal influence on the hydrogen-ion concentration. These buffer systems in the plasma and red cells are HCO_3^-/H_2CO_3 and $HPO_4^{2-}/H_2PO_4^-$. In addition, the plasma proteins act as buffers, as well as the hemoglobin in the red blood cells. The third neutrality mechanism involves the direct excretion of the metabolites—the elimination of excess CO_2 in the lungs (a process which is regulated involuntarily by the respiratory center) and the selective excretion of excess cations and anions by the kidney. This organ excretes a urine of varying pH (4.8 to 8.0) in an effort to maintain the blood pH constant; it also synthesizes and excretes NH_4^+ to combine with excreted acidic anions to conserve the body's sodium and potassium stores. The constant excretion of acidic anions by the kidney nevertheless makes for some drain of accompanying basic cations, mainly sodium and potassium. The supply of basic elements in the metabolic pool is limited and must thus be refurnished from an outside source, the food.

Acid-Base Balance

Foods are said to be *acid-forming* or *base-forming* (or acid-residue foods and base-residue foods) on the basis of their influence on the pH of the urine. Phosphorus, sulfur, and chlorine are elements which form acids on ashing or oxidation; the base-forming elements are sodium, potassium, calcium, and magnesium. Upon oxidation, meat, fish, eggs, cereals, and many other protein-rich foods leave an acidic residue of phosphate, sulfate, and chloride which must be disposed of in the urine; conversely, most fruits and vegetables leave a residue rich in the alkaline cations sodium and potassium. The former are thus referred to as acid-forming foods, the latter as base-forming because of their mineral elements. There are some noteworthy exceptions; because of its high calcium content, milk leaves a basic residue despite its high protein content. Plums, prunes, and cranberries contain relatively large amounts of benzoic and quinic acid. In contrast to most other organic acids which enter the carbohydrate metabolic cycle and are either oxidized to carbon dioxide and water or stored as glycogen or fat, benzoic acid and quinic acid are converted in the liver to hippuric acid and tetahydroxy hippuric acid, respectively, and eliminated as such, lowering the pH of the urine. These fruits are thus acid-forming exceptions to the rule.

   The use of acid- or base-forming diets as an adjunct in the treatment of certain diseases is discussed in the appropriate chapters.

Chapter 4

Energy Metabolism

Man's food furnishes the raw materials for growth and repair; it also provides the energy for mechanical work, for the functional activities of the various organs and tissues, and the heat for maintenance of body temperature. The chemical energy of the various foods is made available to the body as the result of the oxidative breakdown of foods. Carbon and hydrogen are the principal constituents of the molecules of the various foodstuffs from which heat or other forms of energy are derived on oxidation. Carbon and hydrogen are oxidized to carbon dioxide and water, and the sulfur and phosphorus in foods are oxidized to sulfate and phosphate, respectively. The nitrogen of foods is not completely oxidized; this constituent is eliminated primarily in the form of urea. Urea, $(NH_2)_2CO$, contains carbon and hydrogen in addition to the nitrogen; thus not quite all the carbon and hydrogen which are metabolized in the body are completely oxidized to carbon dioxide and water. What should be emphasized is that carbon and hydrogen can be oxidized in the body as completely as outside of it and that the result of this oxidation is the production of heat and energy, essential for the activities of living matter.

In human calorimetry, the unit for the measurement of heat is the large, or kilogram, calorie (kcal), the quantity of heat required to raise the temperature of one kilogram of water from 15 to 16°C.

The Caloric Value of Food Constituents

Substances such as carbohydrates and fats, which contain only carbon, hydrogen, and oxygen, yield approximately the same amount of heat when oxidized in the body as when oxidized in a laboratory bomb calorimeter. Proteins, which also contain nitrogen, yield smaller caloric values when oxidized within the body. This is due to the fact that 12 to 17 percent of the protein molecule is made up of nitrogen which is not oxidized but eliminated principally as urea. At any one time, the oxidation of 1 g of glucose in the body yields approximately 3.7 cal, of starch yields 4.1 cal, and 1 g of sucrose, 4.0 cal. Since the average diet contains more starch than other carbohydrate constituents, the approximate figure of 4 cal has been taken as the caloric value of the carbohydrates in the diet. The complete oxidation of olive oil in the body yields 9.4 cal per gram of oil, and that of butterfat, 9.2 cal. Other fats yield somewhat smaller values, and the approximate figure of 9 cal is generally used as the caloric value of fats in the diet. The average caloric value of protein in the body is 4.1 cal per gram; the round figure of 4 is generally used in dietary calculations.

The Respiratory Quotient

When foods are oxidized in the body, carbon dioxide, water, and heat are produced in direct proportion to the quantity of oxygen consumed in the process. The proportion of carbon dioxide produced to oxygen consumed can, when measured, furnish information as to the kind and quantity of food which is being metabolized. The ratio of the volume of carbon dioxide eliminated by the lungs to the volume of oxygen consumed by the body is termed the *respiratory quotient* (RQ).

When carbohydrates are oxidized, the reaction may be represented as

$$C_6H_{12}O_6 + 6O_2 \rightarrow 6CO_2 + 6H_2O + 675 \text{ kcal (approx.)}$$

Here

$$RQ = \frac{6 \text{ vol } CO_2}{6 \text{ vol } O_2} = 1.0$$

Fats contain less oxygen in their molecules than carbohydrates and thus require more oxygen from the atmosphere for complete oxidation:

$$2C_{51}H_{98}O_6 + 145O_2 \rightarrow 102CO_2 + 98H_2O + 15,314 \text{ kcal}$$
Tripalmitin

Here

$$RQ = \frac{51 \text{ vol } CO_2}{72.5 \text{ vol } O_2} = 0.7$$

The average value of 0.71 has been taken for the RQ of fats.

The RQ for proteins is derived indirectly since its oxidation in the body cannot be represented accurately by a chemical equation. When protein alone is metabolized, the RQ is 0.80.

When one determines the values of oxygen consumed and of CO_2 exhaled by an individual at any one time, the RQ obtained indicates the type of oxidative metabolism which takes place. When carbohydrates alone are burned, an RQ of 1.0 is obtained. The lowest obtainable RQ under normal conditions is 0.71, representing the oxidative metabolism of fats only. An RQ intermediate between these figures indicates the combustion of a mixture of foodstuffs. Normally, when a mixed diet is metabolized, the RQ is about 0.85. Under abnormal conditions, the limits of 0.71 and 1.0 may be exceeded in the lower and upper direction, respectively. In uncontrolled diabetes the RQ will be close to 0.7, indicating that much of the combustion is derived from fats. (Normal utilization of carbohydrates would shift the RQ closer to 1.0, the RQ for the utilization of carbohydrates.) In severe uncontrolled diabetes, respiratory quotients as low as 0.63 have been reported. This indicates that some of the absorbed oxygen was not used for the production of carbon dioxide and water and reflects the conversion of amino acids to glucose (for which oxygen is needed, since the glucose molecule contains more oxygen than the amino acid molecule) and the subsequent excretion and loss of this glucose in the diabetic's urine. One of the most striking results of insulin treatment is that the RQ increases, showing that carbohydrates are again being utilized for energy purposes. Respiratory quotients higher than 1.0 may be found in conditions where excessive amounts of carbohydrates are utilized, to the practical exclusion of fats and proteins, and where glucose is converted into fat and deposited as such in the body. In this case a substance rich in oxygen is converted into one containing less, with a net release of oxygen which is available for the metabolic needs of the body without the requirement of obtaining it from the outside by inhalation.

The protein portion of the metabolized food may be computed from urinary nitrogen by assuming that each gram of nitrogen represents 6.25 g of original protein. The oxidation of this quantity of protein requires the consumption of 5.92 liters of oxygen and liberates 4.75 liters of carbon dioxide. From these figures one can compute the volume of these gases involved in the metabolism of protein alone. Subtracting these figures from the total carbon dioxide exhaled and oxygen absorbed yields the RQ for the fat and carbohydrate metabolism. From this quotient one can arrive at the respective amounts

of these foodstuffs which were metabolized by use of the data in Table 2. Once
the amount of oxygen consumed and of carbon dioxide and nitrogen eliminated

**Table 2   Interrelationship between the Nonprotein
Respiratory Quotient, Relative Quantities of
Carbohydrate and Fat Oxidized, and Heat Value of 1
Liter of Oxygen**

Nonprotein respiratory quotient	1 liter of oxygen is equivalent to:		
	Carbohydrates, g	Fat, g	Calories
0.707	0.000	0.502	4.686
0.71	0.016	0.497	4.690
0.72	0.055	0.482	4.702
0.73	0.094	0.465	4.714
0.74	0.134	0.450	4.727
0.75	0.173	0.433	4.739
0.76	0.213	0.417	4.751
0.77	0.254	0.400	4.764
0.78	0.294	0.384	4.776
0.79	0.334	0.368	4.788
0.80	0.375	0.350	4.801
0.81	0.415	0.334	4.813
0.82	0.456	0.317	4.825
0.83	0.498	0.301	4.838
0.84	0.539	0.284	4.850
0.85	0.580	0.267	4.862
0.86	0.622	0.249	4.875
0.87	0.666	0.232	4.887
0.88	0.708	0.215	4.899
0.89	0.741	0.197	4.911
0.90	0.793	0.180	4.924
0.91	0.836	0.162	4.936
0.92	0.878	0.145	4.948
0.93	0.922	0.127	4.961
0.94	0.966	0.109	4.973
0.95	1.010	0.091	4.985
0.96	1.053	0.073	4.998
0.97	1.098	0.055	5.010
0.98	1.142	0.036	5.022
0.99	1.185	0.018	5.035
1.00	1.232	0.000	5.047

has been determined in the metabolic laboratory, it is thus possible to compute, for any given period, the exact amounts of carbohydrate, fat, and protein which were metabolized.

Basal Metabolism

The metabolism of the body varies with the conditions to which it is subjected. The total energy output reflects two factors, one of which is normally a fairly constant one under certain specified conditions. This factor represents primarily the energy needed to maintain the temperature of the body, to maintain the pumping action of the heart at rest, and to supply the minimal energy requirements of the tissues at rest. The other factor fluctuates widely, depending on the extent of exercise and on the amount of food consumed. The condition under which the metabolism is least subject to other influences is 12 to 18 hours after the ingestion of food, when the individual is awake but at complete rest, at a comfortable temperature, and in a restful state of mind. Under these basal conditions the energy output of the body is relatively constant and low, and the heat output or energy metabolism is termed the *basal metabolism*. The total basal metabolism depends on the mass of cellular protoplasm which takes part in resting respiration; for all practical purposes the latter is proportional to the surface area of the body.

The basal metabolic rate (BMR) is defined as the number of calories given off by the body per square meter of body surface per hour. The average BMR for normal adult males varies from 36 to 41 cal/m^2/hr and for normal adult females, from 34 to 36 cal. Any deviation of the individual BMR from the normal is expressed in terms of percent. For instance, if the BMR of a 40-year-old male is found to be 43.7 cal per square meter of body surface per hour, while the mean normal BMR for this age is 38.0, his BMR is said to be plus 15 percent.

For the practical determination of the BMR a number of apparatuses have been developed. The simplest type (McKesson, Sanborn, or Benedict-Roth) measures the oxygen consumption of the individual while he is in the basal state. Under the conditions of the experiment, each liter of oxygen consumed represents 4.8 cal of heat generated by the body. The surface area of the individual is obtained from the DuBois height-weight chart (Fig. 1), which is based on the formula

$$\text{Area (cm}^2\text{)} = \text{weight (kg) } 0.425 \times \text{height (cm) } 0.725 \times 71.84$$

Given the oxygen consumption during a specified time and the height-weight data, the individual's BMR can thus be obtained in terms of calories generated per square meter of body surface per hour.

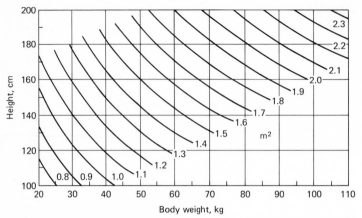

Figure 1 Chart for determining surface area from weight and height data according to the formula of DuBois and DuBois. (*By permission from, "Fundamentals of Biochemistry," by Schmidt and Allen. Copyright, McGraw-Hill Book Company, New York,* 1938.)

Variations in Basal Metabolism

The basal metabolism is subject to variation by a number of physiologic and pathologic conditions. The normal physiologic conditions which modify the BMR are age, sex, climate and/or race, thyroid activity, and environmental temperature; sleep, diet, and premenstrual period also exert an influence. Figure 2 gives the normal variation due to age. The rate is high in infancy and decreases with advancing age. This downward slope is modified during puberty when the rate accelerates somewhat. The rate for women is about 10 percent lower than for men. Inhabitants of tropical regions exhibit lower metabolic rates than those of temperate regions; Eskimos, on the other hand, possess the highest rates. During sleep the oxygen requirement of the tissues is lower, and the BMR as ordinarily determined is decreased by about 10 percent. During emotional states of elation, the rate of metabolism is increased; mental depression decreases it. During the premenstrual period there is a slight increase in basal metabolism. At the onset of the menses, the rate drops slightly below normal and continues at the lower level throughout the period. High environmental temperatures make for a lower BMR.

The pathologic conditions which increase the BMR include hyperthyroidism, fever, hypertension, polycythemia, the leukemias, and others. The pathologic states which may decrease the BMR include hypothyroidism, starvation or chronic undernutrition, extreme obesity states, and others.

The Specific Dynamic Action of Food

When food is ingested, the body's heat output increases above that of the basal level. This stimulus which food gives to metabolism is referred to as its *specific*

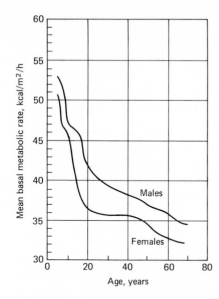

Figure 2 Average basal metabolic rates at different age levels. (*Modified from original data of Boothby et al., Am. J. Physiol.,* **116:**468, 1936.)

dynamic action. The ingestion of carbohydrates and fats increases the body's resting energy output by about 5 percent. After the ingestion and breakdown of proteins (unaccompanied by fats or carbohydrates) the energy output is increased 20 to 30 percent above that of the intake. Certain of the amino acids, notably phenylalanine, glycine, alanine, and glutamic acid exert a very marked calorigenic action, in contrast to arginine and histidine, which produce a low dynamic action.

The specific dynamic action of protein is related to the metabolism of its constituent amino acids. A number of theories have been presented to explain this phenomenon. The traditional opinion is that the calorigenic action of amino acids is the result of the extra energy required by the liver for deamination of the amino acids and the formation of urea. Additional energy is needed to metabolize the carbon-containing residues of the deaminated amino acids if they are not immediately oxidized to carbon dioxide and water (as would be the case in caloric undernutrition). If these residues are converted into glucose, glycogen, or fat, additional energy is required for this transformation. The specific dynamic action is not exerted when the ingested protein is used for growth and structural purposes only. The low specific dynamic action of carbohydrates is probably due solely to the synthesis of glycogen from glucose; that of fats has not yet been explained satisfactorily.

Recent experimentation has cast doubt on the traditional interpretation of the increased heat production following a protein-containing meal. Rather than being related to the energy cost of amino acid degradation and urea synthesis, it is proposed that the observed thermogenesis is related to the energy cost of protein synthesis. From a practical standpoint, heterogeneous diets and not single food constituents are consumed and oxidized, and as a result the differences in the overall energy utilization of equicaloric human diets of different protein content are less significant than is generally assumed on the basis of experimental results obtained for brief periods with intakes of pure proteins, fats, and carbohydrates.

Temperature Regulation

Warm-blooded animals maintain an almost constant body temperature even though their environment may undergo relatively gross temperature changes. Basically, two mechanisms are involved in this heat regulation: (1) heat production, a metabolic or chemical process based on the oxidative breakdown of foods in the body, and (2) heat elimination through a number of physical body processes. Civilized man has introduced additional mechanisms through the use of clothing and environmental temperature control.

The oxidation of foods results in the production of heat. When unlimited food is available, heat production increases as long as the caloric need exists for maintenance of the body temperature and for physical activity; beyond this point, the excess food is converted into fat and stored as such. When the temperature of the environment is low and body heat is lost excessively, a reflex contraction of the blood vessels of the skin decreases the flow of blood through it in order to minimize radiation, convection, and conduction of heat to the outside. Simultaneously, the body's metabolic activity is stimulated, resulting in an increased heat production to make up for heat loss to the cold environment. If the heat loss to the surrounding medium is great, involuntary shivering stimulates further metabolic activity and concomitant heat production. The same mechanism is involved in voluntary muscular activity when the individual resorts to flapping with his arms and stomping with his feet. The insulation provided by the subcutaneous fat layer and the air held in fur, hair, and clothing serve to decrease heat loss through convection and radiation at all times.

The dissipation of body heat takes place by way of four mechanisms:

1   About 70 percent is normally lost to the environment through radiation, convection, and conduction.
2   Evaporation of water from the external surface of the skin and internal surface of the lungs accounts for about 25 percent.
3   About 3 percent of the total heat is used to bring the inspired air and ingested cold foods to body temperature.
4   From 1 to 2 percent is lost with excreta.

When the environmental temperature is high, a reflex dilatation of the blood vessels of the skin increases blood flow through it, increasing the loss of heat from this outer integument to the surrounding medium through radiation, convection, and conduction. Simultaneously, there is an increased production of sweat, which serves to cool the skin upon evaporation. If the air is dry, dissipation of heat through evaporation from the skin and lungs is efficient; under extremely humid conditions this mechanism may become almost inoperative. On the whole, barring abnormal heat production (as during fever and in hyperthyroid states), the normal body temperature of 37°C is maintained surprisingly well even in environmental extremes.

Chapter 5

Caloric Requirements

The amount of energy required to maintain human life is the sum total of the calories needed to satisfy the requirements for basal metabolism and the specific dynamic action of food (Chap. 3), as well as for growth, repair, and physical activity. It has been shown that the energy needed to maintain the average adult at bed rest in a temperate climate is about four-thirds of his basal metabolism; thus the individual basal metabolic rate can be used to calculate rough basic caloric maintenance requirements. Mental activity is usually ignored in estimating energy requirements since it has been shown that it accounts for a metabolic increase of only 3 to 4 percent. In contrast, physical work increases the energy expenditure very materially.

Energy Requirements for Physical Activity

Even minor physical activity adds to the caloric expenditure above the basal requirement; this includes postural effort, something which is usually not regarded as exercise. It has been estimated that the total caloric requirement of a sitting adult is about 15 percent higher than his maintenance energy expenditure when supine; assuming a standing position adds another 15 percent

Table 3   Approximate Energy Expenditure with Different Activities*

Activity	Cal/h	Activity	Cal/h
Dressing and undressing	33	Mental work	7–8
Sitting at rest	15	Mixed carpentry work	180
Standing relaxed	20	Sawing wood	420
Standing stiffly	20–30	Rapid typing	16–40
Walking	130–200	Coal mining (average)	320
Running	500–930	House painting	160
Singing	37	Tailoring	44
Reading aloud	20	Bookbinding	51
Dishwashing	59	Riveting	276
Ironing	59	Cycling	180–300
Sewing	25–30	Swimming	200–700
Sweeping	110	Climbing	200–960
Writing	10–20	Rowing	120–600
Knitting	31	Wrestling	980

*Average 70-kg man or 58-kg woman.

Note: To arrive at the daily caloric requirement of the individual, add his basic metabolic requirement for 24 h, plus a 10 percent increment for the specific dynamic action of food, to the caloric cost of his daily activities as detailed in this table.

to the caloric requirements. The act of walking on level ground at 2.5 mi/h requires an expenditure of about 180 cal/h on the part of the average adult; walking uphill on a 5 percent grade requires 270 cal/h, and on a 15 percent grade, 490. Watch repairing "costs" about 96 cal/h, rapid typing, 108; scrubbing floors, 216; bricklaying, 240; and felling trees, 480. Table 3 details the caloric cost of a variety of physical activities. Such data permit the calculation of fairly accurate individual daily caloric requirements. This is done by adding up the basal metabolic requirement, a surcharge of 10 percent for the specific dynamic activity of food, and the caloric cost of the various activities throughout the day. For convenience, physical activities may be graded as very light, light, moderate, and heavy as described in Table 3A, which details examples of daily energy expenditures as influenced by a mix of different occupations or activities during the waking hours.

The Canadian Dietary Standards (Table 24 in Chap. 13) also incorporate such a system of caloric allowances graded according to physical activity and size. An additional discussion of caloric requirements and their estimation on the basis of standards set by the National Research Council and the Food and Agriculture Organization of the United Nations is found in Chap. 13.

Energy Allowances for Growth, Pregnancy, and Lactation

The body substance gained during growth represents an increased energy requirement since only a food intake greater than that which provides the caloric needs for maintenance and activity will provide the extra protein, fat,

Table 3A   Examples of Daily Energy Expenditures of Mature Women and Men in Light Occupations

Activity category	Time, h	Man, 70 kg		Woman, 58 kg	
		Rate, cal/min	Total, cal	Rate, cal/min	Total, cal
Sleeping, reclining	8	1.0–1.2	540	0.9–1.1	440
Very light Seated and standing activities, painting trades, auto and truck driving, laboratory work, typing, playing musical instruments, sewing, ironing	12	Up to 2.5	1300	Up to 2.0	900
Light Walking on level, 2.5–3 mi/h, tailoring, pressing, garage work, electrical trades, carpentry, restaurant trades, cannery workers, washing clothes, shopping with light load, golf, sailing, table tennis, volleyball	3	2.5–4.9	600	2.0–3.9	450
Moderate Walking 3.5–4 mi/h, plastering, weeding and hoeing, loading and stacking bales, scrubbing floors, shopping with heavy load, cycling, skiing, tennis, dancing	1	5.0–7.4	300	4.0–5.9	240
Heavy Walking with load uphill, tree felling, work with pick and shovel, basketball, swimming, climbing, football	0	7.5–12.0		6.0–10.0	
Total	24		2740		2030

Source: Food and Nutrition Board, National Research Council.

and carbohydrate required for the synthesis of additional tissue mass. In infants the energy increment due to growth has been estimated at 15 to 20 cal per day per kilogram of body weight.

Like growth, pregnancy also calls for an increase in maternal food supply. Additional nutrients are required to support fetal growth, to allow for uterine enlargement and placenta formation, and for the accumulation of extra protein in the maternal tissues to act as a reservoir for emergencies. It is customary to

Table 4   Approximate Calorie Expenditure of Boys

(Calories per Day)

Age	Basal metabolism	Very quiet boy	Active boy	Very active boy
0	200			
1	500	750		
2	800	1200	1600	2350
4	900	1400	1860	2800
6	1100	1600	2160	3230
8	1200	1800	2400	3630
10	1300	2000	2640	3950
12	1440	2130	2870	4300
14	1470	2200	2950	4400
15	1550	2300	3100	4620

Source: Modified from original data by G. Lusk, Requirements for Nutrition, *JAMA*, **70**:821 (1918).

recommend an additional allowance of 300 cal per day, above and beyond normal maintenance and activity requirements, during the second half of pregnancy (Food and Nutrition Board, National Research Council). This increment is subject to the judgment of the attending physician, who is best qualified to judge the caloric allowance on the basis of the individual rate and extent of increase in body weight.

During lactation, the synthesis of milk and its subsequent withdrawal from the mother call for the allocation of additional nutrients with a definite energy value. It is customary to increase the caloric intake of the actively nursing mother by up to 500 cal per day. In actual practice, "ideal weight" and adequacy of breast milk production are the determining factors.

Energy Requirements of Children

The caloric requirements of growing, active boys (and to a lesser extent, girls) are very high. The basal metabolic requirement of children is up to 25 percent

Table 5   FAO Estimate of Caloric Requirements of Adult Population Groups according to Body Size

(Calories per Day; Mean Temperature 10°C)

Weight, kg	Men	Women	Pregnant women	Lactating women
40	. . . .	1823	2273	2823
45	2447	1987	2437	2987
50	2643	2146	2596	3146
55	2833	2300	2750	3300
60	3019	2451	2901	3451
65	3200	2599	3049	2599
70	3379	2743	3193	3743
75	3553			
80	3725			

Table 6 FAO Estimate of Caloric Requirements of Adults according to Age

(Calories per Day;
Mean Temperature 10°C)

Age	Men	Women
20–30	3200	2300
30–40	3104	2231
40–50	3008	2162
50–60	2768	1990
60–70	2528	1817
70	2208	1587

higher than that of adults, and their superimposed incessant muscular activity calls for a surprising caloric expenditure. Table 4 illustrates the energy requirement of boys from birth to the age of 15, at different levels of activity.

Total Energy Requirements

The Committee on Caloric Requirements of the Food and Agriculture Organization of the United Nations (FAO) has set forth caloric requirements based on a standard reference man and woman, adjusted for deviation from the standard with respect to age, body weight, occupation, environmental temperature, and physiologic state. Caloric allowances for children were identical with those recommended by the Food and Nutrition Board, and allowances for pregnancy and lactation follow the recommendations discussed above. Tables 5 and 6 illustrate some of the FAO recommendations.

Table 22 in Chap. 13 details the recommended daily caloric allowances set by the Food and Nutrition Board of the National Research Council, which are essentially the same as the FAO values (adjusted for average United States body size and temperature).

The Canadian Dietary Standards (Table 24) stipulate energy allowances for individuals on the basis of body weight and degree of physical activity. The caloric allowances recommended by the FAO, Food and Nutrition Board, and Canadian Dietary Standards are essentially the same for comparable persons.

Chapter 6

The Physiology and Psychology of Hunger, Appetite, and Food Intake

Hunger and Satiety

The well-known feeling of hunger consists of a series of intermittent, brief, cramping sensations of pressure and tension in the epigastric region. This may be accompanied by the gradual onset of a feeling of generalized weakness and even irritability. The early theories concerning hunger, appetite, and the regulation of food intake centered around the stomach. It was known that an empty stomach caused pangs of hunger, and the sensation was correlated with the strange, repeated gastric contractions characteristic of this organ when empty. Though nobody disputes the relationship between hunger pains and an empty stomach, this mechanism alone is inadequate as an explanation of the regulation of food intake as a whole. Experience has shown that the physical gastric sensations of hunger can be decreased or abolished by smoking, drinking of cold water, and cinching of the belt, though none of these maneuvers involves the intake of solid food. Moreover, partial gastrectomy or even total removal of the stomach does not interfere with the food intake of laboratory animals' or man's drive to eat. Section of the vagus nerve, the splanchnic nerves, and the spinal cord, though severing the motor and sensory connection between the stomach and the central nervous system, does not impair the desire for food intake. Animals thus denervated still respond to the administration of insulin with increased food consumption and decrease their intake when given amphetamine drugs.

The gastric hunger sensation certainly serves as a powerful stimulus for the initiation of feeding; however, it does not regulate the amount eaten during any one feeding period since, as a rule, hunger pangs cease with the onset of the meal. Gastrointestinal mechanisms have also not been able to account for variations in the amount of food eaten when the nature of the diet is changed. The extent of gastric filling per se apparently does not govern the total food intake either, since most people do not gorge themselves *ad nauseam* but stop before the absolute physical capacity of the stomach is reached. Thus gastric mechanisms alone fail to explain adequately the regulation of food intake.

Hypothalamic Regulation

Experiments with laboratory animals and observations in man have led to the now commonly accepted belief that the hypothalamus houses the central nervous system center or centers which govern the urge to eat. Hypothalamic lesions in human beings may cause abnormal obesity produced by extreme overeating. A similar pathological hyperphagia with subsequent obesity can be precipitated in laboratory animals through mechanical destruction of minute areas in the hypothalamus or by electric stimulation of certain hypothalamic regions. In contrast to the abnormality produced through destruction of medial areas in the hypothalamus, which results in the animal ravenously attacking its food, destruction of more lateral areas on both sides of the brain will leave the animal without any urge to eat, and it will die of starvation. This has been interpreted to mean that two distinct regulatory centers are involved, a facilitatory center which governs appetite, or the urge to eat (*appetite center*), and an inhibitory center which acts on the appetite center to prevent overfeeding and thus determines satiety (*satiety center*).

It has been suggested that the hypothalamic regulatory centers react to changes in the composition of blood in a fashion not unlike the respiratory centers in the medulla, which are receptive to changes in the blood carbon dioxide levels and which either stimulate or depress respiration, depending on the need to clear the accumulating carbon dioxide from the blood. A similar mechanism has been postulated for the hypothalamic appetite regulating centers. The level of glucose in the blood is increased after absorption of a meal. The tissue cells utilize blood glucose continuously, and as a result of this withdrawal, a difference exists between the concentration of blood glucose in the arterial and venous blood. This difference is likely to be great in the absorptive state when food is still present in the intestine. In the postabsorptive state, the utilization of glucose in the body continues as heretofore, but the supply of additional glucose from food absorption is gone and smaller measured quantities of glucose are now made available from liver and muscle glycogen reserves. At this point the difference in glucose concentration in arterial and venous blood is likely to be quite small. It has been suggested—and this hypothesis is not accepted by all investigators in the field—that special glucose receptor cells in the hypothalamic centers are responsive to the arteriovenous glucose difference; presumably they initiate the craving for food when this difference is small and inhibit this urge when the difference becomes large again, that is, after food has been ingested and when active absorption of fresh nutrients into the bloodstream takes place. Other investigators feel that the importance of the glucostatic explanation of the regulation of food intake has been overemphasized as the dominant factor; blood levels of amino acid and fats are probably equally important.

Recent findings in monkeys indicate that hunger-satiety control points exist not only in the hypothalamic portion of the brain but also in portions of the limbic system and thalamus.

There is no doubt that a multiplicity of additional factors is involved in the regulation of food intake which may override involuntary, automatic regulatory mechanisms. These factors are associated with man's environment, habits, social customs, and conscious or unconscious emotional drives, none of which are very closely tied to basic physiologic phenomena like gastric contractions or blood glucose levels.

Psychologic Aspects of Appetite and Food Intake

Appetite and hunger are far from synonymous. Man's urge to continue eating an excellent meal may still exist long after the initial hunger sensation has ceased. The factors which make up appetite are to a large degree psychologic. The components of appetite are based on our past experiences and associated memories and go back to our early childhood days, whether they are consciously remembered or not. The nature of our memories concerning early exposures to food and associated or coincident experiences will determine our likes and dislikes and establish individual food patterns which are not necessarily based on any logical consideration. Early training with respect to quantity and quality of food intake tends to be carried over into adulthood. Families which encourage eating of large amounts of "good home cooking" may well set a tendency for later food indulgence and perhaps eventual obesity. On the other hand, spartan environments which discourage excessive physical gratifications, including the pleasures of food, tend to mold a more ascetic and often more athletic type of personality, with less liberal food habits.

Normally, a child who receives adequate emotional gratification of its need for familial love and affection, along with satisfactory fulfillment of its physical need for food, has a good chance to develop mature attitudes toward foods and food intake in later life. In many cases, disorders of appetite in infancy or adulthood serve unconscious purposes connected with inner personality conflicts. The physical hunger of the child for food and its emotional hunger for love and affection are not always kept apart, or compartmentalized, in the personality structure of the growing individual, and substitution mechanisms may develop where food becomes a physical expression for love and acceptance. The poorly adjusted adolescent girl who feels rejected by her group may find solace in oral gratification and develop a pattern of overeating as a crutch for her neglected ego. Many adults who are hungry for acceptance and recognition and whose need for affection is not adequately met try to resolve this conflict by increased food intake; finding no better outlet for this frustration, the person may overeat to compensate for his unmet needs. Eating good food entails experiencing sensory pleasure; oral gratification serves well to decrease tension and reduce anxiety and compensates for frustrations and a sense of dissatisfaction with one's fate. This background for overeating and obesity must be taken into consideration if a weight reduction program is to be successful beyond the initial success due to strict adherence on the part of the patient to a reducing diet. Psychologic supportive therapy may be needed to give the patient enough insight to make a permanent change in his food intake pattern.

Psychogenic hypophagia is not as prevalent as emotionally induced hyperphagia; nevertheless it exists in more instances than is suspected. A person with an unrequited need for love and recognition who suffers from the unhappy sense of social isolation may become depressed and withdrawn and may progressively lose his natural desire to eat to a point where anorexia, low food intake, and borderline malnutrition become a problem. The disease entity anorexia nervosa is an extreme example of a condition where self-induced starvation, leading to cachexia and even death, is a physical manifestation of unresolved psychologic conflicts. Fortunately, the severity of this disease picture is not approached by the majority of persons with decreased appetite and food intake conditioned by conscious or unconscious emotional problems. However, it is easily understood how an emotionally deprived child—to use a frequently occurring example—can express its frustration and sense of loss in a decreased appetite and refusal of food and a pattern of low food intake which is carried into adulthood.

Just as the early psychologic background may influence appetite and food intake patterns, early food experiences may leave their stamp on the developing personality. A child reared in an atmosphere where food is not plentiful and where it must put up a strenuous fight to receive it may carry over into its adult life attitudes of suspicion, insecurity, and doubt, even after its circumstances are such that the supply of food is not in question. In the adult, long-term deprivation of food may bring forth personality changes of a more temporary nature. The characteristic picture of semistarvation neurosis found among starved prisoners of war or inmates of concentration camps includes depression and irritability, resentment of physical activity, a loss of personal initiative and sexual drive, social introversion, and an overlying mental preoccupation with food. A less marked but similar emotional trend is developed when a person is placed on a reducing diet. It is a well-known fact that the subject will be able to endure his fight to eat less much better when he can compensate for the self-induced or physician-imposed loss with some other gratification, such as the mood-improving amphetamine drug prescribed by his physician. Conversely, many smokers who embark on a rigid program of self-denial with regard to smoking develop an active appetite and increase their food intake far above their usual norm.

Any discussion of disorders of appetite would be incomplete without the mention of *pica*, the desire to ingest bizarre items such as chalk, sand, insects, clay, slate, etc. In the case of pregnant women, the sudden craving for particular foods—pickled onions or candied lemon peel—is unexplainable on a physiologic basis and is looked upon as psychogenic. The bizarre cravings or sudden spurts of appetite are interpreted as attention-getting mechanisms or expressions of frustration because of inadequate recognition or love from the immediate family, particularly the husband. The cravings of pregnancy are self-limited and invariably disappear after delivery.

The ingestion of clay and dry cornstarch is not uncommon among pregnant and nonpregnant women belonging to the poorer strata in certain regions in rural Alabama. Although it has been suggested that pica is an intuitive effort on the part of the practitioner to compensate for nutritional deficiences, a careful study of this particular group characterized this type of clay and cornstarch consumption as a sociocultural phenomenon originally founded in superstition and perpetuated by tradition—especially during pregnancy.

The ingestion of bizarre food items by children—plaster, chalk, and the like—is being interpreted by some as representing an instinctive fulfillment of a physiologic need for particular nutrients, especially calcium. This, as well as the broader subject of instinctive choice of the "right" foods by man in modern times, is best left open to question.

Food Patterns

The formation of food habits begins in early childhood. Well before puberty, children tend to imitate adult habits to which they are exposed daily. A variety of factors—family influence, economic necessity, religious or national customs—all impinge on the individual and mold his food pattern. By the time adulthood is reached, personal food habits are apt to be fairly rigid; long-standing habits and a reluctance to venture into untried fields add rigidity to the individual's choice of foods, and the pattern becomes even more set with advancing age. If this pattern happens to meet the nutritional requirements of the individual, adherence to it ensures physiologic well-being; too often the tenets of optimal nutrition have little to do with the development of personal food habits, to the subsequent detriment of the individual. Nutrition education in childhood, through both the teacher and the parent, can direct the developing food pattern into nutritionally desirable channels; the earlier this is done, the better the results. The most important immediate target for such efforts is probably the postpubescent girl, who may soon bear children and whose possible future role in managing food for the family and as educator of her young thrusts her into the key position in developing food habits.

Climate, geography, and soil conditions play a large part in determining the availability and therefore the choice of foods. Agricultural necessity makes corn the staple food of Mexico, rice that of China, and wheat that of the United States, Canada, and Europe, and basic national food adherences are formed accordingly. Modern methods of food technology coupled with the availability of transportation, population shifts, and the worldwide influence of media of communication and information tend to make a wider choice of foods available throughout the year. Thus oranges are no longer a rarity in Scotland or Minnesota, while canned cow's milk may be found in the tsetse belt in Africa. Spaghetti, and before that tomatoes, were once looked upon as strictly Italian foods, but the tomato has established itself as an American staple and spaghetti is gradually doing the same. Economic factors determine food choice by necessity and make for an unequal distribution of the more nutritious (and usually more expensive) food items not only within each country but in the world at large, where dairy products and meats are much more prevalent in the more prosperous countries and rare in the undeveloped areas. Social mores have a bearing on food choice as well as on mealtimes, and religious customs have always had a profound influence on food patterns. Last but not least, fashions and fads may set food patterns, though happily they usually do not attract large sections of the population for long periods.

In summary, it may be said that man's food intake, both qualitative and quantitative, is subject to a large number of determining factors, any one of which may impede his well-being to some degree. It is one of the functions of applied nutrition to adjust these factors so as to assure his maximum physiologic welfare.

Part Two

The Food Elements

Chapter 7

Proteins and Amino Acids

The Nature of Proteins

Proteins are indispensable and normal constituents of every living cell. They are essential components of both the nucleus and cell protoplasm and are found in most extracellular animal tissue fluids. Proteins exist as very large molecules which are composed of great numbers of basic building units, α-amino acids. Although these compounds vary considerably in molecular structure and size, they have one characteristic in common: the presence of an amino group (NH_2) and a carboxyl group (COOH) linked to the same terminal carbon of the molecule. The structure of the remainder of the molecule varies; amino acids may be aliphatic compounds like alanine (α-amino propionic acid) and norleucine (α-amino caproic acid), or more complex aromatic and heterocyclic compounds. The molecular weights of natural amino acids vary from 75 for the smallest (glycine) to 240 for the largest (cystine).

Twenty-two different naturally occurring α-amino acids are known. In the protein molecule, hundreds and even thousands of amino acids are joined to one another in a characteristic linkage, where the amino group of one amino acid is linked to the carboxyl group of the other, one molecule of water being split off in the process. Whenever such a peptide linkage combines two amino acids into one single molecule, the resulting compound is a dipeptide. Polypeptides are composed of a larger number of amino acids connected by peptide linkages. Proteins with molecular weights which vary from 16,000 up to several millions may be looked upon as extremely large "superpolypeptides." The simplest protein may be pictured as a chain of amino acids held together by peptide bonds. However, in addition to the primary peptide linkages in the protein molecule, which hold the chain of amino acids together, secondary linkages exist between the various amino acid moieties. The secondary, nonpeptide linkages make possible a multiplicity of structural differences between proteins. Thus a protein molecule may exist in the form of a coiled chain or helix, a branched structure, or a hollow sphere or basket.

The properties of different proteins vary, depending on their qualitative and quantitative amino acid makeup and on the order and structural arrangement of these building units in the molecule.

By virtue of their molecular size, proteins cannot traverse semipermeable membranes. They possess the characteristic physical qualities of large-sized colloidal molecules; they also exert osmotic pressure, exhibit membrane potentials at semipermeable membrane interphases, etc. Extreme heat will coagulate them, and heavy metal salts precipitate them out of solution.

By virtue of free acidic and basic groups belonging to their constituent amino acids, proteins are amphoteric; i.e., they may act as acids or bases, depending on the pH of the surrounding medium. At a specific pH—the isoelectric point for the particular protein—the amphoteric molecule is least dissociated as an acid or base and the protein exhibits a minimum of solubility, viscosity, and electrophoretic tendency.

Proteins form true salts; in a dilute sodium hydroxide solution much of the protein will be present as *sodium proteinate*. In addition to true salt formation with cations, proteins will also combine with metals in nonionic complexes. Such metal-protein complexes are common in the body tissues.

Proteins are also found conjugated with more complex compounds: glucoproteins are combinations of proteins with complex carbohydrates, as in mucin from the mucous glands of the gastrointestinal tract; lipoproteins are combinations of proteins with fatty compounds (Chap. 9); nucleoproteins, found in nuclear cell chromatin materials, are combinations of proteins with nucleic acids; hemoglobin, the oxygen-carrying red blood cell pigment, consists of the relatively small, active iron pyrrole group *heme* conjugated with a large globin protein molecule. In a similar fashion, all enzymes apparently are proteins often consisting of a large protein "carrier" molecule, which determines the specificity of the enzyme for a particular substrate, conjugated with a structurally smaller, catalytically active moiety such as a metal or vitamin unit.

Absorption

Food proteins are large-sized molecules which are not absorbed by the intestinal mucosa to any appreciable degree; they must be digested and broken down into individual amino acids for absorption. This degradation is brought about by the hydrolytic enzymes of the gastrointestinal tract. (A detailed discussion of digestion and the digestive enzymes is found in Chap. 1.) Occasionally some polypeptides or even proteins may pass the mucosal barrier to be absorbed directly into the bloodstream; in susceptible individuals such unchanged proteins may give rise to immunologic sensitizations and appear thus to be responsible for the development of allergy to specific food proteins. The importance of this phenomenon, especially in the somewhat permeable gastrointestinal tract of the very young infant, is discussed in Chap. 17, Nutrition in Infancy, and Chap. 39, Food Allergy.

The absorption of the individual amino acids which are liberated from food proteins by the digestive process is not a simple, passive diffusion, but a selective process in which individual amino acids appear to compete for a place in the transport system. There are wide differences in the rates of absorption of the various amino acids. Furthermore, the naturally occurring L-amino acids are preferentially more rapidly absorbed than their respective D isomers, a fact which strongly suggests an active mechanism of transport across mucosal cell membranes. It is of interest that the rates of absorption observed for single amino acids do not apply to complex amino acid mixtures of varying composition.

It has become increasingly apparent that a physiologic mechanism exists to ensure the presence in the intestine of an amino acid mixture of approximately constant and optimal composition at the time of absorption of dietary amino acids. The ingestion of food protein stimulates the digestive tract to secrete an appreciable amount of endogenous proteins into the intestinal lumen. This secretion, in the form of gastrointestinal mucoproteins and digestive enzymes, presumably provides enough endogenous protein of relatively "desirable" composition to dilute the food amino mixture in the intestine sufficiently to obscure any amino acid pattern peculiar to the ingested food protein. This mixing of amino acids in the intestinal lumen is thus thought to regulate the relative concentrations of the amino acids available for absorption. Teleologically speaking, such a homeostasis in the intestine during the period of absorption is there to assure the simultaneous absorption (and subsequent presence in the bloodstream) of an amino acid mixture which conforms to a pattern optimal for protein synthesis in the liver and body tissues at large. It has been observed, however, that when large quantities of an incomplete amino acid mixture are presented to the gastrointestinal tract, they are not well utilized in the liver for protein synthesis.

After absorption, most of the amino acids are carried to the liver via the portal vein; some may also pass into the lymphatics.

As can be expected, the general level of amino acids in the bloodstream increases during the postabsorptive stage. However, there is *no* exact relationship between absorption of a specific amino acid and its serum concentration. The concentration of any free amino acid in the blood is subject to a circadian rhythm which appears to be related to the periodicity of many other metabolic body processes. This periodicity persists even for several days after onset of dietary protein restriction or even starvation. On the other hand, blood amino acid rhythmicity is readily altered by the onset of an acute illness or by a change in an individual's pattern of sleep and wakefulness.

Metabolism

Some of the amino acids from the portal circulation are retained by the liver to satisfy the specific requirements and functions of this organ; the rest enter the general circulation, from which they are rapidly removed by the various tissues. The liver is responsible for the formation of the wide spectrum of human plasma proteins. All tissues utilize the available amino acids for the synthesis of specific cell proteins needed for the formation of new cells or the repair and maintenance of existing ones and, in the case of secretory cells, for specialized secretions of a diverse nature. This anabolic activity thus not only pertains to structural proteins and constituents of the cell protoplasm, including intracellular enzymes, but also involves extracellular enzymes, hormones, and the synthesis of a host of other nonproteinaceous amino acid derivatives of greater or lesser physiologic importance.

After the anabolic needs of the body have been met, an excess of amino acids may still remain. These amino acids are catabolized for the production of energy and heat or converted to carbohydrate and fat, and if the energy need is exceeded, there may be storage as fat. Under conditions of shortage of calories or starvation, amino acids are utilized as sources of heat and energy since maintenance of essential body functions has a priority over anabolic activities.

Deamination is usually the first step in the catabolism of amino acids. In this process the amino group is split off and the remaining molecule is transformed into an α-keto acid. The liberated amino group may be utilized for the production of another more necessary amino acid from a suitable precursor, a process referred to as *transamination.* When the amino acid supply is generous, most of the amino nitrogen enters the metabolic channel of urea formation, where two amino groups and one molecule of carbon dioxide combine to form one molecule of urea. The conversion of amino nitrogen into urea takes place in the liver and occurs through the ornithine cycle (Fig. 3).

A small amount of amino nitrogen derived from deamination of amino acids is incorporated into blood glutamine and carried to the kidney, where under certain conditions ammonia can be liberated from the glutamine molecule and excreted in the form of ammonium salts.

In the catabolic breakdown of amino acids, the deaminated carbon-chain residue enters the pathway of carbohydrate or ketone body metabolism. Under conditions of serious caloric need, they are broken down principally into the ultimate end products, carbon dioxide and water, the oxidative degradation yielding the required energy. On the other hand, under normal circumstances the keto acids produced by deamination of amino acids may also participate in

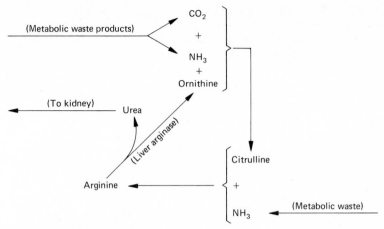

Figure 3 Urea formation in the ornithine cycle.

the formation of storage fat or of glycogen (the form in which carbohydrates are stored in the liver and muscles).

Another catabolic change which an amino acid may undergo is decarboxylation, which involves the splitting off of carbon dioxide from the carboxyl group of the amino acid to yield a number of physiologically active, essential, and sometimes unessential and even toxic amines.

Essential and Nonessential Amino Acids

Some of the amino acids required for protein synthesis in growth, maintenance, and repair (including synthesis of enzymes, hormones, and hemoglobin) must be supplied by the ingested food, while others can be synthesized in the body as the need arises. The amino acids which must be supplied by the food are referred to as *essential* (indispensable). The *nonessential* amino acids are not necessarily of less biologic importance, but this distinction implies the necessity of supplying the essential amino acids in ready-made form from external sources. The nonessential amino acids may be provided per se by the ingested food, or, if missing in the diet, they may be synthesized from precursors available in the metabolic pool of the body. Their carbon skeletons are derived from intermediate products of carbohydrate or fat metabolism, usually in the form of α-keto acids. An amino group becomes attached to this molecule, converting it into the needed amino acid. The amino group is derived either from another amino acid through transamination or from the ammonia available from deamination of dietary amino compounds.

Twenty-two different naturally occurring α-amino acids are known; of these, nine are essential for growth and maintenance in children, and eight are essential for maintenance of nitrogen equilibrium in adults (Table 7). If one or more of the essential amino acids is not present in sufficient quantity when a

Table 7   Amino Acids in Human Nutrition

Essential amino acids	Recommended daily intake, g	Minimum daily intake (men), g	Minimum daily intake (women), g
L-Phenylalanine	2.2	1.10	0.220
L-Methionine	2.2	1.10	0.290
L-Leucine	2.2	1.10	0.620
L-Valine	1.6	0.80	0.650
L-Lysine	1.6	0.80	0.500
L-Isoleucine	1.4	0.70	0.450
L-Threonine	1.0	0.50	0.310
L-Tryptophan	0.5	0.25	0.160

Nonessential amino acids

Glycine	Proline
Alanine	Hydroxyproline
Serine	Citrulline
Cystine	Histidine*
Tyrosine	Arginine*
Aspartic acid	Norleucine
Glutamic acid	Hydroxyglutamic acid

*Arginine is not an essential amino acid for children, while histidine is essential for children but probably not for healthy adults.

body protein is being synthesized, this synthesis is limited quantitatively by the availability of the essential amino acid lowest in supply. On the other hand, if some of the nonessential amino acids are not supplied by the diet and they are needed in the structural makeup of the protein molecule about to be synthesized, they will be formed in the quantity required in the manner outlined above.

Under conditions of marginal amino acid supply from external sources, simple nitrogen-containing compounds like urea, ammonium salts, and glutamic acid exhibit a sparing effect with respect to the nonessential amino acids. These simple compounds are able to provide nonessential nitrogen for both human growth and maintenance. Apparently, under conditions of severe nitrogen deprivation, nonessential amino acids can be synthesized in the body from suitable multicarbon precursors present in the body's metabolic pool and nitrogen fed in the form of urea and ammonium salts.

Table 7 is based on the classic observations of Rose. Because of the variations reported for individual amino acid requirements by a number of investigators, it is, perhaps, practical to take into consideration the reported ranges of daily requirements for the essential amino acids shown in Table 7A.

The question regarding the essential role of histidine in adults is not resolved; its external supply has been shown to be critical in certain disease states (uremia, rheumatoid arthritis).

Table 7A Reported Ranges of Daily Requirements of Essential Amino Acids

Amino acid	Low (mg/day)	High (mg/day)
	Men and Women	
Phenylalanine	400	1,180
Methionine	175	1,100
Leucine	170	1,100
Valine	230	800
Lysine	400	1,200
Isoleucine	70	700
Threonine	103	1,500
Tryptophan	82	630
	Infants	
Histidine	16 mg/kg	34 mg/kg

Biologic Value of Food Proteins

The term *biologic value* is used to express the percentage of absorbed nitrogen which is retained by the organism for maintenance and growth. The biologic value of food proteins depends to a large degree on their amino acid composition. Proteins which do not provide all the essential amino acids upon digestion, or which provide some of them in suboptimal quantities, are not as valuable in supporting body protein anabolism as other proteins which can supply a full complement of the essential and nonessential amino acids.

Proteins are thus classed as having a high or low biologic value primarily on the basis of their ability to supply all the amino acids required for the formation of body tissues, enzymes, and hormones. However, in addition to structural "completeness," other factors influence the value of a given protein. Probably the most important factor is digestibility. In the human adult, a protein must be digested completely and hydrolyzed into its component amino acids before these can be absorbed into the bloodstream and made available to the body's metabolic pool. In the event of incomplete hydrolysis of the protein, only part of the constituent amino acids become available, while others remain locked up in the nondigested protein molecules or in partially hydrolyzed polypeptide fragments and are eventually eliminated without contributing to the nutrition of the individual. The method of preparation (cooking, baking, toasting, etc.) of the protein food has a distinct bearing on its subsequent digestibility. Overheating, particularly in the absence of water (dry heat or frying), can reduce the nutritive value by destruction of essential amino acids such as lysine, which is heat-labile, or by tying them up in new chemical linkages not susceptible to enzymatic digestion. On the other hand, it has been shown that cooking with water increases the digestibility and improves the

Table 7B   Estimated Amino Acid Requirements of Man*

Essential amino acids	Requirement (per kg of body weight), mg/day			Amino acid pattern for high-quality proteins, mg/g of protein
	Infant (3–6 mo)	Child (10–12 yr)	Adult	
Histidine	33	?	?	17
Isoleucine	80	28	12	42
Leucine	128	42	16	70
Lysine	97	44	12	51
Total *S*-containing amino acids	45	22	10	26
Total aromatic amino acids	132	22	16	73
Threonine	63	28	8	35
Tryptophan	19	4	3	11
Valine	89	25	14	48

*Two grams per kilogram of body weight per day of protein of the quality listed in column 4 would meet the amino acid needs of the infant.
Source: Food and Nutrition Board, National Research Council.

nutritive value of wheat protein, possibly by altering the protein structure. As a result, methionine and other amino acids are liberated more rapidly, providing a better overall pattern for absorption.

At the top of the list of proteins of high biologic value is egg protein. Close to it ranks the protein of milk (chiefly casein, with smaller quantities of albumin). Egg or milk proteins can furnish all the amino acids essential for normal growth and healthy life processes provided they are administered in adequate amounts. The incomplete protein gelatin is at the other extreme of nutritive rank. It fails to supply two essential amino acids, valine and tryptophan, and it contains inadequate amounts of tyrosine and cystine. Gelatin cannot sustain normal life or support growth when it is the sole source of protein, even when given in large amounts. However, when the missing amino acids are added to the gelatin in adequate amounts as the pure chemicals or in foods containing them, this nutritional inadequacy is corrected and normal growth and maintenance become possible again.

Fish, meat, and poultry proteins are very high in the scale of biologic value. Of distinctly lower value are the plant proteins such as those of wheat, corn, rice, beans, and nuts. These proteins may contain all the necessary amino acids, but in each one of them one or more of the essential amino acids are present in such inadequate amounts that the entire protein is of low biologic value when it represents the only source of amino acids in the diet. Such incomplete plant proteins must be supplemented with other foods supplying the missing amino acids in order to provide good nutrition.

Table 8 illustrates the essential amino acid composition of various protein foods, listed in decreasing order of biologic value. Table 8A, in turn, illustrates the way selected foods vary in their total essential amino acid contribution in relation to their nitrogen content.

Actually it is possible to be well nourished while consuming only proteins of plant origin provided the diet contains a number of properly selected plant proteins of divergent composition, a fact which would tend to ensure the supply of the entire spectrum of essential amino acids. An excellent example of a nutritionally adequate diet containing only proteins of plant origin is a mixture of corn, sorghum, cottonseed meal, and torula yeast, developed in Central America to combat protein deficiency in young children (Chap. 22).

Mutual Supplementation of Proteins

A given protein may be of low biologic value because of its failure to supply one or more of the essential amino acids; nevertheless, it may still be a useful food when it is supplemented with another protein which provides the missing constituents. If the second, high-quality protein supplies adequate additional quantities of the missing amino acids, the mixture of both proteins will be of high biologic value.

Many of the vegetable proteins are low in essential amino acids, such as lysine, tryptophan, methionine, or threonine, and will therefore neither promote optimal growth nor maintain maximum vigor when one of them alone constitutes the only protein source. In practice, however, most meals contain a mixture of proteins of different origin and dissimilar amino acid composition, and there is a tendency in our food pattern to combine some high-quality proteins with the less complete, less expensive plant proteins (as exemplified by macaroni and cheese, bread and milk, chili beans and meat, breakfast cereal with milk, etc.). Mutual supplementation of proteins has thus been practiced for ages instinctively, though its biochemical mechanism and nutritional importance have been recognized only in this century.

The time factor is of utmost importance in mutual supplementation. There exists no physiologic mechanism for the storage of individual amino acids in the body for periods when they may be required for the synthesis of a special tissue protein. Therefore effective supplementation occurs only when the deficient and supplementary proteins are fed simultaneously or within a brief time interval. Improvement in the utilization of ingested, incomplete proteins through simultaneous feeding of a supplementary high-quality protein has been demonstrated not only in proteins which are quite dissimilar in their biologic quality, such as a breakfast cereal and milk, but also when the proteins involved are of less divergent nature; for instance, the proteins of the staple food of many Central American people, corn and beans, are better utilized when they are ingested together. One practical, dietetic implication of such findings is that in feeding primarily proteins of low biologic value, whatever high-quality proteins are available should always be fed simultaneously.

Table 8 Essential Amino Acid Composition of Protein Foods

(Listed in Decreasing Order of Biologic Value)

Foods and their biologic value	Arginine	Histidine	Threo- nine	Valine	Leucine	Iso- leucine	Lysine	Methio- nine	Phenyl- alanine	Trypto- phan
Egg, whole	700	240	560	790	1,015	700	690	360	640	130
	(6.2)	(2.1)	(4.9)	(7.0)	(9.0)	(6.2)	(6.1)	(3.2)	(5.6)	(1.1)
Milk, whole, human	50	23	59	87	154	80	75	22	64	22
	(4.2)	(1.9)	(4.9)	(7.2)	(12.8)	(6.7)	(6.2)	(1.8)	(5.3)	(1.8)
Milk, whole, cow's	122	72	152	233	398	221	243	93	181	46
	(3.7)	(2.2)	(4.6)	(7.1)	(12.1)	(6.7)	(7.4)	(2.8)	(5.5)	(1.4)
Egg albumin	5,310	2,140	4,430	6,630	7,790	5,740	6,390	3,690	5,270	1,020
	(6.0)	(2.4)	(4.9)	(7.5)	(8.8)	(6.4)	(7.2)	(4.2)	(6.0)	(1.2)
Corn germ, defatted	1,310	475	710	860	1,145	680	940	260	810	210
	(8.1)	(3.0)	(4.4)	(5.3)	(7.1)	(4.2)	(5.8)	(1.6)	(5.0)	(1.3)
Liver, animal	1,090	410	875	990	1,390	790	1,150	530	1,000	246
	(6.6)	(2.5)	(5.3)	(6.0)	(8.4)	(4.8)	(7.0)	(3.2)	(6.1)	(1.5)
Meat, beef	1,220	620	845	975	1,480	980	1,630	515	740	300
	(6.5)	(3.3)	(4.4)	(5.1)	(7.8)	(5.2)	(8.6)	(2.7)	(3.9)	(1.0)
Fish, muscle	1,410	500	890	1,140	1,800	1,235	1,710	610	835	228
	(7.4)	(2.6)	(4.7)	(6.0)	(9.5)	(6.5)	(9.0)	(3.2)	(4.4)	(1.2)
Wheat germ	1,510	630	1,590	1,130	1,690	1,130	1,390	330	760	250
	(6.0)	(2.5)	(6.3)	(4.5)	(6.7)	(4.5)	(5.5)	(1.3)	(3.0)	(1.0)
Soybean meal, low fat	3,270	1,300	1,750	2,370	3,580	2,690	3,050	760	2,370	625
	(7.3)	(2.9)	(3.9)	(5.3)	(8.0)	(6.0)	(6.8)	(1.7)	(5.3)	(1.4)
Rice, whole	440	100	230	380	500	320	195	205	300	80
	(7.2)	(1.7)	(3.8)	(6.2)	(8.2)	(5.2)	(3.2)	(3.4)	(5.0)	(1.3)

Food										
Casein	3,720 (3.9)	2,900 (3.0)	4,280 (4.5)	7,000 (7.4)	9,500 (10.0)	6,050 (6.4)	7,740 (8.1)	3,100 (3.3)	5,150 (5.4)	910 (9.6)
Wheat, whole	560 (4.3)	275 (2.1)	430 (3.3)	560 (4.3)	910 (7.0)	520 (4.0)	350 (2.7)	325 (2.5)	665 (5.1)	155 (1.2)
Potatoes, white, raw	100 (5.0)	44 (2.2)	140 (6.9)	110 (5.3)	190 (9.6)	75 (3.7)	170 (8.3)	50 (2.5)	120 (5.9)	40 (2.1)
Wheat, gluten	3,300 (3.7)	1,790 (2.0)	2,500 (2.8)	3,820 (4.3)	6,450 (7.7)	4,080 (4.6)	1,810 (2.0)	1,500 (1.7)	4,520 (5.0)	690 (0.5)
Oats, whole	775 (6.8)	260 (2.3)	410 (3.6)	615 (5.4)	910 (8.0)	560 (4.9)	410 (3.6)	230 (2.0)	625 (5.5)	150 (1.3)
Barley	610 (5.1)	260 (2.2)	480 (4.0)	610 (5.1)	840 (7.0)	510 (4.3)	420 (3.5)	190 (1.6)	620 (5.2)	190 (1.6)
Yeast, dried brewers'	2,140 (4.3)	1,400 (2.8)	2,740 (5.5)	2,490 (5.0)	2,690 (7.4)	2,930 (5.9)	3,730 (7.5)	1,395 (2.7)	2,040 (4.1)	650 (1.3)
Cottonseed meal	3,450 (11.3)	830 (2.7)	920 (3.0)	1,470 (4.8)	1,830 (6.0)	1,230 (4.0)	1,080 (3.5)	520 (1.7)	1,840 (6.0)	400 (1.3)
Corn, whole	380 (4.8)	200 (2.5)	300 (3.7)	425 (5.3)	1,200 (15.0)	510 (6.4)	180 (2.3)	250 (3.1)	400 (5.0)	48 (0.6)
Rye, whole	590 (5.3)	250 (2.2)	370 (3.3)	560 (5.0)	670 (6.0)	440 (3.9)	450 (4.0)	180 (1.6)	470 (4.2)	140 (1.2)
Buckwheat flour	1,050 (8.9)	250 (2.1)	480 (4.0)	660 (5.6)	740 (6.2)	450 (3.8)	700 (5.9)	220 (1.9)	500 (4.2)	200 (1.7)
Peanut flour	7,440 (11.3)	1,465 (2.1)	1,830 (2.8)	3,000 (4.6)	4,650 (7.1)	2,730 (4.1)	2,390 (3.5)	550 (0.8)	520 (4.9)	520 (0.8)
Peas and beans, dried	1,610 (7.0)	500 (2.2)	895 (3.9)	1,265 (5.5)	1,610 (7.0)	1,270 (5.5)	1,490 (6.5)	460 (2.0)	1,150 (5.0)	185 (0.8)

Note: Figures in parentheses represent percentages of the amino acids in the food proteins (corrected on the basis of an ideal protein containing 16 percent of nitrogen on a moisture- and ash-free basis). Plain figures give the milligrams of essential amino acids provided by 100 g of the food listed.

Table 8A   Ratio of Total Essential Amino Acids to Nitrogen Content in Selected Foods

Source of protein	Ratio of total essential amino acids to total nitrogen, g/g
Casein	3.25
Egg, hen's	3.22
Milk, cow's	3.20
Milk, human	3.13
Beef liver	2.94
Beef heart	2.85
Beef muscle	2.79
Navy bean	2.79
Cornmeal	2.78
Millet	2.75
Sweet potato	2.70
Pork tenderloin	2.67
Fish	2.66
Rice	2.61
Peas	2.59
Soy flour	2.58
Spinach	2.50
Sesame seed	2.47
Oats	2.30
Rye	2.17
Cottonseed	2.15
Sunflower seed	2.11
Peanut flour	2.08
White wheat flour	2.02
1957 FAO reference protein	2.02
Wheat gluten	1.99
Gelatin	1.31
Cassava	1.05

As the global supply of expensive, complete animal proteins becomes increasingly short in the face of a rapidly growing population, the economic significance of the concept of mutual supplementation of proteins is evident. In underdeveloped areas, where protein deficiencies are endemic, it would be folly to preach a diet based primarily on desirable, but expensive, high-quality meat and milk proteins. There a well-planned vegetarian diet which utilizes a properly selected variety of plant protein sources, or which is fortified through a simultaneous supplementation with small quantities of the harder-to-come-by animal proteins, appears to be a logical solution of the problem of adequate protein supply.

Practical experience of recent years has borne out that supplementation of the predominantly consumed cereal staples in underdeveloped countries with small amounts of animal proteins (skim milk powder, fish flour, or fish protein concentrate) or even with indigenous vegetable proteins of higher biologic value (soy flour, peanut flour, several varieties of peas, beans, and hybrid corn) or combinations thereof (soy flour and skim milk powder) results in improved linear growth, weight gain, nitrogen retention, and serum protein levels in growing preschool children.

One of the chief disadvantages of such supplements is that they may interfere with desirable organoleptic properties of food—a factor of particular importance in older children and adults. Lowering the level of such supplements or fortification with individual essential amino acids which are present in the basic cereal staple in deficient quantities may provide a solution in some cases.

Protein Supplementation with Specific Amino Acids

In recent years supplementation of low-quality proteins with individual amino acids in which they are deficient has received increasing attention. In view of the fact that the biologic quality of wheat and rice proteins is limited by their low lysine content, proposals have been made for the fortification of these cereal proteins with lysine in an effort to improve their amino acid balance.

On the basis of present-day knowledge and experience, it is possible to generalize that diets which are limited in lysine can be improved by lysine supplementation and that proper quantitative use of this supplement does not introduce a significant hazard of toxicity or amino acid imbalance. In all probability, people who derive a large proportion of their protein intake from animal sources are not likely to respond to lysine supplementation of the cereal products they consume. Population groups in this or any other country which derive a substantial part of their protein intake from cereals, particularly wheat, will benefit from supplemental lysine if total lysine intake is lower than desirable. To date, experience with infants, preschool children, and schoolchildren in different underdeveloped countries has shown that supplementation of wheat flour with lysine (at a 0.2 percent level) or of other cereals of suboptimal protein quality with lysine and methionine or threonine brought about a statistically significant increase in height, weight, nitrogen retention, serum protein levels, and serum amino acid profiles. New hybrid varieties of wheat, corn, rice, and legumes are also promising.

Anabolism, Catabolism, and Nitrogen Balance

Protein anabolism and *catabolism* are terms used to denote protein synthesis and breakdown in the organism. Thirty to fifty percent of the body protein is in constant flux. Within the individual there occurs a steady, simultaneous tissue protein breakdown and synthesis involving up to half of the total metabolic pool of protein at any one time. For instance, the carbon skeleton of an amino acid which is a constituent of the cell protein in a liver cell may well be found at another time incorporated into the molecule of a digestive enzyme secreted into the lumen of the intestine, later to be reabsorbed and incorporated into a muscle protein molecule, or perhaps to be deaminated and burned for energy gain. The sum total of all the simultaneous gains and losses of nitrogen in the different compartments of the body is reflected in the overall nitrogen balance and is "zero"—neither positive nor negative—in adults under normal conditions of health and adequate diet.

The term *nitrogen balance* refers to the long-term relationship between incoming and outgoing food nitrogen in an organism. Nitrogen equilibrium exists in an individual when the nitrogen (chiefly protein nitrogen) intake equals the waste-nitrogen output. If the dietary protein of a healthy, normal adult with good body reserves is adequate and he does not form new tissues or break down existing ones (except in normal, balanced replacement—a dynamic exchange is always functioning), he will be in nitrogen equilibrium; the absorbed dietary nitrogen (total ingested food nitrogen less the unabsorbed portion recovered in the feces) will equal the excreted nitrogen (chiefly urea nitrogen in the urine). If increased amounts of protein are fed to such a person, an increased absorption of nitrogen takes place, followed by a corresponding increase in the excretion of nitrogenous waste products; and within a short time nitrogen equilibrium is reestablished.

In conventional brief nitrogen balance experiments, nitrogen balance is taken to be the difference between the amount given in the diet and the sum of urinary and fecal nitrogenous wastes. Exacting long-term overall nitrogen balance determinations must also take into account small, but in toto significant, nitrogen losses from sweat and desquamated epidermal cells (protein losses from intestinal secretions and desquamated cells from the gastrointestinal mucosa will be found in the feces), semen, blood, sputum and saliva, hair cut or shed, nail clippings, tooth brushing, toilet tissue, and exhaled ammonia. The total amount of nitrogen lost during excessive sweating under conditions of sustained hard labor and high temperatures is still being debated; the work of some investigators indicates that an acclimatization to such conditions takes place and that subsequent nitrogen losses even during profuse sweating are marginal.

During growth, pregnancy, and lactation, or during rehabilitation after a debilitating disease or malnutrition, total anabolism exceeds total catabolism. More dietary nitrogen is retained to support body protein synthesis, and less is excreted as nitrogenous waste. Such a subject is said to be in positive nitrogen balance.

When total catabolism exceeds total anabolism, body protein is broken down in excess; more nitrogen is excreted in the urine than is absorbed and utilized from food, and a negative nitrogen balance results. A nitrogen loss from dietary causes occurs primarily when the dietary protein intake is inadequate or when the diet does not meet the body's caloric requirement. The energy requirement of the organism has to be satisfied first, and when the diet does not provide sufficient energy sources such as carbohydrates and fats, the necessary energy is obtained by breakdown of tissue substances. In such a case, liver and muscle glycogen and tissue fat are being utilized, as well as the most easily mobilizable protein fractions of the body. The breakdown of tissue proteins for the creation of energy is a wasteful and undesirable process from the standpoint of metabolic body economy.

Excessive breakdown of body protein also occurs during systemic diseases (especially febrile ones), after injuries, burns, and surgery. A diet very rich in good-quality proteins and protein-sparing calories is desirable both before and after elective surgery, as well as after major disease or injury, to counterbalance this loss of protein from the body which may continue for days and be quite extensive.

Deficiency

Insufficient intake of proteins and calories, or consumption of proteins which do not provide an adequate supply of all the essential amino acids, is without doubt the major malnutrition problem in the world today. Because protein plays a vital role in all life processes, the symptoms of protein deficiency in man are varied and not necessarily specific and characteristic. The early symptoms of protein deficiency include loss of weight, lassitude, easy fatigability, decreased resistance to disease, prolonged convalescence and, in children, slow, stunted growth. Continued protein deprivation results in consequences which are of a more specific nature: low blood protein levels (including hemoglobin), edema, and liver damage. The edema is apparently not the direct result of the hypoproteinemia (i.e., the lowering of the intravascular osmotic pressure) alone; apparently hormonal interference with diuresis plays an etiologic role as well. The liver damage is presumably the result of depletion of all mobilizable liver protein, increased susceptibility to toxic injuries, and abnormal liver function with accumulation of fat in the liver parenchyma. The fatty infiltration may eventually progress to destruction of parenchymal tissue with fibrous replacement (cirrhosis).

As a result of studies made subsequent to World War II, a specific protein malnutrition syndrome has been recognized as being widely distributed among infants and children in underdeveloped regions or underprivileged population strata in Africa, India, Central America, and other parts of the world. This disease entity, kwashiorkor, is discussed in Chap. 22, Malnutrition and Deficiency Diseases.

Recommended Protein Allowances

The standards recommended by the Food and Nutrition Board of the National Research Council provide for 56 g of protein per day in the diet of adult men weighing 70 kg and 46 g of dietary protein for women weighing 58 kg (Table 22 in Chap. 13). This allowance of 0.8 g of protein per kilogram of body weight appears to provide a margin of safety when applied to healthy persons with adequate caloric intake, normally vigorous, and living in a temperate climate. Estimates of the increased allowances for protein during pregnancy and lactation vary greatly. The Food and Nutrition Board recommends 76 g of protein daily for pregnant women in the second half of pregnancy and 66 g daily for the period of lactation. Other recommended allowances: children and adolescents, from 23 to 54 g of protein daily, depending on the specific age.

The protein requirements as proposed by the Food and Agriculture Organization of the United Nations are unique in that they are based on a hypothetical reference protein of a desirable amino acid composition. These FAO standards are found in Chap. 13; the same chapter also discusses the basic differences in the aims of the various standards, thus explaining any apparent quantitative differences between them.

These calculated standards suffer identical, unavoidable shortcomings: (1) they do not fully take into account individual biologic variations; and (2) they do not give full consideration to differences in biologic value of the various food proteins, or give full consideration to the effect of mutual supplementation of simultaneously ingested proteins. As for the second point, practical considerations and economic necessity rule out the exclusive use of high-quality proteins of animal origin, and experience has shown that a mixture of both animal and plant proteins or a carefully selected mixture of protein foods entirely of plant origin will support healthy life processes and normal vigor.

Sources

The proteins of the human diet are obtained from both animal and vegetable sources. The most important proteins of animal origin are milk and milk products, meats, fish and seafoods, poultry, and eggs. Plant proteins are readily available in cereals (wheat, rice, corn, barley, rye), legume seeds (beans, peas, grams), and nuts. In the more prosperous countries the proportion of proteins of animal origin, which are more expensive than plant proteins, is relatively high. Wherever such a food pattern prevails, there is assurance that the supply of protein is adequate both quantitatively and qualitatively, since most natural animal proteins furnish the essential amino acids in liberal amounts. The least expensive source of complete proteins is skim milk powder, and its use should be encouraged whenever economic considerations limit the availability of the conventional sources of high-quality proteins. Soybeans are a cheap source of protein of good nutritive value; however, attempts to introduce their use into the countries of the Western world have largely run counter to established gastronomic preferences.

In regions which are characterized by a low standard of living, the protein supply is likely to be derived chiefly from plants, and the protein intake, even if it is quantitatively adequate, may be substandard with regard to essential amino acid content unless the food sources are properly chosen. (For a more detailed discussion, see Chap. 22, the section on kwashiorkor.) If at all possible, one-third or more of the dietary protein should come from foods of animal origin.

Detailed information on the protein content of common foods is found in the Tables of Food Composition in the Appendix.

Chapter 8

Carbohydrates

Chemistry

Carbohydrates are compounds which contain carbon, hydrogen, and oxygen, the latter two in the same proportion as in water. All carbohydrates conform to the same basic empirical formula, $C_n H_{2n} O_n$. With but few exceptions, the carbohydrates are of plant origin. The most important exceptions are glycogen, the animal equivalent of starch; lactose, animal milk sugar; and ribose, a five-carbon sugar associated with animal nucleic acids. Carbohydrates are synthesized in nature by green plants from carbon dioxide of the atmosphere and water, in the presence of sunlight. Life as we know it depends on this photosynthetic process, since the carbohydrates of the plant kingdom are the major energy fuel on which the animal kingdom exists.

The carbohydrates are classified according to molecular structure into a number of groups, of which the following three are of primary importance in nutrition:

1   Monosaccharides: Simple hexose (six-carbon) sugars which cannot be broken down into smaller units by hydrolysis during gastrointestinal digestion. (Example, glucose.)

2 Disaccharides: More complex sugars, formed by the condensation of two monosaccharides; disaccharides can be split into their component hexose sugars by hydrolysis. (Example, sucrose.)

3 Polysaccharides: Larger, complex molecules which are the result of the condensation of a large number of monosaccharides; they too may be hydrolyzed to their component hexose sugars. (Example, starch.)

Only three monosaccharides are of significance in human nutrition: glucose, fructose, and galactose. Of the disaccharides, sucrose (cane or beet sugar) and lactose (milk sugar) are of primary importance, as well as maltose, which is formed during the digestion of starches. Starch, cellulose, and the animal equivalent of starch, glycogen, are examples of polysaccharides which are important in human physiology and nutrition.

The hydrolysis of a molecule of sucrose yields one molecule of glucose and one of fructose; the hydrolysis of lactose, one molecule of glucose and one of galactose. Maltose may be hydrolyzed into two molecules of glucose. When starch is digested, it is degraded primarily by the repeated splitting off of maltose units, which in turn are hydrolyzed into glucose. The large partially degraded glucose polymer units which are intermediates during this process are dextrins. These partially degraded polysaccharides undergo progressive attrition by hydrolysis, glucose being the eventual end product.

Glycogen is the form in which the animal cell stores carbohydrate. It is a polymer of glucose and yields glucose on hydrolysis. Cellulose is a polysaccharide which serves as the structural component of plant tissues. The human digestive tract does not secrete an enzyme which is capable of digesting cellulose; when ingested with fruits, with vegetables, or as the undigestible residue of whole grains, most of it remains unchanged and provides the roughage and bulk which is essential for optimal functioning of the lower intestinal tract and the formation of the feces. Intestinal bacteria may break down and utilize a small part of the cellulose and thus indirectly contribute additional nutrients.

Cereals, vegetables, and fruits are the major natural sources of carbohydrates. The refined carbohydrates sucrose and starch are ingested in considerable quantities in compounded foods (soft drinks, pies, candy, puddings, ice cream, sherbet) and foods based on cereals (bread, rice, spaghetti, noodles), and starchy vegetables such as potatoes account for a major share of our carbohydrate intake. Milk and its derivatives contribute lactose to the diet, the only major carbohydrate of animal origin in our food supply.

Digestion and Absorption

When ingested, carbohydrates are mostly in the form of poly- and disaccharides which must be hydrolyzed into simple hexose sugars before absorption can take place. The process of digestion is initiated in the mouth through the starch-splitting action of the salivary enzyme ptyalin. This digestive action continues to some degree in the stomach (Chap. 1). In the intestinal tract, pancreatic amylase hydrolyzes the remaining starch to maltose. Although the carbohydrases of the intestinal juice can split the disaccharides maltose, lactose, and sucrose into their respective monosaccharide components, liberating glucose, galactose, and fructose, which may then be absorbed in the small intestine, this mechanism applies apparently only to a small fraction of disaccharides present in the intestinal tract. It has been demonstrated convincingly that the major portion of disaccharides is not hydrolyzed to monosaccharides in the lumen of the intestine; rather, the disaccharides are absorbed as such into the cells of the mucous membrane of the small intestine which are known to be rich in disaccharide-splitting enzymes. Hydrolysis then takes place within the cells, and the resulting monosaccharides are secreted into the portal bloodstream. Different disaccharides are absorbed optimally at different sites along the small intestine; lactose is absorbed most efficiently in the duodenum and proximal jejunum, maltose in the jejunum and proximal ileum, and sucrose in the distal jejunum and ileum.

Two types of absorption of monosaccharides take place in the small intestine: (1) a nonspecific, passive physical process of diffusion which is governed by the concentration gradient between the sugar in the intestinal lumen and that in the cells of the intestinal mucosa, and (2) an active absorption of specific disaccharides and monosaccharides which involves phosphorylation of the sugar in the cells of the intestinal mucosa and hydrolysis of the disaccharides. In contrast to other five- and six-carbon sugars, glucose, fructose, and galactose are subject to both types of mechanism; they are therefore taken into the bloodstream more rapidly and their specific absorption rates are independent of their concentration in the intestinal lumen. If we arbitrarily assign an absorption rate of 100 for glucose, the corresponding absorption rates for other sugars are galactose 110, fructose 30, sorbose 30, mannose 19, xylose 15, and arabinose 9.

Carbohydrate Metabolism

The monosaccharides which have been absorbed from the intestinal tract are carried to the liver by the portal circulation. There fructose and galactose are quantitatively converted into glucose. The liver cells may release this glucose into the bloodstream to be distributed to the body tissues where it serves as a source of energy. Any excess of glucose is polymerized in the liver cells into insoluble glycogen, the storage form of body carbohydrate. This conversion of glucose to glycogen is reversible; as the need arises, the liver mobilizes glucose from its glycogen stores and releases it into the bloodstream in sufficient quantity to maintain an optimal blood sugar level. During the immediate absorptive state, when hexose sugars (mostly glucose) are actively absorbed from the digested food in the intestinal lumen, the blood sugar level rises. This postprandial blood sugar tide is being counteracted not only by the active glycogenesis in the liver, but also by withdrawal of glucose from the circulation by the various tissues for purposes of energy metabolism and for storage against future need. Thus the early postprandial rise in blood sugar is followed by a gradual return to the normal blood sugar levels of 80 to 100 mg per 100 ml in the postabsorptive period.

Tissues other than liver are also capable of synthesizing glycogen from glucose. Thus skeletal, cardiac, and smooth muscles maintain their own glycogen stores when at rest or under minor work loads; glycogen is also found in smaller quantities in practically all organs of the body. It is beyond the scope of this chapter to discuss the detailed physiology and biochemistry of muscular contraction; suffice it to say that the energy for muscular work is obtained from high-energy phosphate compounds (adenosine phosphates and creatine phosphate). These are capable of yielding immediate energy on demand and restore themselves to their previous high energy state by acquiring the energy liberated by the oxidation of glucose to carbon dioxide and water inside the muscle cell, and by the oxidation, by muscle, of fatty acids. The basic steps involved in carbohydrate utilization are illustrated in Fig. 4, which summarizes the Embden-Meyerhof-Parnas scheme of glycolysis. During this main pathway of

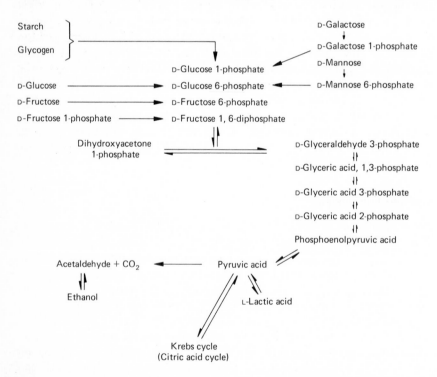

Figure 4   The Embden-Meyerhof-Parnas scheme of carbohydrate utilization.

carbohydrate metabolism, glycogen is degraded to glucose, which in turn breaks down into two molecules of pyruvic or lactic acid. In the presence of sufficient oxygen, lactic acid does not accumulate and the pyruvate is oxidized to carbon dioxide and water through the mechanism of the Krebs citric acid cycle (Fig. 5). During continuous muscular exercise, lactic acid is formed in the working muscle and diffuses thence into the circulation. It is then gradually withdrawn from the bloodstream by the liver, which converts it into glycogen. This liver glycogen may, in turn, serve as a source of blood glucose if additional glucose is needed to maintain the blood glucose level.

The amount of reserve glycogen stored in the liver and muscle depends largely on the nature of the diet and the amount of exercise. The glycogen reserves are progressively depleted during continuous or violent exercise. Cardiac muscle is unique in that it preserves tenaciously its diminishing reserves of glycogen, using blood glucose preferentially to furnish energy for its muscular contraction. Brain tissue utilizes carbohydrates (blood glucose)

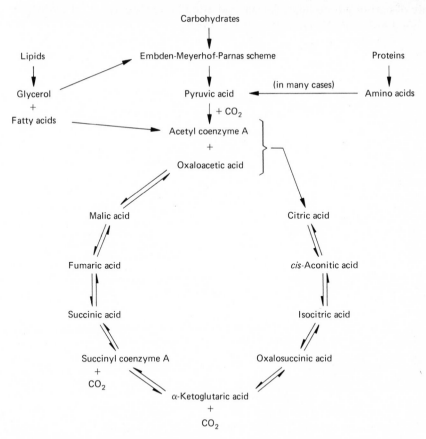

Figure 5 The Krebs citric acid cycle.

almost exclusively for its energy metabolism, in contrast to skeletal muscle, which may utilize carbohydrates or fatty acids to obtain fuel for ordinary exercise.

The chemical pathway outlined above probably represents the major route of carbohydrate metabolism in the body, particularly in muscle tissue. However, there also exists an alternate pathway of carbohydrate utilization, the *hexose monophosphate shunt* ("oxidative, or pentose shunt") (Fig. 6), which serves important functions, at least in certain tissues. Though apparently of no importance in muscle tissue, this pathway operates in the liver to a varying degree (concurrent with the classic Embden-Meyerhof-Parnas reaction), as well as in other organs and in the fatty tissues of the body. An important chemical by-product (reduced triphosphopyridine nucleotide, or TPNH) generated by the shunt pathway—in contrast to the conventional scheme of carbohydrate utilization—is essential for and employed in the synthesis of fats and cholesterol. The possible significance of the operation of this alternate pathway of carbohydrate degradation, and attendant, concurrent fat synthesis, is discussed in Chap. 21, Obesity and Leanness.

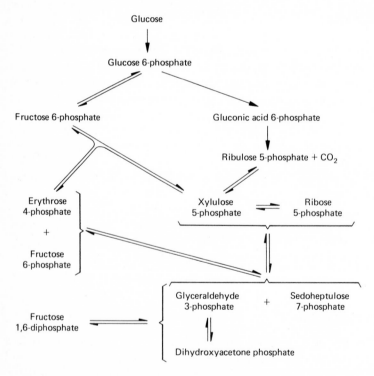

Figure 6   The hexose monophosphate shunt scheme of glucose degradation.

Relations to Fat and Protein

The body has a limited capacity for storing glycogen; however, its ability to store fat is not nearly so restricted. Thus when carbohydrates are supplied by the diet in excess of the capacity of the various tissues for oxidation or glycogen storage, they are converted into fat and stored as such in the adipose tissues. (This maxim holds true for any food ingested in excess of caloric expenditure and applies to dietary protein and fat as well.) Conversely, when carbohydrate is no longer available for energy production, the body begins to draw on its other components and breaks down tissue fat and protein. A certain minimal amount of carbohydrate must be supplied by the diet at all times to prevent the wasteful use of dietary protein or, worse yet, protein from the body's metabolic pool or structural components, for purposes of energy supply. This preventive action of carbohydrates is referred to as *protein sparing.* Experience has shown that a maximum protein-sparing action is obtained if carbohydrate and protein are ingested simultaneously.

It has already been mentioned that the production of carbohydrate from protein which is ingested in excess of specific amino acid and nitrogen needs is a normal process (Chap. 7). Not all amino acids lend themselves to sugar formation; nevertheless, up to 58 percent of dietary protein may follow this metabolic pathway. Conversely, nonessential amino acids may be synthesized in the body from keto acids derived from carbohydrate metabolism.

In the absence of carbohydrates in the diet (or in severe, uncorrected diabetes when the body does not utilize carbohydrates effectively), when fat—derived from the diet or from the body's fat depots—is the primary energy source, end products of incomplete fatty acid breakdown soon accumulate. These "ketone bodies" (see Chaps. 9 and 24) will not be formed and accumulated if a small proportion of carbohydrate is metabolized simultaneously. Carbohydrates are thus said to be *antiketogenic.* Carbohydrates also have the ability to conserve water and electrolytes during temporary starvation, even when supplied only in small daily quantities.

From the foregoing it is apparent that the metabolic pathways of carbohydrates, proteins, and fats are not exclusive and distinct; they interact at many points, and this permits a flexibility in the supply of nutrients and mutual substitution within wide limits without serious injury to the metabolizing tissues.

Carbohydrates and the Diet

Carbohydrates generally make up the bulk of man's energy supply. Nevertheless, wide variations in the percentage of carbohydrate in the diet are still consistent with normal health. In practice, the proportion of energy supplied by dietary carbohydrate is governed by ecologic and economic factors. Whereas in the tropics carbohydrates are likely to contribute up to 80 percent of the daily caloric needs, herdsmen and Eskimos may exist tolerably well on an animal diet which is high in protein and fat and in which carbohydrates supply only 20 percent or less of the daily caloric requirement. Economic status and agricultural practices greatly influence the proportion of carbohydrates in the diet. Rice, potatoes, cereals, flour products, legumes, and vegetables, all predominantly carbohydrate foods, are considerably cheaper than meat, eggs, poultry, and dairy products, which are primarily sources of proteins and fats. It is a well-known fact that the proportion of carbohydrates in national diets varies inversely with the standard of living of the countries compared. A similar inverse relationship between carbohydrate consumption and income exists within each country and determines to a large extent the carbohydrate intake of different population groups. Current nutritional opinion in the United States tends to favor a level of carbohydrates in the diet which supplies roughly 50 percent of the total energy requirement. This need not be considered a hard-and-fast rule. Economic considerations and regional factors may force a higher proportion of carbohydrates in many diets; such a food pattern will still be consistent with optimal nutrition provided that the diet assures an adequate vitamin and mineral intake, that it contains sufficient fat to supply the essential fatty acids and fat-soluble vitamins, and that it contributes a level of protein sufficient to fulfill the needs for growth, defense mechanisms, tissue repair, and maintenance.

Chapter 9

Fats

Chemistry

The lipids constitute a somewhat heterogeneous group of compounds which are related to one another by the fact that they are insoluble in water and soluble in the so-called fat solvents (ether, benzene, chloroform, and others). They either contain one or more fatty acids in the molecule or are combined with a fatty acid in their natural state. For the nutritionist's purposes the term *lipids* is limited to compounds which occur in biologic material.

The lipids may be classified as follows:

I   Simple lipids: esters of fatty acids with various alcohols. Fats are esters of fatty acids with glycerol. Waxes contain alcohols other than glycerol; this includes cholesterol esters, which are combinations of fatty acids and sterol alcohols such as cholesterol.

II   Compound lipids: esters of fatty acids and glycerol which are combined with other chemical groups. For instance, the phospholipids are substituted fats in which phosphoric acid and a nitrogenous base take the place of one fatty acid radical.

III Derived lipids: substances derived from the first two groups by hydrolysis.
A Fatty acids: butyric, oleic, palmitic, stearic, linoleic, etc.
B Alcohols: glycerol, cetanol, lanol.
C Sterol alcohols: cholesterol, ergosterol, sitosterol.

Fatty acids vary with respect to molecular size and with respect to the number and position of double bonds found in the molecule. Those with one or more double bonds in the carbon chain which makes up the molecule are termed *unsaturated* (polyunsaturated if two or more double bonds are present); those devoid of double bonds are *saturated*. Unsaturated fatty acids may be artificially modified by the saturation of the double bonds with additional hydrogen atoms, which converts them into single bonds. This process is referred to as *hydrogenation*.

The following are some examples of fatty acids of biologic importance which are commonly found in foods:

Saturated fatty acids	Source
Empirical formula $C_nH_{2n}O_2$	
Acetic acid	Vinegar
Butyric acid	Butter
Palmitic acid	Vegetable oils, animal fats
Stearic acid	Animal fats, vegetable oils
Unsaturated fatty acids	
One double bond; empirical formula $C_nH_{2n-2}O_2$	
Oleic acid	Vegetable oils, animal fats
Two double bonds; empirical formula $C_nH_{2n-4}O_2$	
Linoleic acid	Vegetable oils (corn, soy, cottonseed, wheat germ, linseed)
Three double bonds; empirical formula $C_nH_{2n-6}O_2$	
Linolenic acid	Vegetable oils (linseed)
Four double bonds; empirical formula $C_nH_{2n-8}O_2$	
Arachidonic acid	Found in small quantities in selected animal fats

Natural fats and oils are usually mixtures of triglycerides with the basic formula

$$
\begin{array}{l}
CH_2OR_1 \\
|\\
CHOR_2 \\
|\\
CH_2OR_3
\end{array}
$$

where R_1, R_2, and R_3 represent identical or different fatty acids. In natural fats the component fatty acids of the various triglycerides are usually not identical. If the mixture is solid at room temperature, it is called a fat; if liquid, it is considered to be an oil. The melting point of a natural fat depends on the fatty acids of which it is composed. Hard fats contain mostly saturated fatty acids, while liquid oils are made up predominantly of unsaturated fatty acids. Saturation of these by hydrogenation will convert a liquid oil into a hard fat (solid, white vegetable shortenings, margarine). The chief sources of food fat are vegetable oils (cottonseed, corn, peanut, soy, sesame, olive), butter, margarine, lard, milk, cheese, eggs, meats, fish, and nuts.

Cholesterol is widely distributed in the animal body, especially in nervous tissue, blood, and bile. It occurs in the free form or esterified with fatty acids. Free cholesterol is the chief constituent of gallstones. Cholesterol is the precursor of bile salts and probably of the steroid adrenal and sex hormones. In the skin it serves as a precursor of vitamin D. When the skin is exposed to sunlight or ultraviolet irradiation, cholesterol and closely related compounds are converted to active vitamin D. Cholesterol facilitates the absorption of fatty acids from the intestine and their transportation in the blood by combining with them in the form of cholesterol esters, which are more soluble and emulsifiable than the free fatty acid molecules. Cholesterol is found only in foods of animal origin and is supplied by diets which contain animal meats, glandular organs, and fats, but the human body is not dependent on dietary sources for its cholesterol supply. It is constantly being synthesized in the body, the main site of synthesis being the liver. The amount produced daily endogenously is probably two to three times the usual dietary intake (in the United States, the usual dietary intake is on the order of 500 to 800 mg daily, and the amount synthesized is the neighborhood of 1.5 to 2 g a day), and the rate of synthesis varies inversely with the amount of dietary cholesterol available. Synthesis and degradation of cholesterol occur simultaneously and continuously. It is excreted either through conversion to bile salts, which are subsequently released into the small intestine, or through conversion to neutral sterols. The cholesterol level in the various tissues is kept fairly constant. The subject of cholesterol and other lipid levels in blood and their relation to atherogenesis and circulatory disease is discussed in Chap. 29.

The three types of phospholipid which are of greatest biologic importance are the lecithins, cephalins, and sphingomyelins. The first two groups are composed of glycerol, two fatty acids, phosphoric acid, and a nitrogenous base. Sphingomyelins contain a fatty acid, phosphoric acid, and two nitrogenous bases. The phospholipids appear to be essential constituents of all living cells; they serve as structural components of the cell wall and the mitochondria within the cells. They also function as metabolic intermediates in transportation and utilization of fatty acids and constitute a readily mobilized and metabolized form of fatty acid reserve.

Digestion, Absorption, and Transport

Hydrolysis of ingested fats is *initiated* when masticated food comes in contact with pharyngeal lipase in the throat. Lipolytic degradation of triglycerides to

Table 8B Fatty Acid Content of Food Fats

(Grams per 100-g Ether Extract or Crude Fat)

Food fat or oil	Saturated fatty acids			Total	Unsaturated fatty acids			Other	Unsaponifiable matter	Iodine value
	Total*	Palmitic C_{16}	Stearic C_{18}		Oleic $C_{18}(-2H)$	Linoleic $C_{18}(-4H)$	Linolenic $C_{18}(-6H)$			
Animal products										
Meats:										
Beef	48	28	19	47	44	2	Trace†	1	...	47
Buffalo	66	34	28	30	24	1	...	5	Trace	31
Deer	63	24	34	32	24	3	2	3	Trace	36
Goat	57	26	24	37	33	2	...	2	2	33
Horse	30	24	5	60	30	6	13	11	6	75
Lamb	56	29	25	40	36	3	1	Trace	...	40
Luncheon meats	36	24	11	59	45	7	Trace	7	...	61
Pork:										
Back, outer layer	38	26	12	58	46	6	...	6	...	64
Bacon	32	21	9	63	48	9	Trace	6	...	67
Liver	34	13	18	61	27	5	...	29	...	64
Other cuts	36	21	13	59	42	9	Trace	8	...	64
Rabbit, domesticated	38	28	4	58	35	11	2	10	...	66
Milk fat:										
Buffalo, Indian	62	29	15	33	26	1	...	6	Trace	30
Cow	55	25	12	39	33	3	1	2	Trace	33
Goat	62	27	8	33	25	5	...	3	Trace	37
Human	46	22	7	48‡	34	7	Trace	7	...	37

Poultry and eggs:									
Chicken	32	24	7	64‡	38	20	2	4	...	92
Turkey	29	22	6	67‡	43	21	1	2	...	84
Chicken eggs	32	25	7	61	44	7	1	9	3	84
Fish and shellfish:									
Eel, body	23	17	2	73	...	36(-2.6H)	...	37	...	119
Herring, body	19	11	1	77	...	19(-3.5H)	...	58	...	140
Menhaden, body	24	15	3	71	15	3	2	51	...	151
Salmon, body	15	12	2	79	...	26(-2.8H)	...	53	1	
Tuna, body	25	18	3	70	...	25(-3.2H)	...	45	1	
Turtle	44	16	7	51	...	31(-2.6H)	...	20	1	74
Separated fats and oils:									
Butter	55	25	12	39	33	3	1	2	Trace	33
Lard	38	31	7	57	46	10	1	Trace	Trace	64
Shortening, see under Plant Products									
Codfish liver	15	12	1	81	...	25(-3.3H)	...	56	...	178
Halibut liver	17	13	Trace	72	31	...	...	41	7	120
Whale blubber	15	9	1	41	...	21(-2.4H)	...	20	40	87

*Includes other saturated fatty acids in addition to palmitic and stearic.

†Trace is used to indicate values of 0.5 or less.

‡Includes 1 g arachidonic acid.

§Varies widely depending on the fats used.

Source: From V. R. Goddard and L. Goodall, *Home Economics Research Report No. 7,* Agricultural Research Service, U. S. Department of Agriculture.

(Continued on following pages)

Table 8B Fatty Acid Content of Food Fats (Continued from pages 72–73)

(Grams per 100-g Ether Extract or Crude Fat)

Food fat or oil	Saturated fatty acids			Unsaturated fatty acids						Unsaponifiable matter	Iodine value
	Total*	Palmitic C_{16}	Stearic C_{18}	Total	Oleic $C_{18}(-2H)$	Linoleic $C_{18}(-4H)$	Linolenic $C_{18}(-6H)$	Other			
Plant products											
Cereals and grains:											
Cornmeal, white	11	8	1	82	34	44	1	3		3	123
Millet (foxtail)	31	10	14	61	20	35	6	...		3	120
Oats, rolled	22	13	4	74	32	41	1	Trace			100
Rice	17	12	2	74	39	35	...	...		5	
Sorghum	12	7	5	81	37	44	...	...		3	122
Wheat flour, white	14	10	4	76	31	42	3	...		6	120
Wheat germ	15	11	4	77	23	48	6	...		4	129
Fruits and vegetables including seeds:											
Avocado pulp	20	18	2	69	45	13	1	10		6	88
Cantaloupe seed	15	10	4	79	26	53	...	...		1	126
Chick-pea	9	4	2	87	50	36	...	1		...	114
Chocolate	56	23	33	39	37	2	...	...		Trace	37
Olives	11	9	2	84	76	7	...	1		1	84
Pigeon-pea	33	...	...	57	6	46	5	...		6	104
Pumpkin seed	17	9	8	78	37	41	...	...		1	119
Rape seed	6	2	2	89	16	14	9	50		...	104
Sesame seed	14	8	4	80	38	42	...	Trace		2	114
Soybeans	20	11	7	75	16	52	7	Trace		...	128
Squash seed	18	12	6	77	35	42	...	...		1	121
Watermelon seed	17	10	6	78	18	59	...	1		1	128

Nuts and peanuts:

Item										
Almond	8	7	1	87	67	20	...	...	Trace	101
Beechnut	8	5	3	87	54	31	2	...	1	112
Brazil nut	20	14	6	76	48	26	...	2	Trace	
Cashew	17	6	11	78	70	7	...	1	1	9
Coconut	86	10	2	8	7	Trace	...	1	Trace	95
Filbert (hazelnut)	5	2	2	91	54	16	...	21	Trace	94
Hickory	8	6	1	87	68	18	...	1	1	101
Peanut	22	11	4	72	43	29	...	...	1	100
Peanut butter	26	11	6	70	45	25	...	...	Trace	105
Pecan	7	6	1	84	63	20	1	Trace	5	95
Pistachio	10	8	2	85	65	19	...	1	1	
Walnut, black	6	3	2	90	35	48	7	...	Trace	135
Walnut, English	7	5	2	89	15	62	8	4	Trace	162

Separated fats and oils:

Item										
Cacao butter	56	23	33	39	37	2	...	...	Trace	37
Corn oil	10	8	2	84	28	53	1	2	2	127
Cottonseed oil	25	22	2	71	21	50	...	...	...	109
Margarine§	26	21	3	70	57	9	Trace	4	1	72
Olive oil	11	9	2	84	76	7	...	1	1	84
Palm oil	45	39	4	49	40	8	Trace	1	1	51
Peanut oil	18	8	6	76	47	29	Trace	1	1	101
Safflower oil	8	3	4	87	15	72	...	...	1	146
Sesame oil	14	8	4	80	38	42	...	Trace	2	114
Shortening (animal and vegetable)§	43	27	12	53	41	11	1	Trace	1	59
Shortening (vegetable)§	23	14	6	72	65	7	Trace	Trace	Trace	75
Soybean oil	15	9	6	80	20	52	7	1	1	133
Sunflower oil	12	6	5	83	20	63	...	...	Trace	134

*Includes other saturated fatty acids in addition to palmitic and stearic.
†Trace is used to indicate values of 0.5 or less.
‡Includes 1 g arachidonic acid.
§Varies widely depending on the fats used.
Source: From V. R. Goddard and L. Goodall, *Home Economics Research Report No. 7*, Agricultural Research Service, U.S. Department of Agriculture.

, fatty acids and mono- and diglycerides starts in the esophagus and
ntinues in the stomach.

The primary site of digestion and absorption of fats is the small intestine.
Pancreatic lipase is the most important enzyme concerned with fat digestion;
intestinal lipase plays a lesser role. Steapsin, or pancreatic lipase, hydrolyzes
fats to glycerol and fatty acids. Apparently, the triglyceride molecule is not
attacked equally at all three linkages with the component fatty acids, but the
hydrolytic action proceeds in stages, producing first diglycerides, then monoglycerides, and eventually splitting the molecule into glycerol and fatty acids.
Di- and monoglycerides are efficient emulsifying agents, and with their aid a
considerable proportion of yet unhydrolyzed triglyceride fat is finely emulsified and may be absorbed directly in this form.

The presence of bile is essential for normal digestion and absorption of
lipids. The bile salts reduce the surface tension of large globules of yet-
unhydrolyzed fat and thus facilitate their subdivision into minute globules
under the constant churning action of the intestine. Consequently, the food fat
is reduced into an ultrafine emulsion which exposes an enormously increased
surface of fat molecules to the saponifying action of the pancreatic lipase and
the alkaline intestinal juice. In addition, the bile salts facilitate the solution of
the otherwise insoluble, partially hydrolyzed glycerides and of the liberated
fatty acids in the aqueous medium, and thus make possible their absorption by
the mucosal cells, or their traversing the mucosal barrier directly into the blood
and lymph vessels of the small intestine. Bile is also responsible for the
solubilizing of the carotenes and the fat-soluble vitamins and is essential for
their normal absorption. It has been shown that monoglycerides, free fatty
acids, and bile salts form micellar solutions within the intestinal lumen. From
this solution, monoglycerides and free fatty acids are absorbed. The 2-
monoglycerides (glycerides where the single fatty acid is esterified to the
number 2, central carbon) are absorbed directly without further hydrolysis, but
not 1-monoglycerides which require preliminary hydrolysis, probably in the
outer brush border of the mucosal cells.

After the fatty acids or finely emulsified glycerides have entered the cells
of the intestinal mucosa, the water-soluble bile salt–fatty acid (or fat) complex
breaks up and the free fatty acids or partially hydrolyzed glycerides are
converted into neutral fat in the mucosal cell. The bile salts are returned to the
intestine to continue their ferrying action; a certain proportion may also be
carried back to the liver by the portal circulation. The neutral fat which was
synthesized in the mucosal cells is extruded into the lacteals, aided by
contraction of the cell protoplasm. More recent thinking tends to deemphasize
the importance of the formation, in the mucosa, of neutral fat from the
absorbed products of complete fat hydrolysis. Presumably a fair proportion of
finely emulsified fat traverses the mucosal cell lining directly through fine
openings and gains entrance into the lacteals without undergoing complete
hydrolysis. In either case, the fat appears in the lacteals as a milky emulsion
called chyle. This chyle passes through the lymphatics to the thoracic duct and
pours into the venous bloodstream at the junction of the left jugular and

subclavian veins. About 60 to 70 percent of ingested fat is accounted for by this pathway. The remainder enters the capillaries of the small intestine and is carried to the liver via the portal circulation. It has been shown that the more water-soluble free fatty acids leave the intestine by way of the portal blood circulation while the more fat-soluble fatty acids and water-insoluble glycerides are transported by way of the lymphatics and the thoracic duct.

Other fat-soluble substances, such as fat-soluble vitamins and cholesterol, are also absorbed with the triglycerides. Dietary cholesterol, usually esterified with fatty acids, is absorbed to the extent of about 50 percent and is largely converted to bile acids in the liver. These bile acids are excreted into the small intestine as needed and are reabsorbed with the various products of fat digestion. This enterohepatic cycle of cholesterol and bile acids serves to regulate, through a negative feedback, the synthesis of cholesterol in the liver. This will also explain why elimination of cholesterol from the diet is not effective by itself in completely regulating blood cholesterol levels.

In normal individuals, ingested fat is absorbed to an extent of 95 percent or more. In the absence of bile, as in the case of obstructive jaundice, and in certain other diseases such as cystic fibrosis with pancreatic impairment, or celiac disease, and in severe malnutrition, fat absorption is poor and fatty stools (steatorrhea) result.

The triglyceride structure of the fat (the position of the fatty acids in the triglyceride molecule), the length of the individual component fatty acids, and their degree of unsaturation, all affect the digestibility and absorption of different fats. A fat molecule will be absorbed more readily if it contains medium- or short-chain fatty acids rather than long-chain fatty acid components. Similarly, triglycerides with a higher proportion of unsaturated fatty acids are absorbed more rapidly than those containing two or three saturated fatty acids per molecule.

The melting.point of fats is largely governed by these factors and thus is an excellent indicator of the digestibility and absorption of the different edible fats.

Fats which melt below 50°C (122°F) appear to be more efficiently digested and absorbed than those which are quite hard at ordinary temperatures. Most natural edible fats—vegetable oils, butter, lard—are digested and utilized without difficulty. Mutton fat, which melts at 50°C, seems to represent the turning point; deer tallow, oleostearin, and fully hydrogenated peanut and other vegetable oils are distinctly less well utilized. Commercial margarine, made from partially hydrogenated vegetable oils, is digested and absorbed as easily as butter.

Lipids in the Circulation

The various lipids which are found in body tissues are also present in blood plasma, in different concentrations. These include triglycerides, free (unesterified) fatty acids, cholesterol, phospholipids, cerebrosides, carotenoids, and the fat-soluble vitamins A, D, E, and K. Body lipids are in a highly dynamic state; in the blood they are carried to fat depots to be stored, or they are transported to other tissues (such as the liver) and working cells (muscle) to be metabolized for energy. Following a meal, fat is moved to adipose tissues for storage of excess energy. This stored fat includes absorbed dietary lipids as well as fat derived from dietary carbohydrate and protein consumed in excess of the body's energy and tissue synthesis requirements. During fasting, lipid transport is away from the fat depots to actively metabolizing tissues where energy is required.

Since lipids are insoluble in water, they require special vehicles to effect their transport in blood. Thus, most or probably all of the plasma lipids are combined with proteins, and in many instances with other lipids, to produce a variety of lipoprotein complexes. Lipoproteins are endowed with some of the physical characteristics of protein which enable them to exist in suspension (or simulated "solution") in plasma for effective transport throughout the body and which facilitate passage into cells and contact with enzymes for metabolism in tissues. Four classes of lipoproteins accomplish the transport of fat in the circulation: (1) chylomicrons produced in the intestinal wall, (2) high-density α-lipoproteins and (3) low-density β-lipoproteins (both produced in the liver), and (4) free or nonesterified fatty acids bound to plasma albumin, which arise principally from the fatty tissues. Other lipids, such as the fat-soluble vitamins and carotenoids, sterols, and hormones, are also transported in the blood in combination with specific plasma proteins.

Several hours after a fat-containing meal, the plasma has a milky appearance because of the presence of finely divided and emulsified neutral fat particles, termed *chylomicrons*. They have a diameter of 1μm or less and are stabilized by an ultrafine, enveloping film of protein. These chylomicrons constitute the vehicle for the transport of exogenous fat from the intestinal wall through the lymphatic system and thoracic duct into and throughout the blood circulation. The peak of this postprandial lipemia is reached at about the fourth to sixth hour after ingestion. The chylomicrons are gradually cleared from the bloodstream with the aid of a specific enzyme, lipoprotein lipase, but the precise mechanism of how ingested fat leaves the blood has not been completely elucidated. A portion of the fatty acids derived from chylomicron degradation seems to become incorporated directly into the fat depots, and about 60 percent is taken up by the liver.

In the liver, the triglyceride is resynthesized and combined with other constituents, notably cholesterol, into β-lipoproteins and secreted into the circulation. It is probable that the β-lipoproteins transport triglycerides from the liver to adipose tissue. They are made up of about 20 percent protein and 80 percent lipid, of which about 30 percent is in the form of phospholipids, 45 percent represents cholesterol esters, and the rest, free cholesterol and triglycerides. The cholesterol, cholesterol ester, and phospholipid constituents of the β-lipoproteins exchange rapidly with the lipids of the liver and are used many times in the transport of triglyceride to the periphery. The level of β-lipoproteins in the blood is subject to fluctuation. Under normal fasting conditions, the β-lipoproteins account for up to three-fourths of the total plasma lipids. The liver also synthesizes high-density α-lipoproteins which are distinguished by a considerably higher protein and higher phospholipid content than the β-lipoproteins and by a smaller molecular weight (approximately 200,000 versus 130,000). Normally, α-lipoproteins are maintained at a rather constant level, accounting for about one-fourth of the total plasma lipid. Their precise role in fat transport has not been fully elucidated as yet.

Although fatty acids enter the adipose tissues from triglycerides of β-lipoprotein or clearing chylomicrons, they leave the depots as nonesterified fatty acids. These free fatty acids are found in the circulation combined with plasma albumin. The free fatty acid fraction represents a very small part of the total plasma lipid; however, its turnover is very rapid. This fraction constitutes the form in which fat is carried from adipose tissue to working cells and represents the primary source of energy for cells burning fats.

In addition to the ingestion of fats, which results in the postprandial hyperlipemia mentioned above, other conditions affect major alterations in blood lipid levels, in health. During extensive fasting, the body mobilizes its fat reserves to serve as sources of energy. This results in an outpouring of fat from adipose tissues, in the form of nonesterified fatty acids. A similar situation obtains after the administration of epinephrine, which accelerates the oxidation of fat by working cells, during severe emotional stress (fear, anger), after several cups of strong coffee, and in untreated diabetes mellitus when normal glucose metabolism is impaired and the body compensates by increasing the utilization of fat for energy purposes. Conversely, the administration of glucose or insulin decreases the blood levels of free fatty acids in a manner suggesting a reduction of fat flow from adipose tissue.

Another condition, age, affects the blood cholesterol levels in particular. In the United States, the average cholesterol level increases from about 170 to 175 mg per 100 ml at the age of 19 to about 240 to 250 mg at the age of 60. The nature of the ingested fat also has an important bearing on blood lipid levels; the amount and kind of dietary fat are among the most important factors controlling β-lipoprotein concentrations, and related cholesterol concentrations, in serum. When the proportion of "saturated" fats (fats rich in saturated fatty acids) is high on the diet, β-lipoprotein and cholesterol blood levels tend to increase. When other fats, higher in polyunsaturated fatty acids, are fed, blood β-lipoprotein and cholesterol levels decrease. Thus a high intake of milk fat, lard, and coconut oil makes for higher blood cholesterol levels than are seen when a high proportion of dietary fat is composed of corn oil, soybean oil, or certain fish oils. The significance of the blood lipid picture and its possible relation to degenerative circulatory disease is discussed in detail in Chap. 29.

Fat Metabolism

The metabolism of the glycerol and fatty acid moieties of ingested fat follows independent pathways. The glycerol which was set free by the hydrolysis of fat is phosphorylated in the liver and converted into glucose. From this point on, its metabolism becomes merged with that of other carbohydrates.

Much of the metabolism of the fatty acids takes place in the liver. Fatty acids originating from absorbed fat, or released from the adipose tissues, are converted into phospholipids through phosphorylation and combination with glycerol and choline (or similar nitrogenous bases). If insufficient choline is available, phospholipid formation is interrupted and fatty acids tend to accumulate in the liver, since fatty acids are transported from the liver to other tissues largely in this (phospholipid) form. Ordinarily, sufficient choline is ingested in the form of dietary phospholipids (eggs and foods of animal origin). Choline may also be synthesized in the body from the amino acid methionine. Choline and methionine are referred to as *lipotropic factors* since they promote transport and utilization of fats and since in their absence phospholipid synthesis in the liver is impaired and fatty acids accumulate in this organ, resulting in an abnormal fatty liver.

Fatty acids are oxidized in the liver and muscle tissue and yield energy during this process. Although muscles *seem* to utilize carbohydrates preferentially for generation of work energy, it has been shown in recent years that during extensive or prolonged exercise fats play an important role as an energy fuel for muscular work. The fatty acids utilized for this purpose are provided through hydrolysis of fats from fat depots. These had been laid down during periods of positive caloric balance when any excess of dietary carbohydrate, fat, or protein was converted to body fat, and they are constantly ready to act as energy reservoirs when the demand exceeds supply—as during muscular exercise.

Several theories have been advanced to explain the actual mechanism of fatty acid oxidation. The omega oxidation theory holds that the terminal methyl group of the fatty acid molecule is oxidized to a carboxyl group, after which beta oxidation (see below) proceeds from both ends of the molecule. The multiple alternate oxidation theory suggests that oxidation occurs not only at the β carbon, but that simultaneous oxidations occur at other alternate carbon atoms in the fatty acid chain, resulting in the formation of two- and four-carbon compounds. The beta oxidation theory is probably the most accepted hypothesis. According to this mechanism, the fatty acids are oxidized at the β carbon (the second carbon from the carboxyl end group on the molecule). Subsequently, a two-carbon fragment is split off from the newly formed β-keto acid. This process is repeated, yielding a progressively shorter fatty acid molecule, until the four-carbon stage is reached. The keto acids acetoacetic acid and β-hydroxybutyric acid are formed when the remaining four-carbon fragment (butyric acid) is oxidized. These "ketone bodies" are not oxidized further in the liver; instead they are carried to the other body tissues where they participate in the oxidative metabolism of carbohydrates in the Krebs cycle (Fig. 5 in Chap. 8) and are eventually oxidized to carbon dioxide and water.

Whenever large amounts of fat are metabolized and the rate of ketone body formation exceeds the rate at which they can be metabolized, the concentration of nonoxidized ketone bodies in the blood increases, the blood pH is shifted to the acid side (acidosis), and eventually "ketosis" ensues. Some of the acetoacetic acid is decarboxylated, liberating carbon dioxide and yielding a third ketone body, acetone. Some of the excess of ketone bodies is excreted into the urine (ketonuria). Such abnormal fat metabolism may be seen to a greater or lesser degree whenever large amounts of fat are ingested in the absence of carbohydrates, or during prolonged starvation when the carbohydrate stores of the body are exhausted and fat alone, from the fat depots, is burned for energy. A similar but even more severe situation exists in uncontrolled diabetes, when fat metabolism is increased (since the energy needs of the diabetic are not satisfied through normal carbohydrate breakdown) and when the rate of ketogenesis exceeds that of oxidative disposal of the accumulating ketone bodies.

Synthesis and Storage

The fat depots of the body are found under the skin, in the peritoneal cavity (mesenteric and omental fat), around kidneys and ovaries, and interspersed with the muscles. The subcutaneous fat is the most labile and responds first to dietary deprivation. Surplus quantities of fats and carbohydrates, ingested in excess of the individual's caloric needs, or proteins supplied in excess of specific amino acid needs and energy requirements are incorporated into the adipose tissues; in the case of carbohydrates and amino acids this process is preceded by a conversion to fat.

There are two chemical routes of fat synthesis. One is the reversal of the classic beta oxidation pathway mentioned above; it takes place within the mitochondria of the cell and is based on the sequential addition of two-carbon fragments (acetyl coenzyme A) yielding a progressively longer fatty acid molecule. The second pathway appears to be the quantitatively more important route for long-chain fatty acid synthesis, and takes place outside of the mitochondria in the cytoplasmic portion of the cell. This pathway involves first the carboxylation of acetyl coenzyme A with carbon dioxide to form three-carbon units of malonyl coenzyme A. Subsequently, palmitate is formed from a further combination of several malonyl units and acetyl coenzyme A.

Fat synthesis takes place in the liver and mammary glands, in many other tissues, and in the adipose tissue itself. The depot fat which is formed in the adipose tissues consists primarily of neutral fat (triglycerides) in contrast to the phospholipids and cholesterol, which are synthesized in the more actively functioning organs. The fatty acid composition of the depot fat varies. That portion which is synthesized from carbohydrate and protein, in the adipose tissue and liver, is characteristic of the species, and its fatty acid composition tends to be fixed. That portion which is derived from ingested fat, some of which can be stored without modification, tends to vary with the nature of the dietary lipids.

In general, seven fatty acids, lauric ($C_{12}H_{24}O_2$), myristic ($C_{14}H_{28}O_2$), palmitic ($C_{16}H_{32}O_2$), palmitoleic ($C_{16}H_{30}O_2$), oleic ($C_{18}H_{34}O_2$), stearic ($C_{18}H_{36}O_2$), and linoleic ($C_{18}H_{32}O_2$), account for 97 percent of the fatty acids in human depot fat. The adipose tissue fatty acid composition of normal lean subjects, and of obese individuals and patients with coronary heart disease, diabetes, and hypothyroidism, only shows minor differences. There is a sex difference in the depot fat composition, men having a greater total of saturated fatty acids and fewer unsaturated ones.

Adaptive changes in human depot fat have been found in individuals after prolonged adherence to diets high in polyunsaturated fats; in such cases the mean amount of linoleic acid in the adipose tissue rose significantly. The fat stored in the body's adipose depots is in a highly dynamic state, with newly absorbed or synthesized fat deposited to replace that which has been removed and oxidized. Quantitatively, this constant interchange and its final balance depend on the extent of dietary caloric inflow and on the concurrent energy requirements. There is no demonstrated upper limit in the capacity of the body to form and store fat when caloric intake exceeds expenditure.

Essential Unsaturated Fatty Acids

Apparently not all fatty acids can be synthesized de novo in human and animal tissues. Early experimental work has shown that complete exclusion of fat from an otherwise adequate diet induces cessation of growth, scaliness of skin, impaired reproduction, and kidney damage in young rats. These abnormalities are cured, or prevented, by the feeding of small amounts of linoleic or arachidonic acid. It has been shown since that these fatty acids are essential for a wide range of animals, most of whom respond to the specific dietary deficiency by histologic abnormalities in the skin. It appears that although animal tissues are capable of synthesizing most saturated and unsaturated fatty acids, they cannot produce unsaturated fatty acids of the linoleic series, which have a double bond in the number 6 position (counting from the methyl end of the molecule), unless a dietary precursor is furnished. Specifically, linoleic acid cannot be synthesized de novo; if linoleic acid is supplied in the diet, the tissues can synthesize arachidonic acid from it. Arachidonic acid alone or arachidonic and linoleic acids are essential for maintenance of a normal skin structure in the young. This need is less readily demonstrated in the adult animal, perhaps because of accumulated body stores of these essential fatty acids. Early speculations that the essential fatty acids form an essential part of the actual structure of certain cells have been confirmed by recent investigators. A number of vital structures of the cell are rich in phospholipids containing unsaturated fatty acids (particularly phosphatidyl ethanolamine), including the nucleus, cell membranes, mitochondria, and microsomes.

During recent years evidence has been obtained that the above holds true for man as well. Infants experimentally deprived of the essential fatty acids develop an eczematous dermatitis which responds specifically to the administration of linoleic and/or arachidonic acid. A decrease in the plasma levels of these fatty acids parallels the skin lesions. In adults, skin lesions do not appear on deprivation, and only the change in plasma levels is demonstrable.

The ideal intake for infants has not yet been established. Breast milk contains 6 to 9 percent of calories as linoleic acid. The clinical symptoms of induced essential fatty acid deficiency clear when a diet is furnished which contains *not less* than 1.3 percent of the calories as linoleic acid. On this basis it has been estimated that in the growing infant the minimum linoleic acid requirement probably lies between 1.3 and 2 percent and that an intake of 3 to 4 percent would be desirable. Since linoleic and arachidonic acids are known to be essential structural elements for synthesis of tissue, it seems wise to provide more than the minimum requirement in the diet, particularly to the fetus and the young. According to the Food and Nutrition Board, the minimum human requirement is near 2 percent of the total caloric intake. Amounts of the essential fatty acids greatly in excess of 4 percent of total calories are not recommended, but can be metabolized. A number of factors influence the requirement for essential fatty acids. The younger the animal, the higher its requirements, possibly because of lack of body stores. The requirement also increases with increasing dietary levels of saturated fatty acids and of cholesterol.

The essential fatty acids are found in natural vegetable oils, in the fat of mammalian organ tissues (and to a lesser extent in that of muscle tissue), in poultry fat, and in fish oils. Since the chances of ingesting essential unsaturated fatty acids are inversely related to the proportion of ordinary saturated fats in the diet, it would probably be wise to add to the existing concept of a balanced diet (i.e., protein, fat, carbohydrate, minerals, and vitamins) a new proviso concerning a (yet-unspecified) balance between the intake of saturated and unsaturated fats.

Physiologic and Nutritional Role of Fats

The current emphasis on a possible relationship between dietary fat and atherosclerosis should not obscure the fact that fat is a necessary component of living tissues and essential in human nutrition.

A number of general functions of fat are well known. Fat is the prime reserve fuel of the body. It is the most concentrated energy source which the diet can provide. Weight for weight, it furnishes more than twice as much energy as proteins or carbohydrates, and combines a high caloric value with very little bulk. This is an important consideration not only from the standpoint of the volume of food taken in, but also from the point of view of body economy and physical dimensions, since fat is the sole source of energy which the body can store in quantity. Stored fat is readily mobilized when needed as a fuel, and it (as well as concurrently ingested and absorbed fat) is metabolically very labile. Carbohydrate is the preferred substrate for oxidation in the body, but there exists a close reciprocal relationship between the metabolism and carbohydrate and fat as sources of energy.

Fat per se lends palatability to the meal, and a certain amount of it is essential to make the diet acceptable to most individuals. Many of the substances responsible for the flavor and aroma of foods are fat-soluble and are found associated with the fat in the diet.

Fat slows the emptying time of the stomach and decreases intestinal motility. This deceleration of the digestive process delays the onset of the sensation of hunger. Thus fat-containing meals have a high satiety value; they "stick to the ribs" longer.

Last but not least, fat exerts a sparing action on protein, and a balanced fat intake is essential to ensure the dietary supply of the essential fatty acids and of the fat-soluble vitamins.

Levels of Fat in the Diet

Just as the proportion of carbohydrate in the human diet is influenced by the standard of living, economic factors seem to govern the level of fat in many food patterns. However, whereas the proportionate intake of carbohydrates varies inversely with economic status, the intake of fat varies directly with the ability to pay for food. In underdeveloped, overpopulated parts of the world fats may contribute 6 to 10 percent of the total calories provided by the diet. This contrasts sharply with the United States and Canada, where about 35 to 44 percent of the dietary calories are obtained from fat. A similar principle applies to individuals within a given country; the percentage of fat in the family diet tends to increase with increased availability of money for the purchase of more fat-containing foods like meats, eggs, and dairy products.

The 1948 recommendations of the Food and Nutrition Board of the National Research Council suggested that enough fat be included in the diet to account for at least 20 to 25 percent of the total calories and that at least 1 percent be contributed by the essential fatty acids. The Canadian Dietary Standards favor a low level of 25 percent of total calories. Current thinking favors a judicious examination of the prevalent United States level, and attention is being focused on a higher intake of unsaturated fatty acids through a more equitable balance of saturated and unsaturated fats in the diet. (These aspects are discussed further in Chap. 21, Obesity and Leanness, and Chap. 29, Nutrition and Diet in Cardiovascular Diseases.) However, to date it has not yet been possible to state definitely what is an optimum allowance for fat in the diet or to indicate the characteristics of a fatty acid mixture most favorable for the support of health. Accordingly, no definite allowance for fat in the diet was suggested in the 1974 revision of the Food and Nutrition Board's Recommended Dietary Allowances.

Chapter 10

The Vitamins
I: Fat-soluble

The vitamins constitute a group of organic compounds which are essential in small quantities for the normal metabolism of other nutrients and maintenance of physiologic well-being. These compounds cannot be synthesized by the body and must be obtained from the diet. The various vitamins differ greatly in chemical composition and in their ultimate functions in the body. They are found in varying quantities in different foods; most foods contain a variety of vitamins, but no one food contains all of them in sufficient quantity to satisfy the human requirements under normal conditions of food intake. In contrast to macronutrients like proteins, carbohydrates, fat, and water, vitamins are required in relatively small quantities. This is explained by the fact that the function of many vitamins is primarily catalytic; they are components of enzyme systems which facilitate essential metabolic reactions. While major quantities of the macronutrients and their metabolic intermediates and derivatives are involved in these reactions, only minor quantities of the essential organic catalysts are required to facilitate and accelerate them, and ordinarily the enzyme system involved is used up only to a minor degree.

Vitamins have come into prominence by virtue of the deficiency diseases which are caused by their prolonged absence from the diet. Much of the early investigative work was concerned with the search for the unknown accessory dietary factors which would prevent classic deficiency diseases like rickets, scurvy, and beriberi, which used to accompany man's existence for long periods on a limited or artificially altered diet. Much of the more precise knowledge of vitamin action was later obtained from animal experiments with purified diets to which specific nutrients were added in a search for "vitamin activity." The most significant attainment of modern research in this field is the chemical identification and synthesis of the vitamins and the recognition of their specific, distinct, biochemical roles in human metabolism. The recognized vitamins have all been isolated in pure, crystalline form. They are now identified by specific chemical names, and their human requirement, so far as known, is expressed in terms of milligrams of the pure substance or in terms of *units,* which in turn are based on specified quantities of the pure chemical.

Nomenclature and Grouping

Original designation	Present-day terminology
Vitamin A	Vitamin A
Vitamin B	Thiamin (vitamin B_1, aneurin)
Vitamin B_2, G	Riboflavin
Pellagra-preventive factor	Niacin (nicotinic acid) or niacinamide (nicotinamide)
Water-soluble vitamin B complex	Pyridoxine (vitamin B_6)
	Vitamin B_{12}, cyanocobalamine
Vitamin M	Folic acid, folacin
	Pantothenic acid
	Biotin
Vitamin C	Ascorbic acid
Vitamin D	Vitamin D (calciferol)
Vitamin E	Vitamin E (α-tocopherol)
Vitamin K	Vitamin K (menadione)

Traditionally, the vitamins have been divided into two groups on the basis of their solubility. Actually, a certain usefulness is derived from such a grouping since it aligns the vitamins according to certain common physiologic characteristics. Thus the fat-soluble vitamins A, D, E, and K are found in foods in association with lipids. These fat-soluble vitamins are absorbed along with dietary fats, and conditions unfavorable to normal fat uptake also impair their absorption. They are not normally excreted in the urine; they tend to be stored in the body in moderate quantities, and given such reserves, man is not absolutely dependent on their day-to-day supply in the diet. In contrast, the water-soluble vitamins are not associated with dietary lipids and derangement of lipid uptake does not interfere with their own absorption. They are normally excreted in small quantities in the urine. Most of the water-soluble vitamins are proved components of essential enzyme systems. They are not stored in the body in appreciable quantities, and a constant dietary supply of these vitamins is desirable to avoid their depletion and the attendant derangement of normal physiologic functions.

VITAMIN A

Chemistry

Vitamin A is a pale, viscous, fat-soluble alcohol with the empirical formula $C_{20}H_{29}OH$. Its molecular structure is as follows:

Vitamin A alcohol or retinol

The name retinal denotes the oxidized, aldehydic form of vitamin A alcohol ($C_{20}H_{27}OH$) which has a special function in the visual cycle (see below).

Vitamin A—retinol—is fairly heat-stable but easily destroyed by oxidation. Vitamin A is found in nature to a large extent in the form of its precursors, the carotenoid provitamins α-, β-, and γ-carotene, lycopene, and cryptoxanthine (the yellow and orange pigments of most fruits and vegetables). Vitamin A is formed in the body of man or fish from these precursors after a hydrolysis which yields one or two molecules of vitamin A per carotene molecule, depending on the number of β-ionone rings present. β-Carotene, which incorporates two β-ionone rings in its molecular structure, yields two molecules of vitamin A on hydrolytic splitting and is thus quantitatively the most important provitamin A. The conversion of the precursors to the physiologically active vitamin takes place chiefly in the cells of the intestine.

Physiology

Vitamin A plays an important role in normal vision. It is found in the normal retina, associated with specific proteins in the form of visual pigments in the two distinct photoreceptor systems—the rods and the cones. The rods are especially sensitive to light of low intensity, and the cones perceive light of high intensity and colors. Retinal is an active component of the photosensitive pigment in both rods and cones. During the visual process retinol is oxidized to retinal; in the dark, retinal is present in the 11-cis form, and when activated by light quanta, it is converted into the 11-trans form. The energy for this conversion is furnished by light, and the process produces nervous excitations which are transmitted to the brain and result in visual sensations.

In the rods, for instance, retinal is found associated with a specific protein (opsin) in the form of the visual pigment rhodopsin (visual purple). On exposure to light, rhodopsin is converted, in steps, to visual white. This reaction is reversible, and visual purple is later reconstituted. However, restoration of visual purple is only partially complete, and a fresh supply of vitamin A must be available to permit complete regeneration of the normal complement of visual purple. Incomplete regeneration, as is found in vitamin A deficiency, results in impairment of vision in subdued light when this follows previous exposure to bright light. This type of night blindness, or lack of dark adaptation, is rapidly amenable to vitamin A administration.

Another function of vitamin A, outside of the visual cycle, is believed to be related to ensuring the normal structure and function of biologic membranes, be they components of intracellular organelles or peripheral cell membranes. Such a hypothesis is reasonable since many physiologic functions in man are affected by vitamin A and a large number of pathologic lesions appear in vitamin A deficiency, indicating that it must play an essential role common to many biochemical systems and tissues.

We know that vitamin A is essential for the integrity of epithelial tissues and normal growth of epithelial cells. Deficiency of vitamin A results in atrophy of the normal epithelial cell layer followed by proliferation of the basal cells and metaplasia to a stratified, keratinized epithelium. In mucous membranes, secretory function is deranged and eventually obliterated. These changes may occur in the mouth, the respiratory tract, the urinary tract, the female genital tract, the prostate and seminal vesicles, and the eyes and paraocular glands. In nonsecretory, protective epithelium, vitamin A deficiency results in hyperkeratinization.

A third function of vitamin A is concerned with its effect on growth of developing bony structures and teeth. Apparently vitamin A is essential for orderly activity of osteoblasts and osteoclasts; a deficiency (in animals, at least) results in impaired epiphyseal bone formation and formation of hypoplastic teeth having a thin and defective enamel.

The symptomatology of Vitamin A deficiency is discussed in Chap. 22, Malnutrition and Deficiency Diseases.

Absorption, Transport, and Storage

Unless the diet is rich in liver, eggs, butterfat, or fish-liver oils (which contain large amounts of vitamin A), much of the vitamin is ingested in the form of its carotenoid precursors, of which β-carotene is the most efficient. Conversion of the ingested carotene to vitamin A takes place primarily in the cells of the intestinal mucosa. Vitamin A and the carotenoids require the presence of bile in the intestinal tract and conditions favorable to fat absorption in general. Chronic diarrhea, biliary and pancreatic dysfunction, celiac disease, or sprue will interfere with proper absorption of carotene and vitamin A. The continued ingestion of large quantities of mineral oil (for laxative purposes) may also impede carotene and vitamin A absorption since both dissolve preferentially in the liquid petrolatum which serves as a vehicle that carries them out of the intestinal tract.

Dietary vitamin A (retinol) ester is hydrolyzed in the intestinal lumen prior to its absorption. Free retinol, either ingested as such with foods of animal origin or resulting from the hydrolysis of dietary retinol ester, then passes across the mucosal cell membrane, enters the cell, and together with retinol resulting from hydrolytic splitting within mucosal cells of carotenes from dietary plant sources is esterified inside the mucosal cell, preferentially with palmitic acid. Retinyl palmitate then travels in chylomicrons via the lymphatic system and the thoracic duct to the venous circulation and from there to the liver. When needed (when vitamin A blood levels become abnormally low), retinol is mobilized from the liver storage through enzymatic hydrolysis of the stored retinol ester and travels in the circulation to the tissues where a metabolic requirement exists. In an aqueous medium like blood, retinol and retinol esters are found in combination with a specific transport protein which has a molecular weight of approximately 21,000. Normally, vitamin A blood levels range from 30 to 67 μg per 100 ml.

More recent work indicates that vitamin A in the form of retinoic acid may be absorbed directly via the portal blood circulation (rather than via the lymphatic system) and stored in the liver.

The liver stores roughly 95 percent of the body's vitamin A reserves. Normally this amount is smallest at birth and in childhood and increases with advancing age. In healthy adults, vitamin A is stored in the liver in amounts sufficient to meet the requirements of one or more years. (The normal adult liver may contain from 100 to 300 μg per gram wet tissue.) There is an increased need for the substance during pregnancy and lactation.

Hypervitaminosis A

Excessive carotene intake may produce carotenemia and a concomitant yellow discoloration of the skin (see Chap. 35, Nutrition in Diseases of the Skin). Prolonged, excessive intake of vitamin A (usually due to excessive dosages of vitamin A preparations) may result in a toxicity syndrome which is characterized by excessive bone fragility and deep bone pain, enlargement of the liver and spleen, drying and peeling of the skin, general pruritis, loss of hair, nausea, headache, and elevated blood alkaline phosphatase and vitamin A levels. Vitamin A intoxication is observed in adults taking 50,000 international units of the vitamin daily for a protracted period and in children to whom an overdosage is administered daily by ill-informed, vitamin-conscious parents. Onset of clinical symptoms takes place in inverse relationship to the daily overdose. Withdrawal of excessive vitamin A results in a diagnostically significant, rapid, and complete recovery.

Sources

Vitamin A per se is obtained only from animal sources, while the carotenoid precursors are supplied in abundance by the dark green and deep yellow vegetables and yellow fruits. The following are good dietary sources; liver, egg yolk, dark green leafy vegetables, deep yellow vegetables, tomato and tomato products, liver sausage, butter, fortified margarine, and cheese made from whole milk. The reader is referred to the Tables of Food Composition in the Appendix for specific data on the vitamin A content of foods.

Stability

Heat in itself is not inimical to vitamin A, but oxidation is, and it is more destructive at higher temperatures. Therefore the potential loss of vitamin A in food preparation, cooking, canning, and processing depends on the skill with which air (oxygen) is excluded. Ordinary cooking or processing in closed equipment causes little loss of provitamin A from vegetables and fruits, especially since the fat-soluble carotenoids are not extracted by the cooking water.

Standards and Requirements

The international standards are sponsored by the World Health Organization of the United Nations, and the United States Pharmacopeia units usually follow them closely. Until recently, vitamin A activity in foods was expressed as international units (IU), 1 IU being equivalent to 0.3 μg of retinol, 0.344 μg of retinyl acetate ("vitamin A acetate"), or 0.6 μg of pure β-carotene. The latest standards express vitamin A activity in foods in terms of the equivalent weight of retinol in micrograms ("retinol equivalents"). By definition, one retinol equivalent is equal to 1 μg of retinol, or 6 μg of β-carotene, or 12 μg of other provitamin A carotenoids. In terms of international units, one retinol equivalent is equal to 3.33 IU of retinol or 10 IU of β-carotene.

Because of physiologic inefficiency in conversion of β-carotene to retinol and of widely varying efficiency of intestinal absorption (estimated in man to be only one-third of the provitamins ingested as compared with retinol which is assumed to be completely absorbed), the overall utilization of dietary β-carotene from food is taken as one-sixth that of retinol and the efficiency of other carotenoids as vitamin A sources is taken as one-twelfth that of retinol. In general, the average American diet provides about one-half of its vitamin A activity as carotenes (from plant sources) and the other half as preformed vitamin A (from animal sources).

The Food and Nutrition Board of the National Research Council has adopted a recommended allowance for vitamin A activity (regardless of form) of 5,000 IU per day for men and 4,000 IU for women. For children, the recommended daily intake varies from 1,400 IU for infants to 3,300 for boys and girls at the age of 10. The allowance for pregnant women in the second semester is 5,000 IU, and that for lactating mothers is 6,000 IU per day (Table 22 in Chap. 13). The Canadian Dietary Standards call for a basic requirement of 50 to 55 units of carotene per kilogram of body weight per day; this allocates 3,700 units of carotene for an adult who weighs 70 kg. The minimum requirement for vitamin A is about 6 μg/kg body weight per day.

VITAMIN D

Chemistry

There are several sterol compounds which are capable of preventing or curing rickets. Of these, two are of primary practical importance at present, vitamin D_2 and vitamin D_3. Vitamin D_2, or calciferol, is prepared by ultraviolet irradiation of the plant sterol ergosterol (activated ergosterol); it is a white crystalline material, soluble in fat and fat solvents, and stable to heat, acids, alkalies, and oxidation. Its empirical formula is $C_{28}H_{44}O$, and it has a melting point of 117°C.

Vitamin D_2

Vitamin D_3 is a very similar compound; it is formed in the human skin from 7-dehydrocholesterol on exposure to sunlight or ultraviolet light (at a wavelength of 235 to 315 nm). Its empirical formula is $C_{27}H_{44}O$, and it has a melting point of 82 to 83°C. In contrast to vitamin D_3, vitamin D_2 (calciferol) does not occur naturally. Both forms are of equal biologic value in man.

Physiology

Vitamin D increases the utilization and retention of calcium and phosphorus in the body. It increases the absorption of dietary calcium and phosphorus from the intestine; it also has the specific effect of reducing the excretion of phosphorus in the urine by stimulating its resorption in the renal tubules.

It has recently been found that the process of intestinal absorption of calcium is mediated by a specific calcium-binding protein which is elaborated in the intestinal mucosa under the stimulus of a metabolite of vitamin D—1,25-dihydroxycholecalciferol (see below). In addition to maintaining proper calcium and phosphorus levels in the blood, thus ensuring conditions generally favorable to normal mineralization of growing bone structures and remineralization of mature bone, vitamin D probably has a specific action at the site of mineral deposition in developing bone. Indirect evidence indicates that vitamin D is essential for the conversion of organic phosphorus to inorganic phosphorus in bone.

A deficiency in vitamin D results in inadequate intestinal absorption of calcium and phosphorus and in increased loss of these minerals via the urine and feces; there is an attendant fall in serum calcium and phosphorus levels (the decrease in the latter is especially pronounced), and calcium must be mobilized from bone in order to maintain normal blood calcium levels. This demineralization of bone in adults is referred to as osteomalacia. The features which differentiate vitamin D deficiency in adults (osteomalacia) and children (rickets) are caused by the fact that the ends of children's bones are in a state of active growth. Here the organic cartilaginous matrix which precedes hard bone formation is formed, but calcium and phosphorus salts are not deposited in it. The cartilage cells do not degenerate, so that the growing capillaries which normally push forward in the direction of intended growth cannot expand further. This results in a typical *rachitic metaphysis,* manifested clinically as a beading of the rib ends and a widening of the ends of the long bones. Inadequate mineralization also results in a soft skull (craniotabes) and delayed closure of the anterior fontanelle. The combination of retarded or insufficient mineralization and the normal mechanical stress results in skeletal malformations such as bowleg, knock-knee, curvature of the spine, and pelvic and thoracic deformities. The teeth of rachitic children erupt late, are less well formed, and decay early. A detailed discussion of rickets and osteomalacia in adults is found in Chap. 22, Malnutrition and Deficiency Diseases.

Hypervitaminosis D

Prolonged, excessive intake of vitamin D, such as a daily administration of 10,000 to 20,000 units to children and 100,000 units to adults, may result in a toxicity syndrome which is being diagnosed with increasing frequency. (In fact, daily administration of more than 1,600 units to infants is undesirable.) The effects resemble hyperparathyroidism. The syndrome is characterized by anorexia, vomiting, headache, drowsiness, and diarrhea. Polyuria and polydypsia as well as dysuria may occur. The serum calcium and phosphorus levels are increased, and ectopic calcium deposits may be found in the heart, large vessels, renal tubules, and other soft tissues. The effects of this hypervitaminosis are reversible if the abnormally high administration of vitamin D (usually by the hands of a misguided parent) is stopped. A temporary concomitant low-calcium diet may also be indicated during the period of adjustment.

Absorption, Transformations, and Storage

Being a fat-soluble compound which is associated with fats in food, vitamin D is absorbed in the intestine with the dietary lipids. Conditions which interfere with the absorption of fats—idiopathic steatorrhea, celiac disease, sprue, and biliary and pancreatic dysfunction—decrease the absorption of vitamin D. Ingestion of marked quantities of mineral oil has the same effect (see section on vitamin A). Vitamin D deficiency may result from inadequate intake of the vitamin as well as from lack of sunshine.

Vitamin D is absorbed mainly in the jejunum and transported in lymph chylomicrons. In blood, the vitamin is transported bound to a specific α-2-globulin with which it forms a complex. After it is transported in blood to the liver, it is hydroxylated in the liver to an active, polar metabolite—25-hydroxycholecalciferol—which is carried further, complexed with a similar (or identical) α-2-globulin, to the kidney, intestines, and other tissues. In the kidney, 25-hydroxycholecalciferol is further converted to a more polar metabolite—1,25-dihydroxycholecalciferol—which is the metabolically active molecule which induces the cells of the intestinal mucosa to synthesize in their brush border a specific calcium-binding protein which facilitates active intestinal calcium absorption against a gradient. (This scheme explains why individuals with advanced kidney failure are "vitamin D–resistant" and have severely impaired calcium absorption.) 1,25-Dihydroxycholecalciferol has also recently been shown to be highly active in facilitating bone calcium resorption, and is likely to be the biologically active form of vitamin D both in the intestine and in bone. It has been suggested that a group of relatively rare metabolic disorders known as "vitamin D–resistant rickets" may have its origin in the hereditary inability of the patient to convert the precursorlike conventional vitamin D molecule into its more polar and biologically active metabolites (as is the case in patients with advanced kidney impairment).

After absorption from the intestine or formation in the human skin, any excess of vitamin D is transported to the liver, where it is chiefly stored; other deposits are found in the skin, brain, spleen, and bones. The body can store sizable reserves of vitamin D, just as is the case with other fat-soluble vitamins.

These reserves probably account for the infrequency of vitamin D deficiency in adults; the most common deficiency is in the rapidly growing infant who has had little opportunity to accumulate adequate body stores.

Sources

Most foods contain little or negligible amounts of vitamin D. The natural foods which contain it are of animal origin. Saltwater fish, especially those which are high in body oils (salmon, sardines, herring), supply satisfactory quantities. Fish-liver oils are very rich sources of the vitamin, but they must be considered medicinal preparations. Liver and liver sausage are a satisfactory source. Egg yolks contain substantial amounts, and so does summer milk, since the cows are exposed to a maximum of sunlight during the summer months. Because vitamin D is present in natural foods in small amounts and its content in the few food sources is variable and depends greatly on the season, the requirements for this vitamin are largely met by artificial enrichment of suitable foods, by exposure to sunlight, and, in the case of some infants, by pharmaceutical supplementation. Fresh milk fortified with 400 units of vitamin D per quart is widely available. Virtually all evaporated milk is fortified to supply this amount per reconstituted quart; this is of importance since evaporated milk is very widely used as a base for infant feeding formulas. Some brands of butter and practically all makes of margarine are likewise enriched with vitamin D. (Most brands of margarine are fortified to contain 2,000 or more units per pound.) Other fortified foods include some brands of chocolate mixes, cocoa, and cereals. Enrichment of bread with this vitamin largely ceased with the advent of the thiamin, niacin, riboflavin, and iron enrichment program for bread during World War II.

Table 9   Vitamin D in Foods
(International Units per 100-g Edible Portion)

Beefsteak	13	Liver, beef, raw	34
Beet greens	0.2	Liver, lamb, raw	18
Butter	92	Liver, pork, raw	44
Cabbage	0.2	Liver, veal	9.6
Carrot tops	3	Mackerel, fresh, raw	1,100
Cheese	33	Milk, whole	4.4
Cod-liver oil	10,000	Milk, vitamin D	44
Corn oil	9	Pilchards, canned	745
Cream	17	Salmon, canned	314
Crisco	9	Sardines, canned	1,380
Egg yolk	265	Shrimp	150
Halibut-liver oil	140,000	Spinach	0.2
Herring, canned	330	Tuna	200–320

Standards and Requirements

The international standard of vitamin D is the international unit (IU), which represents the biologic activity of 0.025 μg of vitamin D_3 (1 mg of vitamin D_3 equals 40,000 IU). For all practical purposes the U.S.P. unit and the international unit are identical.

The estimated vitamin D intake of the modern child may vary widely. It will usually be over 300 IU per day and may reach 3,000 IU because of the existence of food fortification. Age and the degree of exposure to sunlight and skin pigmentation determine the true degree to which dietary sources of vitamin D are required (a black infant in Chicago is more prone to develop vitamin D deficiency than a white adult in Arizona).

The daily intake recommended by the Food and Nutrition Board of the National Research Council is 400 IU for infants, children, adolescents, pregnant women (in the second half of pregnancy), and lactating mothers. The vitamin D requirement of nonpregnant, nonlactating adults is minimal and unspecified. The Canadian Dietary Standards also call for 400 units. A quart of reconstituted evaporated milk or of fresh vitamin D–fortified milk supplies the daily requirement for this vitamin (400 units). When these foods are used in infant feeding, additional supplements of vitamin D become superfluous, depending on the quantity of milk or formula consumed.

VITAMIN E

Chemistry

At least four closely related compounds possess vitamin E activity: α-, β-, γ-, and Δ-tocopherol. These are viscous oils, soluble in the fat solvents, stable to heat and acids and unstable to alkalies, ultraviolet light, and oxygen. All are powerful antioxidants, protecting the oils with which they are associated in nature against oxidation (and the attendant rancidification). α-Tocopherol is the physiologically most powerful vitamin E compound. It has a molecular weight of 430, and its empirical formula is $C_{29}H_{50}O_2$. Additional tocopherol and tocotrienol derivatives exist; they exhibit vitamin E–like properties, but of a lower order.

Vitamin E (α-tocopherol)

One international unit of vitamin E is defined as one milligram of synthetic *dl*-α-tocopherol acetate.

Physiology

Vitamin E is an established essential dietary factor for a number of animals and is now being recognized as essential for man. A deficiency in this vitamin results in degeneration of the germinal epithelium and immobility of spermatozoa in the male rat and termination of pregnancy and fetal death in the female rat. In certain other animals, deficiency results in generalized edema, encephalomalacia, or a progressive muscular dystrophy with characteristic lesions in striated and cardiac muscle, and abnormal creatinuria. Though clinical lesions associated with vitamin E deficiency have been sought diligently for years, to date no one definite and clear-cut clinical deficiency syndrome has been found in adult man in the absence of other disease conditions (particularly those causing impaired lipid absorption) or generalized malnutrition. Increased sensitivity to in vivo hemolysis of erythrocytes by hydrogen peroxide, low α-tocopherol blood and tissue levels, and creatinuria have been described in newborn infants and in adults with biliary and pancreatic dysfunction or after long-continued experimental depletion coupled with increased intake of polyunsaturated fats. In *premature* infants a syndrome consisting of edema, skin lesions (papular erythema and seborrhea), and morphologic changes in red blood cells with increased erythrocyte sensitivity to peroxide hemolysis has been induced with a diet high in polyunsaturated fatty acids and devoid of vitamin E. These abnormalities responded rapidly to vitamin E supplementation. This syndrome is not found in full-term infants under similar circumstances.

Neither the function nor the mechanism of action of vitamin E in the living cell has been conclusively established so far. It is known that the vitamin plays a role as an antioxidant, inhibiting the oxidation of unsaturated fatty acids and of vitamin A in naturally occurring fats. It is postulated that in animal tissues, vitamin E prevents peroxidation of unsaturated lipid components of subcellular structures like mitochondria in all tissues, including the brain, and of erythrocyte walls, particularly where the proportion of highly unsaturated fatty acid components has been increased through a high dietary polyunsaturated fat intake. According to such concepts, certain polyunsaturated fatty acids serve essential structural and functional roles in biologic membranes in mitochondria, microsomes, and lysosomes (or in erythrocytes) while vitamin E and other substances with antioxidant properties prevent the peroxidation of these potentially labile fatty acids. Thus possible damage to subcellular and cellular membranes is avoided. While the concept of vitamin E as a biologic antioxidant is consistent with current knowledge, thus far the search for a role for vitamin E or one of its derivatives as a component of an essential enzyme system (similar to many other vitamins) has not been fruitful.

Vitamin E is regularly consumed by man in all practical diets. It is absorbed in a fashion similar to the other fat-soluble vitamins and is stored in the body primarily in the fat depots. In blood, vitamin E is transported in β-lipoproteins. Serum tocopherol levels in normal adults in the United States average 1.06 mg per 100 ml. A complete definition of the role of vitamin E in human physiology and nutrition still awaits the future.

Sources

The richest dietary sources of the tocopherols are the cereal seed oils. Wheat germ oil is particularly rich in α- and β-tocopherol. Other excellent sources are soybean oil (alpha, beta, and gamma forms), cottonseed oil (alpha and gamma), corn oil (mostly gamma), and margarine. Eggs, fish, all meats (especially liver), and butter contribute some α-tocopherol. Fruits and vegetables are not important sources in the quantities ordinarily consumed. Processing and storage destroys some of the vitamin E content of most foods. With the exception of deep fat frying, normal cooking procedures do not reduce vitamin E content markedly.

Requirements

With the wide distribution of vitamin E in foods there is little possibility of a deficiency occurring, especially when the usual American or Western diet is consumed and the individual's absorptive mechanisms are normal. It has been suggested that the human adult requirement varies from a minimum of less than

Table 10 Vitamin E in Foods
(Milligrams of Total Tocopherols per 100 g of Fresh Material)

Apples	0.74	Lamb chops	0.77
Bacon	0.53	Lettuce	0.50
Beans, dry navy	3.60	Liver, beef	1.40
Beefsteak	0.63	Margarine	54
Bread, white	0.23	Milk, whole	0.09
Bread, whole wheat	2.20	Oatmeal	2.10
Butter	2.40	Oranges	0.24
Carrots	0.45	Peanut oil	22
Celery	0.48	Peas, green	2.10
Chicken	0.25	Pork chops	0.71
Coconut oil	8.30	Potatoes, sweet	4
Cornmeal, yellow	1.70	Potatoes, white	0.06
Corn oil	87	Rice, brown	2.40
Cottonseed oil	90	Soybean oil	140
Eggs, whole	2	Tomatoes	0.36
Grapefruit	0.26	Turnip greens	2.30
Haddock	0.39		

10 mg per day to a maximum of about 15 mg—the particular level depending on the amount of polyunsaturated fats in the diet. It is estimated that the average daily intake of vitamin E is about 14 mg. The daily intake recommended by the Food and Nutrition Board of the National Research Council varies from 4 IU for infants to 15 IU for pregnant women and lactating mothers (Table 22).

On the basis of studies with infants it has been recommended that tocopherol supplements be given to premature infants and to children suffering from cystic fibrosis of the pancreas and biliary atresia—conditions characterized by impaired lipid absorption. In general, conditions interfering with fat absorption (biliary tract diseases, pancreatic insufficiency, celiac disease, sprue, and excessive mineral oil ingestion) reduce the amount of vitamin E absorbed. In such conditions, supplementation with vitamin E and, in fact, all the fat-soluble vitamins is advisable.

VITAMIN K

Chemistry

Numerous naphthoquinone compounds with vitamin K activity are known. The simplest and biologically most potent is menadione, or vitamin K_3, a synthetic, yellow crystalline powder. It is fat-soluble, stable to heat, and labile to oxidation, alkali, strong acids, and light. Menadione is 2-methyl-1,4-naphtoquinone; its molecular weight is 172, and its empirical formula $C_{11}H_8O_2$.

There are two major natural sources of vitamin K. Vitamin K_1 is ingested with plant food sources, particularly leafy vegetables (2-methyl-3-phytyl-1,4-naphthoquinone; $C_{31}H_{46}O_2$; molecular weight 451). In contrast, the bacterial flora of the human intestinal tract synthesizes vitamin K_2 (2-methyl-3-difarnesyl-1,4-naphthoquinone; $C_{41}H_{56}O_2$; molecular weight 581).

Vitamin K_1

Physiology

Among the most important factors regulating the clotting of blood are 10 special circulating proteins (factors I to X). Vitamin K is required for the synthesis of four of these, namely, factor II (prothrombin), factor VII, factor IX, and factor X. Though vitamin K plays an indispensable role in the synthesis of these factors from polypeptide precursors by the liver, it is not actually incorporated into the respective protein molecules of prothrombin and factors VII, IX, and X. Deficiency of the vitamin results in reduced prothrombin levels and levels of the other factors with a consequent reduction in the coagulability of the blood and increased bleeding tendency. Not all cases of hypoprothrombinemia are due to a vitamin K deficiency; liver dysfunction or injury may be the cause, and indeed the lack of response of hypoprothrombinemia to vitamin K administration is an effective test of liver function. Further aspects of vitamin K deficiency are discussed in Chaps. 35 and 38. In addition to the need of vitamin K for clotting factor synthesis, an established physiologic function of this vitamin in man, recent findings suggest that it is implicated in electron transport, and a role for vitamin K_1 in oxidative phosphorylation has been proposed.

Absorption and Storage

Vitamin K is fat-soluble. Conditions which impair lipid absorption in the intestine—biliary and pancreatic dysfunction, sprue, celiac disease, and idiopathic steatorrhea—also interfere with normal vitamin K absorption and may lead to a hypoprothrombinemia and bleeding tendency. Long-continued ingestion of mineral oil interferes markedly with proper absorption of the vitamin (see section on vitamin A). Much vitamin K_2 is elaborated by the intestinal microflora and subsequently absorbed from the intestine. Hypoprothrombinemia can be precipitated by sterilization of the intestine with sulfa drugs and antibiotics, and this must be kept in mind in preparing patients for abdominal surgery. In the newborn infant low blood prothrombin levels can be observed for several days after birth until an intestinal flora has been established and serves as a source of vitamin K. The vagaries of absorption and of synthesis by the intestinal flora influence the individual's supply of vitamin K much more than deliberate choice of food sources of this factor. In fact, human vitamin K deficiency due to dietary restriction has yet to be demonstrated.

Vitamin K is apparently not stored in large quantities in the body. The liver serves as the primary site for storage.

Sources

Vitamin K is widely distributed in nature. The richest food sources are green leafy vegetables. Seeds, tubers, and fruit contain markedly less of the vitamin than green leaves. Pork liver is a very rich source, while eggs and milk contain small amounts. Man's most important source of vitamin K appears to be his intestinal bacterial flora, which provides him with adequate amounts of the vitamin under normal conditions. Considering this source of supply, it is clear why no definite dietary requirements have been set for vitamin K under normal circumstances. The synthetic vitamin may be administered to mothers in labor

Table 11   Vitamin K in Foods

(Micrograms of Vitamin K_1 per
100-g Edible Portion)

Cabbage	250
Carrots	10
Cauliflower	275
Corn	10
Liver, pork	115–230
Milk	5
Mushrooms	7
Oats	75
Peas	7
Potatoes	20
Soybeans	190
Spinach	334
Strawberries	13
Tomato, green	49
Tomato, ripe	24
Wheat	36
Wheat bran	80
Wheat germ	37

or to their newborn infants in situations conducive to neonatal hemorrhage (erythroblastosis, prematurity, anoxia) in dosages of 2 to 5 mg for the mother or 1 to 2 mg for the infant.

Recently the Committee on Nutrition of the American Academy of Pediatrics tentatively recommended that milk substitute formulas for infants contain at least 100 μg of vitamin K per liter. In clinical situations associated with malabsorption of fat, a daily oral supplement of 50 to 100 μg is recommended (or if oral feeding is impractical, 1 mg per month parenterally).

Chapter 11

The Vitamins
II: Water-soluble

THIAMIN

Chemistry

Thiamin (vitamin B_1) is a water-soluble, crystalline compound, relatively stable to dry heat and labile to oxidation and an alkaline pH. It has a melting point of 248 to 259°C and a molecular weight of 337; the empirical formula of the hydrochloride is $C_{12}H_{17}N_4OSCl \cdot HCl$.

Thiamin hydrochloride

Metabolic Role and Physiology

The pyrophosphoric ester of thiamin is called cocarboxylase, thiamin pyrophosphate (TPP), or diphosphothiamin (DPT). It is an essential coenzyme in decarboxylation reactions which are catalyzed by specific carboxylases and participates in nearly all oxidative decarboxylations which lead to the formation of CO_2. Cocarboxylase is of primary importance in the oxidative decarboxylation of pyruvic acid, and in its absence this essential step in carbohydrate metabolism does not take place (Chap. 8) and pyruvic and lactic acids accumulate. Most decarboxylating enzymes studied so far consist of thiamin pyrophosphate and magnesium linked to a substrate-specific protein. Apparently all nucleated cells can form the necessary carboxylase systems if supplied with thiamin. Thiamin pyrophosphate is also a coenzyme in the transketolase reaction, which is part of the so-called direct oxidative pathway of glucose metabolism (see Chap. 8, Fig. 6). The thiamin requirements of the body are roughly proportional to the caloric expenditure of the body referable to carbohydrate metabolism and the carbohydrate content of the diet. Thiamin is not stored to any appreciable extent, and the total amount in the body suffices for only a few weeks of normal functioning.

The primary result of thiamin deficiency is a *biochemical lesion,* impaired carbohydrate metabolism at the pyruvate stage due to lack of cocarboxylase, with abnormal accumulation of intermediate compounds. Thiamin deficiency expresses itself clinically as beriberi in several distinct forms: (1) the "dry" type—multiple peripheral neuritis with subsequent muscular atrophy; (2) "wet" beriberi—beriberi with generalized edema and effusions into the body cavities (with or without myocardial lesions and insufficiency); (3) combination of dry and wet beriberi; and (4) infantile beriberi. The recovery from the symptoms of thiamin deprivation is spectacular once adequate amounts of thiamin are administered. It is of interest that bed rest and fasting have an ameliorating effect on the early stages of thiamin deficiency. This observation is consistent with the principle that thiamin is essential for a normal carbohydrate metabolism; exercise will increase the latter (and thus the need for thiamin), while bed rest will spare it; and during fasting, in the absence of carbohydrate intake, fat mobilization and fat metabolism (which requires less thiamin) will supply the body's energy needs.

In the United States thiamin deficiency syndromes occur almost exclusively in alcoholics and are usually attributed to a poor dietary intake. It has recently been demonstrated that in addition to the expected poor diet, in severe alcoholism there is also a specific impairment of intestinal absorption of thiamin which may play a determining role in alcoholic thiamin deficiency. In conjunction with this it should be mentioned that a new form of the vitamin—thiamin propyl disulfide—has intestinal absorption qualities greatly superior to those of the conventional thiamin hydrochloride, which is absorbed by a rate-limiting process and is often not absorbed well in malnourished subjects and alcoholics. (In such individuals oral administration of thiamin propyl disulfide yields superior therapeutic results.)

The symptomatology of thiamin deficiency is discussed in Chap. 22, Malnutrition and Deficiency Diseases.

Sources

The food sources of thiamin are numerous, but comparatively few foods supply it in concentrated amounts. The richest sources are pork, organ meats (liver, heart, and kidney), yeast, liver sausage, lean meats, eggs, green leafy vegetables, whole or enriched cereals, berries, nuts, and legumes. Thiamin is also found in smaller amounts in many other foods. The reader is referred to the Tables of Food Composition in the Appendix for specific data on the thiamin content of foods.

The milling of cereals removes those portions of the grain which are richest in thiamin (the sperm, the aleurone layer, and the bran). As a result, white flour and polished white rice may be practically devoid of thiamin. This explains the prevalence of thiamin deficiency in populations where white polished rice constitutes the backbone of the diet. The situation is not as serious in the Western countries whose food intake is less dependent on white flour alone. Nevertheless, among population groups who depend to a large degree on refined cereal products, the thiamin requirement is rarely met unless good sources of this vitamin are included in the diet. Large-scale enrichment of flour and cereal products in general with thiamin has proved very beneficial in eliminating the risk of thiamin deprivation in countries which practice such fortification. The use of thiamin-enriched rice in certain regions in the Philippines has demonstrated the possibility of virtually eliminating beriberi in these areas.

Losses of thiamin during cooking occur through extraction of the water-soluble vitamin by the cooking water and through oxidation, especially in an alkaline pH. Such potential losses are held down to some extent by the nature of many thiamin-containing foods, which are consumed without excessive cooking (enriched bread, breakfast cereals). Parboiling of rice facilitates retention of some of the thiamin and is a desirable method of preparation of rice which aids in the prevention of beriberi.

In discussing the sources of thiamin, the synthesis of this vitamin by the bacterial flora of the human intestinal tract and its absorption must not be overlooked. It has been estimated that in Japan about one-quarter of the daily thiamin requirement is met by this source. Conversely, in rare cases the intestinal microflora may be responsible for thiamin deprivation (see Chap. 1 under The Intestinal Flora).

Requirements

The thiamin requirement is largely proportional to the caloric content of the diet and is influenced by the amount of carbohydrate metabolized. This is consistent with the fact that in areas in which beriberi is endemic the food pattern is high in carbohydrates (up to 80 percent of the food calories may be derived from carbohydrates) and low in fats and thiamin. The minimum adult requirement, in the case of diets typical of the United States, is reported as 0.23 mg per 1000 cal. The total individual requirement is augmented in conditions which are characterized by increased metabolism such as fever, exercise, hyperthyroidism, and in pregnancy and lactation. In the latter instance, increased caloric intake normally results in a parallel rise in the vitamin requirement.

The Food and Nutrition Board recommends a thiamin intake of 0.5 mg for each 1000 cal for adults on ordinary levels of caloric intake. The minimum recommended daily intake is 1.0 mg, even if the caloric intake falls below 2000 cal. It is generally assumed that the recommendations made for adults (in terms of thiamin per caloric intake) are equally suitable in childhood, adolescence, pregnancy, and old age. The reader is referred to Table 22 in Chap. 13 for specific values.

RIBOFLAVIN

Chemistry

Riboflavin is a yellow, crystalline isoalloxazine compound which shows a characteristic yellow-green fluorescence when dissolved in water. It is relatively stable to heat and sensitive to light and ultraviolet radiation. Riboflavin has a molecular weight of 376; its empirical formula is $C_{17}H_{20}N_4O_6$.

D-Riboflavin

Metabolic Role and Physiology

In combination with specific proteins, riboflavin, in the form of riboflavin mononucleotide (riboflavin 5-phosphate) and the more complex flavin adenine dinucleotides, serves as a catalyst of importance in cellular oxidations. Mammalian tissues contain a number of different flavoprotein enzyme systems, each made up of a riboflavin-containing prosthetic group (coenzyme) and a substrate-specific protein (apoenzyme). Some of these have been identified, to wit, Warburg's old yellow enzyme, cytochrome C reductase, D- and L-amino acid oxidases, succinic dehydrogenases, diaphorases, and xanthine and alde-hyde oxidase.

Deficiency of riboflavin may result in fissures at the angles of the mouth and local inflammation, desquamation, and encrustation (angular stomatitis). However, this lesion is not necessarily specific for ariboflavinosis. Another set of deficiency symptoms concerns the eyes; the cornea becomes abnormally vascularized by a proliferation of capillaries, and a "sandy" feeling, visual fatigue, and photophobia may also be present. Glossitis and seborrheic dermatitis about the nose and scrotum have also been reported. Well-controlled experiments with human volunteers hardly ever display an acute uniform syndrome involving all these deficiency symptoms. In view of the important metabolic role of riboflavin, the paucity of a more serious symptomatology is somewhat surprising. This may perhaps be explained by the fact that synthesis by the intestinal bacterial flora may supply man with small amounts of riboflavin, thus preventing an acute clinical deficiency picture.

Sources

Common foods which supply significant amounts of riboflavin are organ meats (liver, heart, kidney, etc.), liver sausage, milk, cheese, meats, eggs, green leafy vegetables, whole grains, and legumes. It is also found in smaller quantities in many other foods. Specific values are given in the Tables of Food Composition in the Appendix. Fortunately, the relative heat stability of riboflavin (provided light is excluded), coupled with its slight solubility in cooking water, serves to minimize excessive losses of the vitamin during ordinary cooking.

Requirements

Little is known concerning riboflavin requirements in childhood, adolescence, and pregnancy as contrasted with adult needs. The Food and Nutrition Board has correlated its recommended riboflavin allowance with the caloric intake of the individual as well as with body size, metabolic rate, and rate of growth. The recommended daily allowance varies from 0.4 mg for infants to 1.9 mg for lactating women (Table 22). The Canadian Council on Nutrition has tied its recommended riboflavin intake to the caloric intake of the individual. The Canadian riboflavin standards vary from 0.5 mg for infants to 1.8 mg for men (Table 24 in Chap. 13). Both sets of standards call for a basically similar riboflavin intake.

NIACIN

Chemistry

Niacin (nicotinic acid) is a white crystalline compound, soluble in hot water and fairly stable to heat, light, acids, and alkalies. Niacin and its much more water-soluble amide, niacinamide (nicotinic acid amide), have a similar biologic function. Plant tissues contain the vitamin in the form of the acid, whereas animal tissues contain it in the physiologically active form of the amide. In the human, ingested niacin is easily converted to niacinamide.

Niacin
$C_6H_5O_2N$

Niacinamide
$C_6H_6ON_2$

Niacin is a mild vasodilator. Side effects accompanying vigorous niacin therapy may include flushing of the face, an increase in skin temperature, and momentary hypotension with dizziness. For this reason the amide, which does not induce those side reactions, is used in pharmaceutical preparations. It has been shown that very large doses of niacin (nicotinic acid, not the amide) will lower high blood cholesterol levels in man. This appears to be a pharmacologic effect.

Metabolic Role and Physiology

Niacinamide is a component of coenzyme I (niacin adenine dinucleotide, NAD, or diphosphopyridine nucleotide, DPN) and of coenzyme II (niacin adenine dinucleotide phosphate, NADP, or triphosphopyridine nucleotide, TPN).

Coenzyme I

Coenzymes I and II are the functional groups in important intracellular oxidation-reduction enzyme systems which are necessary for the utilization of all major nutrients. DPN, coupled with specific apoenzymes, is the dehydrogenase responsible for the conversion of lactic to pyruvic acid, alcohol to acetaldehyde, β-hydroxybutyric acid to acetaldehyde, and other reactions. TPN, coupled with specific apoenzymes, is the dehydrogenase of hexose phosphate, citric acid, and many other substrates. More than 40 biochemical reactions dependent on these enzymes have been identified, involving glycolysis, pyruvate metabolism, pentose biosynthesis, and the process by which high-energy phosphate bonds are synthesized.

Deficiency in niacin (or niacinamide) expresses itself clinically in the form of pellagra. The exact mechanism is not clear by which the specific biologic lesion, or metabolic impairment, causes the organic symptomatology of this disease. Pellagra may be briefly characterized by its major symptoms of dermatitis, diarrhea, and stomatitis, and mental changes. The tongue is smooth, red, and painful, and there is a burning sensation in the mouth. The recovery from the symptoms of niacin deprivation is quite spectacular once adequate amounts of the vitamin are administered.

In mammalian tissues, niacin can be synthesized from the amino acid tryptophan. The degradation of tryptophan to niacin does not take place in the absence of pyridoxine (vitamin B_6). Roughly 60 mg of the precursor tryptophan is required to furnish 1 mg of niacin by this route. Adequate amounts of tryptophan are as curative in human pellagra as the administration of niacin, the absence of which is directly responsible for this deficiency disease. Pellagra is endemic in population groups that rely on corn as their principal food because corn is a poor source of niacin and because it also lacks adequate amounts of the amino acid tryptophan, which could be used as a precursor for niacin. The clinical picture of niacin deficiency is discussed in Chap. 22, Malnutrition and Deficiency Diseases.

Sources

The following foods are good sources of niacin: liver, meats, fish, whole-grain and enriched breads and cereals, dried peas and beans, nuts, and peanut butter. It has been shown that niacin may occur in untreated cereals, including corn, in a bound form which yields little free, physiologically active vitamin upon ingestion. Alkali treatment of the grain appears to increase the yield of free niacin. The convertibility of tryptophan to niacin in the mammal has a direct bearing on the interpretation of the pellagra-preventive potential of foods. One can no longer think of the niacin content of a food without considering its tryptophan content as well. Thus, though milk is a relatively poor source of niacin, it is pellagra-preventive because of its more than adequate tryptophan content. Information regarding the niacin content (as such) of foods is found in the Tables of Food Composition in the Appendix.

In discussing sources of niacin, one must not overlook evidence that this vitamin may be produced by the bacterial flora in the human intestine. At present little is known about the extent of this "endogenous" synthesis.

Requirements

The human requirement for niacin cannot be simply defined since it is related to the intake of tryptophan-containing food proteins (provided there exists no deficiency in vitamin B_6, which is essential for the tryptophan-niacin conversion). The current recommendations of the Food and Nutrition Board (1974) are expressed as niacin since the contribution from tryptophan is variable and unpredictable. Nevertheless, in estimating the amount of niacin available from foods, the average value of 60 mg of tryptophan should be considered equivalent to 1 mg of niacin. The recommended daily allowance for niacin varies from 5 mg for infants to 20 mg for male adults (Table 22). Even though there is an increased conversion of tryptophan to niacin during pregnancy, an additional 2 mg of niacin daily is recommended during pregnancy because of increased caloric intake. During lactation an added daily allowance of 4 mg of niacin is recommended.

PYRIDOXINE

Chemistry

Pyridoxine, or vitamin B_6, is a water-soluble, white, crystalline compound, fairly stable to heat, and sensitive to ultraviolet light and oxidation. There exist three related compounds with interchangeable potential vitamin B_6 activity: (1) pyridoxine ($C_8H_{11}O_3N$, molecular weight 169), (2) pyridoxamine ($C_8H_{12}O_2N_2$, molecular weight 168), and (3) pyridoxal ($C_8H_9O_3N$, molecular weight 167). All three compounds occur in natural materials and are interconverted during normal metabolic processes. The biologically active form is pyridoxal.

Pyridoxine   Pyridoxal

Pyridoxamine

Metabolic Role and Physiology

Pyridoxal 5-phosphate functions as the coenzyme for a number of enzyme systems essential for normal amino acid metabolism: decarboxylase, transaminase, desulfurase, and many others. The number and variety of reactions involved are so great that pyridoxal can be considered as essential for practically all enzymatic reactions involving the nonoxidative degradation and interconversion of amino acids. This includes the degradation of tryptophan to niacin (see section on niacin), racemization (for instance, conversion of D- to L-glutamic acid), dehydration (serine $\rightarrow H_2O$ + pyruvate + NH_3), and desulfhydration (cysteine $\rightarrow H_2S$ + pyruvate + NH_3). Pyridoxine also appears to be essential for the "active" absorption of the amino acids methionine and tyrosine from the intestine (in contrast to absorption by passive diffusion) and may play a role in the active process of uptake of amino acids by cells in general. Studies on the effect of pyridoxine on fat metabolism indicate a functional relation between vitamin B_6 and unsaturated fatty acids. Apparently pyridoxine is specifically involved in the synthesis of the highly unsaturated fatty acids, such as arachidonic and hexenoic acids, from linoleic and linolenic acids. Vitamin B_6 is also intimately involved in carbohydrate metabolism; pyridoxal phosphate is a constituent of the key enzyme phosphorylase which is responsible for the breakdown of glycogen to glucose 1-phosphate.

Pyridoxine deficiency has been produced in man by a deficient diet and by the administration of deoxypyridoxine, a structural analog and competitive antimetabolite (antagonist) of the vitamin. The most common deficiency symptoms are a seborrheic dermatitis about the eyes, nose, and mouth, behind the ears, and in intertriginous areas. Cheilosis, glossitis, and stomatitis have been reported, presumably indistinguishable from the oral lesions of riboflavin and niacin deficiency. Some patients show signs of a sensory peripheral neuropathy, followed by motor impairment. The appearance of abnormally large amounts of xanthurenic acid in the urine after test doses of tryptophan have been given is a reliable test for pyridoxine deficiency. The administration of pyridoxine in doses as low as 5 mg per day results in prompt regression of all lesions.

Pyridoxine deficiency has been shown to produce convulsive seizures in infants and has been implicated in a convulsive disorder with abnormal electroencephalographic findings, exhibited by infants fed exclusively a proprietary formula in which faulty heat sterilization had partially destroyed the vitamin. A hereditary need for an abnormally high pyridoxine supply may also have played a role in some of these cases. A small number of individuals have a hereditary enhanced need for larger-than-normal quantities of pyridoxine to maintain a normal metabolism ("hereditary pyridoxine dependency"). Such individuals may display a pyridoxine deficiency syndrome characterized in infancy by neonatal convulsions, irritability, and—on a long-term basis— mental retardation. They can be diagnosed with the aid of an intravenous tryptophan load test; since they are incapable of converting tryptophan to n-methylnicotinamide, abnormal quantities of xanthurenic acid will appear in the urine. Routine supplementation with 2 to 10 mg of pyridoxine (15 mg in *some* cases) usually suffices for normal maintenance and to prevent progression of the disease in individuals with inborn pyridoxine dependency. There have also been reports of a pyridoxine-responsive anemia in *adults* with an inherited or acquired higher daily requirement for pyridoxine, but this picture is as yet unclear. A pyridoxine-responsive hereditary cystathioninuria and a form of homocystinuria have also been demonstrated.

Pyridoxine is now used prophylactically in tuberculosis patients subject to long-term chemotherapy with isoniazid (isonicotinic acid hydrazide). Prolonged administration of isoniazid produces a peripheral neuropathy in many cases which responds specifically to vitamin B_6 supplementation. It has been

Table 12   Pyridoxine in Selected Foods
(Micrograms per 100-g Edible Portion)

Food	μg	Food	μg
Apple	26	Milk, human	3.5–22
Asparagus, canned	30	Milk, evaporated	25–41
Banana	320	Milk, dry	330–820
Barley	320–560	Milk, dry skim	550
Beans, green, canned	32	Molasses, blackstrap	2,000–2,490
Beef	230–320	Oats, rolled	93–150
Beer	50–60	Onions	63
Beet greens	37	Orange juice, canned	16–31
Brains, beef	160	Orange juice, fresh	18–56
Cabbage	120–290	Peaches, canned	16
Cantaloupe	36	Peanuts	300
Carrots, raw	120–220	Peas, fresh	50–190
Cauliflower	20	Peas, canned	46
Cheese	98	Peas, dry	160–330
Cod	340	Pork	330–680
Corn, canned	68	Potato	160–250
Corn, yellow	360–570	Raisins	94
Corn grits	200–250	Rice, whole	1,030
Cottonseed meal	1,310	Rice, white	340–450
Eggs, fresh	22–48	Rye	300–370
Flounder	100	Salmon, canned	450
Frankfurter	130	Salmon, fresh	590
Grapefruit juice	8–18	Sardines, canned	280
Grapefruit sections	17–24	Soybeans	710–1,200
Halibut	110	Spinach, canned	60
Ham	330–580	Strawberries	44
Heart, beef	200–290	Tomatoes, canned	710
Honey	4–27	Tuna, canned	440
Kidney, beef	350–990	Turnips	100
Lamb	250–370	Veal	280–410
Lemon juice	35	Watermelon	33
Lettuce	71	Wheat bran	1,380–1,570
Liver, beef	600–710	Wheat germ	850–1,600
Liver, calf's	300	White flour	380–600
Liver, pork	290–590	Yams	320
Malt extract	540	Yeast, bakers'	620–700
Milk, whole	54–110	Yeast, brewers' dry	4,000–5,700

proposed that persons subject to excessive urinary oxalic acid excretion may be benefited by an increased pyridoxine intake.

Penicillamine (dimethylcysteine) is a chelating agent used primarily for treating lead poisoning and Wilson's disease (hepatholenticular degeneration). It has been shown to exert an antipyridoxine effect, which can be reversed by supplementation with vitamin B_6. Such supplementation should be routine whenever penicillamine is used therapeutically for any purpose.

Sources and Requirements

Information on the pyridoxine content of foods is yet incomplete because of difficulties in analysis. Good sources are liver, meats, whole-grain cereals, soybeans, peanuts, corn, and a number of vegetables. Table 12 details some of the available data. The daily requirement of pyridoxine for subjects with a high protein intake appears to be higher than for those on a low protein intake. It has been estimated, in adults, to be 1.25 to 2 mg, an amount which is readily provided by the ordinary mixed diet found in Western countries. For artificially fed infants, 400 μg per 1000 cal probably provides a sufficient safety factor. Patients with constitutionally increased pyridoxine needs have been shown to require 5 to 10 mg daily. The recommended daily allowances of the Food and Nutrition Board vary from 0.3 mg for infants to 2.5 mg for pregnant or lactating women (Table 22).

BIOTIN

Chemistry

The empirical formula of biotin is $C_{10}H_{16}O_3N_2S$, and its molecular weight is 244. It is readily soluble in hot water, sparingly soluble in cold water, stable to heat, and labile to oxidizing agents and strong acids and alkalies.

Biotin

Biotin combines with avidin, a glycoprotein found in raw egg white, to form a stable complex which is not broken down by proteolytic digestion. When biotin is so combined, it is nonabsorbable and nutritionally unavailable.

Metabolic Role and Physiology

Like other B vitamins, biotin acts as a coenzyme. It is thought to be involved in the carboxylation and decarboxylation of oxaloacetate, succinate, aspartate, and malate. Biotin has also been related to the biosynthesis of aspartate and the oxidation of pyruvate, as well as to the biosynthesis of citrulline and fatty acids, where it is a component of the essential enzyme acetyl coenzyme A carboxylase. Biotin has also been assigned, in recent years, a role in protein and purine synthesis, oxidative phosphorylation, deamination reactions, and carbohydrate metabolism.

Normal biotin levels average 32 µg per 100 ml in infants, 26 µg percent in adults. This level decreases to an average of about 13 µg percent during pregnancy, suggesting a possible increased biotin requirement during gestation.

Experimental biotin deficiency in man (induced by a biotin-deficient diet and the use of very large quantities of raw egg white) results in a scaly dermatitis, grayish pallor, extreme lassitude, anorexia, muscle pains, insomnia, some precordial distress, and a slight anemia. This deficiency picture responds promptly to administration of biotin. Spontaneous biotin deficiency in man seems unlikely, as balance studies indicate that this substance is synthesized by the human intestinal flora in sufficient quantities to render an exogenous source unnecessary. It is unlikely that a normal diet contains enough avidin from raw egg white to produce a biotin deficiency; however, individuals with perverted appetites may theoretically succeed, and in fact this has happened. There is no definitive human disease known with biotin deficiency as the underlying etiology.

Sources

Organ meats are excellent sources of biotin. Other good sources are peanuts, chocolate, egg yolk, cauliflower, and mushrooms. The bacterial intestinal flora

Table 13   Dietary Sources of Biotin
(Micrograms per 100-g Edible Portion)

Bananas	4	Milk	5
Beans, dried lima	10	Molasses	9
Beef	4	Mushrooms	16
Carrots	2	Onions, dry	4
Cauliflower	17	Oysters	9
Cheese	2	Peanuts, roasted	39
Chicken	5–10	Peas, fresh	2
Chocolate	32	Peas, dried	18
Corn	6	Pork, bacon	7
Eggs, whole fresh	25	Pork, muscle	2–5
Filberts	16	Salmon	5
Grapefruit	3	Spinach	2
Halibut	8	Strawberries	4
Hazelnuts	14	Tomatoes	2
Liver, beef	100	Wheat, whole	5

apparently can furnish the major share of the human daily requirement for biotin. Cow's milk contains about 50 μg of biotin per liter.

Requirements

Although the minimum daily requirement for biotin has not been established, diets providing 150 to 300 mg per day are considered adequate. This amount is provided by the average American diet, and the associated synthesis by the intestinal flora.

PANTOTHENIC ACID

Chemistry

Pantothenic acid is a water-soluble compound formed by the union of pantoic acid and β-alanine. It has the empirical formula $C_9H_{17}O_5N$ and a molecular weight of 219. It is stable in neutral solution but sensitive to acid and alkali. Panthenol, the hydroxy analog of pantothenic acid, is biologically active; it exists in the form of a viscous oil. The calcium salt of pantothenic acid—a white crystalline solid—is the most widely used form of the vitamin.

Pantothenic acid

Metabolic Role and Physiology

Pantothenic acid is a constituent of coenzyme A, an essential coenzyme involved in many reversible acetylation reactions in carbohydrate, fat, and amino acid metabolism. The complete enzyme system consists of a specific protein (apoenzyme) combined with the coenzyme moiety. Acetyl coenzyme A, the activated molecule, may act as an acetyl donor or acetyl acceptor. It facilitates condensation reactions like the formation of citrate from oxaloacetate in the Krebs cycle (Fig. 5 in Chap. 8). Acetyl coenzyme A acts as a receiver of acetyl radicals formed in the oxidation of fatty acids, pyruvate, and citrate and transfers them elsewhere; it conjugates not only with acetyl but also acyl groups and is active in the synthesis of fatty acids, cholesterol, and other steroids. Pantothenic acid, the key constituent of the coenzyme, is thus of obvious and fundamental importance in cellular metabolism.

There is a close correlation between pantothenic acid tissue levels and adrenal cortex function, and the vitamin (as coenzyme A) is presumed to be involved in the function of this organ. Symptoms have been induced in man with the aid of a specific metabolic antagonist, ω-methylpantothenic acid, and a pantothenic acid–deficient diet. The resulting syndrome is characterized by

Acetyl coenzyme A

torpor, apathy, depression, cardiovascular instability (especially in the erect position), abdominal pains, increased susceptibility to infections—apparently due to impaired antibody production—impaired adrenal function, and a neuromotor disorder with paresthesias and muscle weakness.

Table 14 Pantothenic Acid in Foods
(Micrograms per 100-g Edible Portion)

Bananas	300	Oysters	490
Beans, dried lima	830	Peaches	140
Beef, brain	2,100–2,900	Peanuts, roasted	2,500
Beef, heart	2,100–2,500	Pears	70
Beef, kidney	3,400	Peas, fresh	600–1,040
Beef, liver	5,700–8,200	Peas, dried	2,800
Beef, muscle	1,100	Pineapple	170
Bread, whole wheat	570	Pork, bacon	280–980
Bread, white	400	Pork, ham	340–660
Broccoli	1,400	Pork, kidney	3,100
Cauliflower	920	Pork, liver	5,900–7,300
Cheese	350–960	Pork, muscle	470–1,500
Chicken	530–900	Potatoes, Irish	400–650
Eggs	2,700	Potatoes, sweet	940
Lamb	600	Salmon	660–1,100
Lamb, kidney	4,300	Soybeans	1,800
Milk, whole	290	Tomatoes	310
Mushrooms	1,700	Veal chop	110–260
Oats	1,300	Wheat, whole	1,300
Onions	140	Wheat, germ	2,000
Oranges	340	Wheat, bran	2,400

Sources

As the name ("derived from everywhere") implies, pantothenic acid is very widespread in plant and animal tissues. Good sources are organ meats, egg yolk, peanuts, broccoli, cauliflower, cabbage, whole grains, and cereal brans. Meat, milk, and fruits contain moderate quantities. Ordinary cooking does not seem to lead to excessive losses of this vitamin.

Requirements

The daily requirement for panthothenic acid is about 5 to 10 mg. This requirement is apparently easily satisfied, even by poor diets, since, although the substance plays an important role in human metabolism, a definitive clinical disease entity due to pantothenic acid deficiency is not known. Blood levels of pantothenic acid are lower during pregnancy and for 6 weeks after parturition; on this basis inclusion of 5 to 10 mg of pantothenic acid in a daily prenatal supplement has been suggested by some workers.

FOLIC ACID (FOLACIN)

Chemistry

Folic acid (pteroylglutamic acid, folacin) is a water-soluble, yellow, crystalline compound, labile to heat in acid media, and labile to sunlight when in solution. Its empirical formula is $C_{19}H_{19}N_7O_6$; it has a molecular weight of 441.

Folic acid

Man is unable to synthesize the pteridine ring of folic acid and is totally dependent on extraneous sources—food or synthesis by his intestinal flora—for his essential need of this vitamin. In foods, folic acid is found conjugated with one to seven molecules of glutamic acid which are linked at the γ carbon position. These pteroylpolyglutamates must be enzymatically deconjugated before intestinal absorption can take place.

The mucosa of the duodenum and jejunum is the major site of production of a specific enzyme, conjugase or folic deconjugase, which splits the natural polyglutamic folic acid to monoglutamic folic acid. The precise site of this hydrolysis, whether intraluminal, at the mucosal brush border, or within the intestinal cell, is as yet undetermined.

Within the mucosal cell, monoglutamic folate is converted to the physiologically active form of folic acid by reduction to tetrahydrofolic acid and is released, largely in the form of N^5-methyltetrahydrofolate, into the portal circulation.

Tetrahydrofolic acid

Metabolic Role and Physiology

The precise metabolic action of folic acid has not yet been fully established. Several folacin-containing coenzymes (conjugated with a substrate-specific protein apoenzyme) are known to be metabolically active in man in a manner analogous to the known coenzymes which incorporate other water-soluble vitamins. Their major role is in the transfer of one-carbon units to appropriate metabolites in the synthesis of nucleic acids such as ribonucleic acid (RNA) and deoxyribonucleic acid (DNA), and methionine, serine, and others. Folacin coenzymes are essential for reactions like the methylation of homocysteine to form methionine, the conversion of glycine to serine, and histidine to glutamic acid, the formation of creatine from guanidino acetic acid, and the formation of DNA and RNA, and of porphyrin compounds (hemoglobin). Vitamin B_{12} is believed to be an essential cofactor for the enzyme system involved in the transfer of the methyl group of N^5-methyltetrahydrofolic acid, which yields tetrahydrofolic acid and one-carbon units for synthesis of DNA, RNA, and other essential compounds.

Since folic acid is necessary for synthesis of essential nucleic acids, which in turn are required for normal cell division and replication, a folacin deficiency first manifests itself in the most rapidly growing tissues such as the bone marrow (erythropoiesis), alimentary tract mucosa, or tumor. From a clinical standpoint, the most important activity of folic acid is the role it plays in the orderly production of new red blood cells. In the absence of an adequate supply of nucleoproteins, normal maturation of primordial red blood cells does not take place and hematopoiesis tends to bog down in the megaloblast stage. As a result of this megaloblastic arrest of normal red blood cell maturation in the bone marrow, a typical peripheral blood picture results which is characterized by macrocytic anemia, thrombopenia, leukopenia, and old, multilobed neutrophils.

In man, a dietary folic acid deficiency causes a macrocytic anemia which resembles pernicious anemia without the nervous system involvement. Glossitis, gastrointestinal lesions, diarrhea, and intestinal malabsorption may accompany the macrocytic anemia. A similar syndrome may be produced by administration of a specific folic acid antagonist, aminopterin. These conditions respond to folic acid therapy.

Folic acid is effective in the treatment of the sprue syndrome and in a number of macrocytic, megaloblastic anemias other than pernicious anemia (the megaloblastic anemias of infancy and pregnancy and nutritional macrocytic anemia). A detailed discussion of these disease entities and folic acid is found in Chap. 33, Nutrition and the Anemias.

Sources

Appreciable quantities of folic acid are found in liver, dark green leafy vegetables, asparagus, lima beans, kidney, nuts, whole-grain cereals, and lentils. Oranges and orange juice (including frozen, reconstituted orange juice) appear to be a good source of folate in the monoglutamate form which requires no further hydrolysis before absorption. Another source of folic acid may be the bacterial flora of the human intestinal tract, which is known to synthesize the vitamin. However, the amounts made available to the individual are quite unknown and may vary under different environmental and dietary conditions. Table 15 lists the folic acid content of a number of common foods. Cooking and storage losses of the vitamin may range up to 50 percent.

Requirements

The daily requirement of folic acid in man has not yet been determined with accuracy. The lowest recorded effective therapeutic dose of this vitamin, in the case of megaloblastic anemia of infancy, was 200 μg per day. In anemias which respond to folic acid therapy, the recommended therapeutic oral or parenteral dose is 5 to 15 mg per day. It seems reasonable, therefore, to speculate that 0.5 mg daily will maintain good health under normal conditions. The folic acid requirement is sharply increased by conditions producing an increase in metabolism of one-carbon units, such as hyperthyroidism, hemolytic anemias, and pregnancy. In therapeutic dosage, folic acid may mask the presence of pernicious anemia and permit neurologic lesions to develop while supporting a normal red blood cell picture (Chap. 33). The U.S. Food and Drug Administration has therefore set a daily limit of 0.1 mg of folic acid in vitamin preparations which are sold without prescriptions. The daily allowance recommended by the Food and Nutrition Board varies from 0.05 mg for infants to 0.8 mg for pregnant women (Table 22).

Table 15   Dietary Sources of Folic Acid
(Micrograms per 100-g Edible Portion)*

Meat, eggs		Brussels sprouts	27
Beef:		Cabbage	6–42
Round steak	7–17	Carrots	8
Chuck	15	Cauliflower	29
Hamburger	5	Celery	7.2
Heart	3.1	Corn, sweet	9–70
Kidney	58	Cucumbers	6.7
Liver	290	Eggplant	5–15
Sweetbreads	22.8	Greens:	
Lamb:		Beets	20–50
Stew meat	1.9	Chicory	30
Leg	3.3	Endive	27–63
Liver	280	Escarole	26
Pork:		Kale	50.9
Liver	220	Mustard	17–38
Loin	2.4	Parsley	43
Ham, smoked	7.8	Spinach	49–110
Sausage	12	Swiss chard	32–64
Poultry:		Turnip	83
Chicken, dark	2.8	Watercress	48
Chicken, white	3.1	Kohlrabi	10
Chicken, liver	380	Lentils, dry	99
Turkey	3–15	Lettuce	4–54
Eggs:		Mushrooms	14–29
Whole	5.1	Okra	24
White	0.6	Onions:	
Yolk	13	Green, with tops	13
		Mature	6–14
Nuts		Parsnips	8–37
Almonds	46	Peas	5–35
Brazil nuts	4.5	Peas, dry split	22
Coconuts	28	Peppers, green	4–11
Filberts	67	Potatoes, peeled	4–12
Peanuts	57	Potato peels	14
Pecans	27	Potatoes, whole	2–130
Walnuts	77	Pumpkin	5–10
		Radishes	3–10
Vegetables, fresh		Rutabagas	3–7
Asparagus	89–140	Soybeans, dry	1.91
Beans, lima	10–56	Squash:	
Beans, lima, dry	100	Acorn	16.7
Beans, snap	13–56	Crookneck	7–16
Beans, navy, dry	130	Zucchini	11
Beans, wax	15–39	Sweet potatoes	5–19
Beets	13	Tomatoes	2–16
Broccoli	34	Turnips	4.3

Table 15-Cont'd. Dietary Sources of Folic Acid

(Micrograms per 100-g Edible Portion)*

Fruit		*Cereals and other grain products*	
Apples	0.5	Breads:	
Apricots	3.6	Cracked wheat	27
Apricots, dried	4.7	Rye	20
Avocados	4–57	Vienna	11
Bananas	9.6	White	15
Berries:		Breakfast cereals:	
Blackberries	6–18	Cornflakes	5.5
Blueberries	7.6	Cornmeal	6.5
Cranberries	1.7	Corn and soya	80
Red raspberries	5.1	Oats, ready to eat	22
Strawberries	5.3	Oatmeal	30
Cantaloupes	3–8	Wheat bran	100
Cherries, Bing	6.5	Wheat farina	14
Dates, dry	25	Wheat, shredded	29–87
Figs	6.7	Flour:	
Figs, dry	7–14	Cake	6.6
Grapefruit	2.7	Rye	18
Grapes, green	4.5	White, enriched	8.1
Grapes, red	4.9	Whole wheat	38
Honeydew melon	4.9	Grains:	
Lemons	7.4	Barley	50
Limes	4.6	Corn, yellow	24
Oranges	22–35	Oats, white	23–66
Orange juice	26–40	Rice, brown	22
Peaches, yellow	2.3	Rye	34
Pears	2.5	Wheat	27–51
Pineapple	0.8–6		
Plums, red	0.6–3	*Milk and cheese*	
Plums, yellow	1.2	Milk:	
Prunes, dry	5.4	Buttermilk	11
Rhubarb	2.5	Evaporated milk	0.7
Tangerines	7.4	Cheese:	
Watermelon	0.6	Cheddar	15
		Cottage	21–46
		Processed	11

*Figures rounded off to two digits.

Source: Based on *Agricultural Handbook 29* (1951), U.S. Department of Agriculture, Bureau of Human Nutrition and Home Economics.

VITAMIN B$_{12}$

Chemistry

Vitamin B$_{12}$ (cyanocobalamin) is a water-soluble, red, crystalline compound which is labile to acids, alkalies, and light. The molecular weight is approximately 1,450, corresponding to the composition $C_{63}H_{84}O_{14}N_{14}PCo$. It is unique in being the first cobalt-containing substance which has been found to be essential for life and is the only vitamin that contains an essential mineral element.

Vitamin B$_{12}$

Metabolic Role and Physiology

Vitamin B$_{12}$ is thought to play a role in the transfer of single carbon intermediates, primarily methyl groups. Examples of such transmethylations are the synthesis of choline from methionine and the formation of serine from glycine and of methionine from homocysteine. The vitamin also takes part in the formation of pyrimidine bases and in purine metabolism. It is involved in the synthesis of the deoxyriboside moiety of deoxyribonucleic acid. Vitamin B$_{12}$ affects, directly or indirectly, the metabolism of folic acid and may be essential for the formation of the various folic acid–containing coenzymes. By way of its participation in the metabolism of purines and pyrimidines, vitamin B$_{12}$ is involved in the synthesis of nucleic acids and nucleoproteins, and thereby in normal red blood cell formation (see section on the metabolic role of folic acid). It is certain that vitamin B$_{12}$ plays an important role in the metabolism of nervous tissue, though the precise mechanism is not yet clear.

(In the rat, vitamin B_{12} prevents certain types of experimental liver cirrhosis.)

Vitamin B_{12} is present in food in coenzymatically active forms bound to protein, from which it is freed by cooking or peptic digestion prior to absorption. It is very poorly absorbed from the gastrointestinal tract unless a heat-labile mucoprotein, the *intrinsic factor*, is present concurrently. This glycoprotein is secreted by the normal healthy stomach mucosa. It binds selectively to vitamin B_{12} and delivers it, in the complexed form, to receptor sites on the brush border of mucosal cells of the ileum. Attachment and subsequent absorption of vitamin B_{12} through the ileal mucosal cells takes place in the presence of calcium and an alkaline pH; the intrinsic factor is probably not absorbed under normal conditions. Other specific vitamin B_{12}–binding proteins, the transcobalamines, facilitate transport of the vitamin in the blood and its uptake into the tissues. When ingested in very large amounts (exceeding 25 μg), vitamin B_{12} is partially absorbed even in the absence of the intrinsic factor.

Pernicious Anemia

The classic example of serious vitamin B_{12} deficiency is Addisonian pernicious anemia. The basic defect in patients with this condition is a lack of normal intrinsic factor activity (which is essential for proper intestinal absorption of vitamin B_{12}). At one time it was thought to be exclusively due to a degenerative change in the gastric mucosa which ceases to elaborate and secrete intrinsic factor. More recently, specific antibodies to intrinsic factor have been found in the gastric juice, saliva, and blood of patients with pernicious anemia, which either precipitate intrinsic factor or block its binding of vitamin B_{12}; in such patients, although the secretion of intrinsic factor is normal, its facilitation of vitamin B_{12} absorption is impaired. Total, and sometimes subtotal, gastrectomy can result in inadequate elaboration of intrinsic factor. If any of these conditions is severe enough, vitamin B_{12} from food sources is no longer absorbed and the consequent tissue deficiency of vitamin B_{12} leads to pernicious anemia. The classic picture of Addisonian pernicious anemia is characterized by megaloblastic arrest of erythrocyte maturation in the bone marrow (see section on folic acid), macrocytic anemia, leukopenia, and progressive neurologic degeneration. The nervous system involvement ranges from a peripheral sensory deterioration and peripheral neuritis to damage to the motor pathways and to sclerosis of the posterior and lateral columns of the spinal cord (*combined system disease*). Untreated, the disease is ultimately fatal.

Pernicious anemia responds promptly to parenteral administration of vitamin B_{12}. However, the fundamental absorption defect remains, and the patient must henceforth receive a maintenance dose of the vitamin since it will not be absorbed from food sources in the absence of the missing intrinsic factor. In pernicious anemia, treatment with folic acid causes a prompt remission in the abnormal blood picture but does not benefit the nervous system disorder. Because of the hazard of continued neurologic degeneration, folic acid therapy should not be attempted in this disease. A more detailed discussion of pernicious anemia and vitamin B_{12} therapy is found in Chap. 33, Nutrition and the Anemias.

Other Deficiencies

Vitamin B_{12} deficiency may occur also in persons infested by the fish tapeworm and in those with blind intestinal loops or pouches, jejunal diverticula, chronic pancreatic insufficiency, sprue, and other malabsorption syndromes. In the case of *Diphyllobothrium* tapeworm infestation the parasite competes with the host for the vitamin and is thus capable of producing a macrocytic anemia. Intestinal lesions which cause stasis and consequent bacterial overgrowth include surgical blind loops, jejunal diverticula, strictures, enteric fistulas, and scleroderma. Massive overgrowth of enteric microorganisms in the small bowel (the "blind-loop syndrome" when associated with steatorrhea and malabsorption) is regularly associated with vitamin B_{12} malabsorption and can lead to megaloblastic anemia with or without neurologic defects.

Lastly, persons adhering strictly to an exclusive, lifelong vegetable diet (which contains no vitamin B_{12}) develop a variety of deficiency symptoms which respond to administration of the vitamin. Oddly enough, neurologic symptoms are more frequent in this group than frank megaloblastic anemia (possibly because folic acid prevents the latter).

Sources

Vitamin B_{12} is found almost exclusively in foods of animal origin. The original source of the vitamin is probably bacterial fermentation in the intestinal tract of animals, particularly in the rumen of herbivora. Humans apparently do not derive enough vitamin B_{12} from endogenous bacterial synthesis and are dependent on a supply of the preformed vitamin in the diet. Liver and kidney are excellent sources of vitamin B_{12}, muscle meat and fish supply it in moderate amounts, and whole milk in smaller quantities; most cereals are very poor sources. The vitamin is normally quite stable during cooking, but severe heating of meat and meat products may cause its degeneration.

Requirements

The human daily requirement of vitamin B_{12} has not yet been established with certainty. A dosage corresponding to 1 μg of the crystalline vitamin per day suffices for maintenance of a patient with pernicious anemia. This indicates that absorption of 1 μg per day may meet the normal requirement for adults. A minimal daily dietary intake of vitamin B_{12} of 0.6 to 1.2 μg is adequate to

Table 16   Vitamin B$_{12}$ in Foods

(Micrograms per 100-g Edible Portion)

Beans, green	0–0.2	Haddock	0.6
Beef, kidney	18–55	Ham	0.9–1.6
Beef, liver	31–120	Milk, whole	0.3–0.5
Beef, round	3.4–4.5	Milk, evaporated	0.1–0.3
Beets	0–0.1	Milk, powder, whole	1–2.6
Bread, white	0–0.3	Milk, powder, skim	2.5–4.0
Bread, whole wheat	0.2–0.4	Oats	0.3
Carrots	0–0.1	Peas	0–0.1
Cheese, American	0.6	Scallops	0.7
Cheese, cream	0.2	Sole, fresh fillet	1.3
Cheese, Swiss	0.9	Soybean meal	0.2
Corn, yellow	0.0	Wheat	0.1
Egg, whole	0.3		

maintain health and normal hemopoiesis in normal subjects operating with low body stores. This requirement is provided by the ordinary mixed diet in the United States, even if it is of a "low cost" nature. The daily allowance recommended by the Food and Nutrition Board varies from 0.3 μg for infants to 4 μg for pregnant women (Table 22).

ASCORBIC ACID (VITAMIN C)

Chemistry

Ascorbic acid is a water-soluble, crystalline compound, fairly stable in acid solution but sensitive to oxidation. Its empirical formula is $C_6H_8O_6$, and it has a molecular weight of 176. The L isomer of ascorbic acid is the physiologically active form. Vitamin C is readily oxidized to dehydroascorbic acid, which is still physiologically active though less stable. This oxidation reaction is reversible.

Ascorbic acid   Dehydroascorbic acid

Further oxidation beyond the dehydroascorbic acid stage results in irreversible and total loss of antiscorbutic activity. Iron and copper salts, an alkaline pH, heat, oxidative enzymes, and exposure to air and light facilitate this oxidation and cause loss of vitamin potency in ascorbic acid–containing foods.

Metabolic Role and Physiology

Ascorbic acid plays an important role in the metabolism of amino acids, particularly in the final oxidation of phenylalanine and tyrosine; it may function as a coenzyme in these reactions. Ascorbic acid facilitates the conversion of folic acid to folinic acid and is essential for many hydroxylation reactions. There is evidence that the vitamin acts as a carrier in certain intracellular hydrogen transfer systems and thus regulates oxidation-reduction potentials within the cells, but the exact mechanisms of these reactions are not yet clearly defined. Ascorbic acid in large amounts enhances the absorption of iron from the intestine in normal as well as iron-deficient human beings. This effect is probably the result of the reducing properties of ascorbic acid.

Ascorbic acid is necessary for the formation of the intercellular substance of collagenous and fibrous tissue in the animal organism. It is essential for the normal elaboration of intercellular matrices (collagen and mucoproteins) in teeth, bone, cartilage, connective tissue, and skin, as well as for the structural integrity of capillary walls. Thus it plays an important role in tooth and bone formation (through its influence on elaboration of normal osteoid and chondroid), in the laying down of callus in the union of bone fractures, and in the healing of wounds and burns, where the first step in the repair mechanism is the laying down of a collagenous intercellular matrix which makes for physical union of the traumatized parts. The beneficial and essential effects of ascorbic acid in connective tissue formation and wound healing appear to be based on the fact that vitamin C is necessary for maintenance of normal levels of the enzyme collagen proline hydroxylase and lysine hydroxylase and may act as a specific enzyme cofactor in mercaptanase. The enzyme is needed for synthesis of hydroxyproline, a constituent of collagen, a basic protein component of all connective tissues. Ascorbic acid is similarly essential for maintenance of adequate levels of the enzyme β-hydroxybutyric dehydrogenase, which is very active in bone and tooth tissues during formative stages. Ascorbic acid is also believed to enhance the capacity of the organism to withstand injury from burns and bacterial toxins.

Absorption and Storage

Ascorbic acid is absorbed directly from the small intestine by simple diffusion at a rate which depends on the amount ingested (i.e., the concentration gradient). Through tissue saturation, the human adult stores sufficient amounts of vitamin C to carry him through several months of deprivation. High concentrations of the vitamin are found in the adrenals, pituitary gland, thymus, and corpus luteum, while smaller quantities are found in the viscera, brain, and all metabolically active tissues. The total body saturation of ascorbic acid has been calculated to amount to approximately 5 g.

In human metabolism, an appreciable amount of ascorbic acid is converted to 2-ascorbic acid sulfate as a tissue constituent and normal excretion product. Ascorbic acid available in excess of metabolic requirements and tissue storage capacity is excreted largely in the urine.

Deficiency

Most animal species can synthesize their own supply of ascorbic acid. Man, monkeys, guinea pigs, an Indian fruit-eating bat, and the bulbul bird are exceptions; they must obtain vitamin C from exogenous sources. Scurvy is the classic manifestation of severe ascorbic acid deficiency. The most obvious lesions observed are those related to a weakening of the collagenous intercellular substance. The clinical picture is characterized by weakness; swollen, tender joints; delayed wound healing; spongy, friable gums; loose teeth; and hemorrhages, which may appear anywhere in the body, particularly near bones and joints and under the skin and mucous membranes. In the United States, infantile scurvy is the form most frequently seen. The disease responds rapidly and dramatically to the administration of as little as 50 mg of ascorbic acid daily. The usual therapeutic dose is actually considerably higher.

A detailed discussion of scurvy is found in Chap. 22, Malnutrition and Deficiency Diseases.

Sources and Stability

The common foods which are richest in vitamin C are citrus fruits and their juices, strawberries, cantaloupes, raw or minimally cooked vegetables, especially peppers, broccoli, cauliflower, kale, brussels sprouts, turnip greens, cabbage, tomatoes, and potatoes. The last two vegetables are especially important suppliers of ascorbic acid because of the quantities consumed by the population groups which do not consume much citrus fruit. The reader is referred to the Tables of Food Composition in the Appendix for specific data on the ascorbic acid content of foods.

The vitamin C content of fruits and vegetables varies with the conditions under which they are grown, stored, and cooked. For instance, the amount of sunlight available during ripening determines to a large extent the final ascorbic acid content of tomatoes. Storage and processing methods tend to reduce the amount of vitamin C contributed by foods, since vitamin C is very sensitive to oxidation and, being freely water-soluble, subject to mechanical loss by leaching. Freezing per se and storage in the frozen state are accompanied by little loss, but blanching, washing, and prolonged standing at room temperature make for considerable reduction in vitamin C content. The cutting up, washing, and cooking of vegetables may lead to a 50 percent loss, but losses of such magnitude are not necessary. Holding cooked foods in steam tables—a favorite procedure in institutions and restaurants—encourages rapid destruction of the vitamin. Modern methods of canning tend to preserve ascorbic acid in foods since processing conditions are planned to eliminate conditions which facilitate loss of this vitamin; however, the possibility of losses during preparation for the table still remains.

Requirements

There exist marked differences in the recommendations for a desirable intake of ascorbic acid. The British Medical Research Council has set the allowance for adults at 30 mg per day. The Canadian Dietary Standards call for the same amount. The Food and Nutrition Board of the National Research Council recommends a daily allowance which varies from 35 mg for infants to 45 mg for adults and allocates larger amounts for pregnant and lactating women (Table 22).

The minimum amount required to prevent scurvy in otherwise well-nourished adults is in the range of 6.5 to 10 mg per day. An intake of 50 to 100 mg per day does not saturate the tissues but causes tissue retention and some excretion in the urine. In the United States the average intake of ascorbic acid per day has risen from 69 to 117 mg; however, occasional cases of scurvy occur, usually among infants and the elderly, as the consequence of severely restricted diets.

Chapter 12

Minerals

All forms of living matter require many inorganic elements for their normal life processes. Virtually all the elements of the periodic table have been found in living cells, though not all are necessarily essential to life. The nutrients which are commonly referred to as *mineral elements*, or *inorganic nutrients*, and which have definite demonstrable functions in the human body and metabolism are calcium, phosphorus, magnesium, sodium, potassium, sulfur, chlorine, iron, copper, cobalt, iodine, manganese, zinc, and perhaps fluorine (in addition, molybdenum and selenium are essential, at least for experimental animals). Aluminum, arsenic, nickel, and silicon might be mentioned as elements which occur very consistently in the human body, though for them there exists no proof of human need. The mineral, or inorganic, nutrients are interrelated and balanced against each other in human physiology; they cannot be considered as single elements with circumscribed functions, just as proteins, carbohydrates, fats, and vitamins do not play independent and self-sufficient roles in the general body symphony. For example, calcium and phosphorus are in a definite relationship in the formation of bones and teeth. Iron, copper, and cobalt (in vitamin B_{12}) are interrelated in hemoglobin synthesis and red blood cell formation. Sodium, potassium, calcium, phosphorus, and chlorine serve individual and collective purposes in the body fluids. Calcium and magnesium are necessary for normal soft tissue and nerve cell function. Iodine is an essential constituent of the thyroid hormone, while zinc, molybdenum, and manganese serve as essential activators of a number of enzyme-catalyzed metabolic reactions.

About 13 different minerals are known to be needed by the body, and all must be derived from the diet. The three elements whose supply is most likely to be critical are calcium, iron, and iodine.

CALCIUM

Function

Calcium and phosphorus serve as the main structural skeletal elements. Ninety-nine percent of body calcium is present in bones and teeth and only 1 percent in the soft tissues and body fluids. Calcium is present in bone as a multiple apatite salt composed of calcium phosphate and calcium carbonate arranged in a definite proportion and crystal lattice. Bone may be regarded as more than a structural framework; it also serves as the calcium reservoir of the body. The skeletal calcium is in dynamic equilibrium with the constituents of the body fluids and other tissues, and the rate of exchange is greater than the rate of original deposition of new bone. The most readily mobilized calcium is found in the trabecular portion of bones; it comes into play when the calcium requirement of the individual increases, as during pregnancy and lactation. The dentine and enamel of teeth are metabolically more stable and do not yield calcium with similar ease.

Normal blood contains from 9 to 11 mg of calcium per 100 ml, practically all in the serum and none in the erythrocytes. About 60 percent of this calcium is present in the soluble, ionized form; the rest occurs in a protein-bound form. The blood calcium serves several major functions. It is essential for the normal clotting of blood. Its presence is also required for normal functioning of nerve tissue. A reduced blood calcium level increases the irritability of nervous tissue; very low calcium levels may cause a characteristic tetany with convulsions. Concentrations of calcium above the normal range depress nerve irritability. An optimal calcium range is also essential for a normal pulse and cardiac contraction. The relative concentrations of potassium, magnesium, and sodium are also involved in the effect of calcium on nerve and muscle irritability. Magnesium deficiency may lead to extensive deposition of calcium in soft tissues and distortion of bone structure.

Absorption and Utilization

Dietary calcium is absorbed in the small intestine. The amount absorbed is influenced by a number of factors. It is practically a biologic law that the body utilizes and conserves material more efficiently when in need. This axiom also holds with respect to calcium. The greater the need and the smaller the dietary supply, the more efficient the absorption. Under normal conditions, calcium absorption increases somewhat, though not proportionately, with an increased intake. Absorption of calcium is facilitated in the presence of vitamin D and by a low intestinal pH which keeps the calcium in solution. Normal gastric hydrochloric acid secretion is thus necessary to facilitate efficient absorption. Lactose also stimulates absorption of calcium; the exact mechanism involved is unclear.

Oxalic acid has an adverse effect on calcium utilization since it forms insoluble calcium oxalate which passes through the intestine without being absorbed. This effect is limited because it depends completely on the quantity of oxalic acid which is ingested with foods; ordinarily the amounts of dietary calcium are such that losses through calcium oxalate formation are not serious. However, because of their oxalic acid content, large quantities of specific foods like rhubarb and spinach may interfere with efficient calcium absorption.

Phytic acid, a hexaphosphoric acid ester of inositol which is found in cereal seeds, may form insoluble calcium salts with free calcium in the intestinal contents, thus making some calcium unavailable for absorption. Phytic acid is found mainly in the bran portion of cereals, and a heavy intake of bran or whole cereals can adversely affect calcium absorption. In this case, as in that of oxalic acid in foods, the possible harmful effect depends primarily on the quantity of oxalate or phytate involved, and a sufficiently liberal calcium intake suffices to compensate for it. An excess (or poor digestion) of fat in the intestine may reduce calcium absorption through the formation of insoluble calcium soaps; on the other hand, small amounts of fat appear to improve calcium absorption. Recently it has been shown that a diet rich in protein decreases the efficacy of dietary calcium uptake.

Calcium absorbed from the food is readily transferred through the body by the circulation. It is withdrawn from the body by the bones and teeth during periods of growth, and some calcium is incorporated into bone at all ages. The calcium blood level is regulated by the parathyroid hormone and by the hormone calcitonin, which opposes the effects of parathormone. Calcium may be withdrawn from the bones to maintain normal blood levels during periods of dietary calcium deprivation.

Excretion

Normally, the kidney excretes any excess of blood calcium over 7 mg per 100 ml. The parathyroid hormone appears to regulate urinary calcium excretion through control of the individual renal threshold.

The urine is not the only route by which calcium is excreted; considerable amounts may be found in the feces. Some fecal calcium consists of the unabsorbed dietary mineral, but a large proportion represents calcium which has been lost from the body. A regulated excretion is probably not involved. It appears that calcium is secreted into the intestinal lumen with the digestive juices and becomes intimately mixed with the dietary calcium and intestinal contents; being subject to the factors governing intestinal calcium absorption, it may not be reabsorbed quantitatively. Small amounts of calcium (1 to 20 mg per hour) may also be lost by way of the skin during heavy sweating.

Deficiency

The principal cause of rickets in children is lack of vitamin D. However, insufficient intakes of calcium and phosphorus as well as a marked imbalance in calcium-phosphorus intake may result in this disease. In adults, calcium deficiency may cause osteomalacia, a generalized rarefaction and demineralization of bone. This condition is usually due to a deficiency of vitamin D and calcium and is rare in the United States, where the stigmata of dietary calcium lack in adults are not frequently observed. (See Chap. 22 for a discussion of rickets in children and osteomalacia in adults.) Osteomalacia is often confused with a common disease in older people, osteoporosis, a metabolic disorder resulting in decalcification of bone with a high incidence of pathologic fractures following light trauma. A number of causes contribute to the development of this disorder; among them are faulty metabolism of the proteinaceous bone matrix (secondary to the drop in anabolic hormone levels in old age), disuse demineralization, and a chronic negative calcium balance, over a period of years, due to greater outgo than intake of the mineral. (See Chap. 19 for a more detailed discussion.)

One particular condition which induces calcium loss from the skeleton bears mentioning—namely, prolonged immobilization and bed rest. Immobilization of limbs by orthopedic casts or prolonged body immobilization such as in prolonged hospital bed rest enforced by bone fracture or disease reduces the daily mechanical stress and pressure forces on bony tissues which normally stimulate a constant mineralization of the skeleton in order to permit it to perform its structural tasks in the body. Once this mechanical stress is removed owing to immobilization and disuse (or because of lack of the normal stress of gravity in the case of astronauts in space), skeletal demineralization sets in with considerable losses of calcium and phosphorus from bone. This loss of bone mineral may proceed at a steady rate for prolonged periods, until reambulation and restoration of physical exercise (or, in the case of previously "weightless" astronauts, until gravitational stress and physical exercise are again encountered). Calcium and phosphorus excretion in patients under conditions of enforced, prolonged hospital bed rest not infrequently is large enough to lead to the formation of kidney stones in the urinary tract. It has been claimed that oral phosphate supplements given during periods of immobilization restore a positive calcium balance and prevent excessive bone decalcification and hypercalcinuria.

Requirements

Measurements of the calcium requirement in infants vary widely because of the available methods used and differences in prenatal endowment. Estimates vary considerably, depending on whether the chosen criterion for calcium intake is breast milk or cow's milk. The Food and Nutrition Board of the National Research Council has set its Recommended Dietary Allowances in childhood at 0.8 g, and in the teens, at 1.2 g (Table 22). The Canadian Dietary Standards specifiy smaller amounts (Table 24). There is no doubt that the need for a high intake of milk or other calcium sources is great during the active period of bone growth and skeletal enrichment with calcium in childhood and especially during the pubertal growth spurt.

In contrast to the situation in children and adolescents where a high calcium intake and retention are clearly desirable, the adult has no apparent need for more calcium than that required to maintain body stores. The Food and Nutrition Board recommends a daily intake of 800 mg.

The calcium requirement is obviously increased in pregnancy to satisfy the demand created by growth and development of the fetal skeletal system. Good prenatal calcium nutrition and accumulation of calcium reserves are essential to optimal fetal development. The requirement of the pregnant woman consists of her own as well as that of the growing fetus, and the recommended allowance has been set at 1.2 g in the United States. A very low maternal intake may result in calcium withdrawal from the maternal skeleton to supply the fetus. The recommended calcium allowances for pregnant women prevent such withdrawal in most instances.

The calcium content of human milk varies with the maternal calcium intake and may range from 100 to 300 mg per day. There is no doubt that a lactating woman should have a markedly increased calcium supply to meet her own needs as well as the calcium requirement for milk production. The Food and Nutrition Board recommends a daily intake of 1.2 g.

Sources

The following are good sources of calcium: milk and most dairy products, shellfish, egg yolk, canned sardines and salmon (with bones), soybeans, and green vegetables like turnip greens, mustard greens, broccoli, and kale. In the United States and much of Europe, the principal sources of calcium are milk and cheese.

The reader is referred to the Tables of Food Composition in the Appendix for information regarding the calcium content of different foods.

PHOSPHORUS

Function

Phosphorus has more functions than any other mineral element in the body. A complex calcium phosphate lends rigidity to bones and teeth, and about 80 percent of the body's phosphorus is found in the skeletal tissues. The other 20 percent is located in the body fluids and in every cell of the body and is vitally concerned with their metabolism and function. A complete discussion of phosphorus metabolism would require coverage of practically all metabolic processes in the body. Phosphorus plays an important part in muscle energy metabolism, carbohydrate, protein, and fat metabolism, nervous tissue metabolism, normal blood chemistry, skeletal growth and tooth development, and the transport of fatty acids. Phosphate is a component of many enzyme systems and is involved in the storage and transfer of energy in phosphorylated compounds such as adenosine di- and triphosphate.

Blood contains from 35 to 45 mg of phosphorus per 100 ml. Of this amount, 3 to 5 mg is in the form of inorganic phosphate, the portion which is most readily available for chemical reactions. Normally there is an inverse relationship between the serum calcium and the serum inorganic phosphate.

Absorption and Excretion

Ordinarily about 70 percent of the phosphorus ingested in foods is absorbed. It is assumed that intestinal phosphatases liberate simple phosphorus compounds from the ingesta before absorption takes place. As with calcium, absorption is favored by an acid medium. Excesses of iron, aluminum, and magnesium interfere with phosphorus absorption through the formation of insoluble phosphates. (This is not an important factor in ordinary diets.) For optimum absorption of both calcium and phosphorus, both nutrients should be supplied by the food in roughly equal amounts. An abnormal calcium/phosphorus ratio in food interferes with the absorption of both elements and may result in calcium deficiency. As with calcium, the absorption of phosphorus is considerably increased when vitamin D is available to the individual (Chap 10); this may be due to a secondary effect.

Phosphorus in the feces represents both the unabsorbed mineral and phosphorus secreted into the intestinal tract. Urinary phosphorus is principally inorganic phosphate; the amount fluctuates with the quantity absorbed from foods but is also dependent on other factors. Catabolism of body tissues during starvation releases much phosphorus into the urine. In individuals with a constant phosphorus intake, intense carbohydrate metabolism, which requires phosphorus, tends to decrease urinary phosphorus temporarily.

Requirements

Phosphorus is not often a subject of concern for the nutritionist, since the diet of man is generally adequate in this element and phosphorus deficiency has not been found in human beings. Little precise information is known concerning phosphorus requirements except for a generalization, based on experience, that the phosphorus intake should approximately equal that of calcium (provided the calcium intake is adequate). The Food and Nutrition Board recommends an intake equal to that of calcium for all age groups except young infants. In these, a calcium/phosphorus ratio of 1.5:1 is desirable. (See Table 22 in Chap. 13 for a more detailed listing of the recommended daily allowances.) The common foods which meet the calcium and protein needs of the individual invariably supply the phosphorus requirement simultaneously.

Antacids can impair phosphorus absorption in man, and the long-term use of nonabsorbable antacids containing magnesium-aluminum hydroxides can lead to phosphorus depletion of varying degree. This condition is characterized by low blood and urine phosphate levels with compensatory increased skeletal demineralization and hypercalcemia; very prolonged and excessive ingestion of nonabsorbable antacids can result in extreme phosphorus depletion with clinical osteomalacia.

Sources

Protein-rich foods of animal origin, such as meat, fish, poultry, and eggs, are excellent sources of phosphorus. Milk and cheese are good sources, as well as nuts and legumes. The availability of the phosphorus of cereal grains, especially of the bran portion, is somewhat doubtful since much of this phosphorus is present as phytic acid which is not utilized well. Information regarding the phosphorus content of common foods is found in the Tables of Food Composition in the Appendix.

IRON

Function

Iron is a component of the hemoglobin and myoglobin molecules and of the cytochromes and other enzyme systems, and as such it plays an essential role in oxygen transport and cellular respiration. Hemoglobin, a heme-protein component of the red blood cells, combines reversibly with oxygen in the lungs and normally releases it in the tissues wherever a need for oxygen exists. (Hemoglobin also serves as a return vehicle for some of the carbon dioxide elaborated in active tissues, releasing it in the lungs.) In the muscles, some of this oxygen is taken up by another iron-porphyrin protein, myoglobin, which serves as a temporary oxygen acceptor and reservoir. Iron is also found in the intracellular cytochrome enzyme system which functions in energy production.

Absorption and Utilization

Dietary iron is absorbed primarily by the mucosa of the duodenum. The degree of absorption depends to a large extent on the current iron balance of the body. The iron economy and state of iron storage in the body are maintained at a constant level largely by the ability of the mucosa to reject available but unneeded dietary iron (and not by selective excretion of excess iron from the body).

Except for iron in meat, food iron is relatively poorly absorbed. Ferrous iron is absorbed more efficiently than ferric iron. It is probable that the major part of ingested food iron, once liberated by gastrointestinal digestion, is reduced from the ferric to the ferrous state prior to absorption. Absorption of iron is enhanced when it takes place from an acid medium. It is not clear if this results from improved conversion of ferric to ferrous iron in the presence of the normal acid gastric secretions. It is well known that absorption of iron is more efficient in the presence of ascorbic acid, sulfhydryl compounds, and similar reducing substances. Ascorbic acid and fructose also form soluble complexes with iron, resulting in enhanced absorption. Both the nature of the food mixture ingested and the form in which food iron is presented to the gut exert an influence on the efficiency of dietary iron absorption. An excess of phosphates, oxalates, or phytates in the food may impair iron absorption because of the formation of insoluble iron compounds which pass through the intestinal tract without being absorbed. It is known that iron is absorbed poorly in the presence of egg yolk and certain vegetables. Conversely, iron from foods of plant origin (wheat, corn, beans) is better absorbed when combined with meats than when given alone. In general, iron from animal sources is absorbed more readily and to a greater extent than that from cereals or vegetables.

Normally about 10 percent of ingested food iron is absorbed. This amount increases greatly in iron-deficiency states when up to 26 percent may be taken up by the body. The main factor that affects iron absorption is the body's need for this substance. Thus, absorption is increased during periods of rapid growth in youth, during pregnancy, as a result of blood loss, and in persons living at high altitudes.

A current generally accepted theory (*mucosal blockage*) explains why under normal conditions iron is absorbed only when needed, thus preventing excessive storage in the body. Presumably iron enters the mucosal cell where it combines with a specific protein (apoferritin) to yield an iron-protein complex, ferritin. Ferritin gives up its iron component to the bloodstream whenever new iron is needed by the body. Iron-free apoferritin in the mucosal cell may combine with additional iron absorbed from the intestinal contents. However, no further absorption takes place as long as the mucosal cell is saturated with iron-containing ferritin, and only removal of iron from this ferritin for the purpose of blood hemoglobin formation, or for use in other tissues, will unblock the system and will make further intestinal iron absorption possible.

In the plasma, iron is found in the ferric state, bound to a specific globulin in an iron-protein complex, transferrin. A large percentage of the plasma iron is utilized in the bone marrow in the synthesis of hemoglobin, while some is taken up by other tissues for the formation of intracellular enzymes. The presence of small amounts of copper is required for the synthesis of iron into hemoglobin and the cytochromes. (It has been suggested that copper is an essential component of an enzyme system which facilitates the release of iron from ferritin.)

Storage

The body of an average adult contains about 3.5 to 4.0 g of iron. Of this, approximately 1 g is stored iron, located principally in the liver and spleen. Reservoir iron is found intracellularly in the form of a protein complex, either as hemosiderin or as ferritin. This iron is readily mobilized when the need arises; as a deficiency develops, the ferritin and hemosiderin reservoirs are depleted before an actual anemia develops.

Iron Loss

Red blood cells require about $7^1/_2$ days for their development; they then have an average life-span of about 120 days, after which they break down. The liberated iron is salvaged efficiently, and new hemoglobin is synthesized in maturing erythrocytes, which will then replace the destroyed red cells.

Despite the assiduous conservation of body iron some normal losses occur daily by way of sweat, hair, desquamated epithelial and mucosal cells, leucocytes, and urine and by way of some possible fecal and biliary excretion or occult bleeding. The normal daily loss of iron in the male adult amounts to about 1 mg. Additional quantities are lost to women through menstrual blood (about 14 to 28 mg) and when the pregnant mother furnishes the fetus with iron (a total of 300 to 500 mg of iron throughout the period of gestation). The total daily iron loss of a woman during the period of her active sexual life is estimated at 1 to 2 mg. Injury with bleeding, occult intestinal blood loss, and blood donation all contribute considerably to iron loss from the body.

Deficiency

Iron deficiency in man is expressed as hypochromic anemia (Chap. 33). In this condition the number of circulating red blood cells is either normal or reduced, but the total quantity of circulating hemoglobin is decidedly subnormal. Each erythrocyte has a reduced hemoglobin content, and the red blood cells are pale. The blood has a decreased oxygen-carrying capacity which reflects unfavorably on most body functions. The hematologic manifestations are coupled with a clinical picture common to all anemias: pallor of skin and tissues, weakness and fatigability, dyspnea on exertion, headache, palpitation, and a constant feeling of tiredness.

Iron-deficiency anemia may develop on a purely nutritional basis, as a result of inadequate diet or poor absorption. Occult or overt blood loss accelerates the depletion of body iron. Even though absorption and the diet are adequate, chronic blood loss may lead to a severe exhaustion of the body's iron stores and to subsequent hypochromic anemia. Individuals who harbor intestinal parasites or who suffer from chronically bleeding hemorrhoids, peptic ulcers, or recurrent nosebleeds are particularly prone to iron depletion. Women in their reproductive years may develop a deficiency if their menstrual loss is copious or if repeated and closely spaced pregnancies recurrently exhaust their iron stores. A concurrent poor diet or poor iron absorption puts a strain on the already overburdened iron economy, and frank deficiency symptoms are not infrequent in this group.

Infants constitute another group in which iron-deficiency anemia is frequent. The iron nutrition and iron needs of infants are discussed in Chap. 17, Nutrition in Infancy, and Chap. 33, Nutrition and the Anemias. It is important to remember that availability of iron is not the sole factor determining the hemoglobin economy of the individual; the total dietary is involved, including protein supply, protein-sparing calories, and availability of the B vitamins and ascorbic acid.

For the sake of completeness, any discussion of iron deficiency should include mention of an unusual perversion of appetite (pica; see Chap. 6) characterized by the habitual ingestion of extraordinary amounts of ice. The condition, pagophagia, appears to be related to iron lack (present in all patients) and is completely resolved by the administration of quantities of iron smaller than those required for resolution of iron-deficiency anemia (which many of these patients have) or complete replenishment of iron stores.

Iron Overload

The usual balance between iron intake and iron loss is such that iron deficiency is fairly common while iron overload is rare. Body iron can be increased by excessive iron intake, as in the South African Bantu, who consume large amounts of iron with kaffir beer (which is brewed in iron utensils), which overwhelms the body's innate, but limited, ability to regulate iron balance through diminished absorption.

Excessive amounts of iron can also be absorbed owing to a specific disease entity, hemachromatosis. In this condition, defective limitation of absorption by the intestinal mucosa results in an overload not of the reticuloendothelial cells of the liver, spleen, or bone marrow (which are normal storage areas), but of the parenchymal liver cells. Advanced hemachromatosis is a grave condition characterized by gray skin pigmentation, breakdown of liver function, hepatic enlargement and scarring, pancreatic infiltration with diabetes, and heart failure due to myocardial disease.

Requirements

It has been estimated that the normal adult male must assimilate about 1 mg of iron daily to balance his natural losses; the normal adult woman probably requires 1 to 2 mg of assimilated iron per day. Since normally only about 10 percent of ingested food iron is absorbed, the desired daily iron intake for adult men and women lies between 10 and 20 mg per day. The Food and Nutrition Board recommends a daily intake of 10 to 15 mg for infants, 15 to 20 for children, 10 to 18 for adults and adolescents, and 18 for pregnant and lactating women (Table 22). The Canadian Dietary Standards are lower; they suggest 5 mg daily for children, 12 for adolescents, 6 for male adults, 10 for female adults, and 13 for pregnant and lactating women (Table 24).

These allowances, especially the Canadian Dietary Standards, are conservative estimates and should be increased considerably if there is evidence of blood loss or of conditions which impair the assimilation of ingested iron.

Sources

The following are good sources of iron (in decreasing order of excellence): liver, heart, kidney, liver sausage, lean meats, shellfish, egg yolk, dried beans and other legumes, dried fruits, nuts, green leafy vegetables, whole-grain and enriched cereals and cereal products, and dark molasses. Milk is a poor source of iron, which is the reason for an early use of iron-enriched cereals, egg yolk, meat, and green leafy vegetables in infant feeding.

Information regarding the iron content of the common foods is found in the Tables of Food Composition at the end of the book.

COPPER

Function

Copper is a component of the enzyme tyrosinase (polyphenol oxidase), which is necessary for melanin pigment formation in the body. It is also part of the molecule of uricase and of butyryl coenzyme A dehydrogenase and is probably associated with other oxidation-reduction enzymes in the body such as cytochrome C oxidase and ascorbate oxidase. It is believed that copper stimulates the absorption of iron. Copper appears to play a role in the synthesis of iron into the hemoglobin and cytochrome molecules, but the exact mechanism for this hematopoietic role is not established. Copper is also a constituent of the elastic connective tissue protein, elastin, and is involved in the formation of myelin, the material which sheathes peripheral and central nerve fibers.

Metabolism

In man, copper absorption takes place in the stomach or upper intestine or both. From the intestine, copper moves into the blood, where it is present in two forms: (1) a small fraction of loosely albumin-bound and largely "available" copper which is concerned in the transportation of the mineral from the gastrointestinal tract to the tissues and between the various tissues, and (2) a larger fraction contained in the copper protein ceruloplasmin which originates in the liver. It is currently thought that ceruloplasmin prevents accumulation of toxic levels of copper and that it promotes saturation of transferrin with iron. Another specific copper protein, erythrocupreine, is found exclusively in red blood cells, where it accounts for 60 percent of erythrocyte copper.

The liver is the chief organ of storage; it also serves as the major organ of excretion since copper is excreted primarily in the bile. About 2 to 5 mg of copper is consumed and excreted each day. Approximately 30 percent of the intake is absorbed; of this amount about 80 percent is excreted by way of the bile (and ultimately the feces), about 16 percent diffuses back into the intestinal lumen through the gut wall, and about 4 percent is excreted in the urine.

The copper content of the fetal liver is five to ten times as great as that of the liver of the normal adult. This has been interpreted teleologically as a wise provision of nature to tide the newborn over a period during which the diet consists chiefly of milk, which is notably low in copper.

The relation of diet therapy to abnormal copper metabolism and storage (Wilson's disease, or hepatolenticular degeneration) is discussed in Chap. 32, Nutrition and Diet in Congenital Metabolic Disorders.

Requirements and Deficiency

In infrequent cases of hypochromic anemia in infants, the therapeutic efficacy of iron is augmented by the concurrent administration of copper. Many of these infants have subsisted on almost nothing but cow's milk for periods of up to 10

Table 17   Dietary Sources of Copper
(Micrograms per 100-g Edible Portion)

Almonds	1,210	Halibut	230
Apples	120	Kale	328
Asparagus	141	Liver, beef	2,450
Avocado	690	Lobster	730
Bananas	200	Mackerel	230
Beans, dry	960	Mushrooms	1,790
Beans, lima, dry	915	Oats	738
Beef, round	80	Oranges	80
Bread, white	205	Oysters	3,623
Cabbage	50	Peas, dried	802
Carrots	80	Pecans	1,360
Cheese, American	180	Pork chops	310
Chicken, dark meat	410	Prunes, dried	291
Chicken, white meat	270	Rye, whole	656
Chocolate, bitter	2,670	Shrimp	430
Cocoa	3,340	Spinach	197
Corn	449	Sweet potatoes	184
Eggs	253	Turkey, dark meat	200
Flour, whole wheat	435	Turkey, white meat	150
Flour, white	170	Walnuts	1,000
Grapes, Malaga	90	Wheat	787

months, and it has been suggested that these may be rare cases of a true copper deficiency.

Demonstrable instances of primary copper deficiency have yet to be recognized in adult man. Cases of copper depletion can be found where the hypocupremia is secondary to increased loss of plasma copper protein due to protein-losing enteropathies or due to renal plasma protein leakage into the urine in kidney disease. The human diet ordinarily contains more than enough copper to maintain balance. The daily requirement of copper is 2 mg. Even poor diets contain at least this amount, and copper is widespread enough in foods so that death from caloric starvation is likely to occur prior to the appearance of an overt clinical deficiency of copper.

IODINE

Physiology

Iodine is an essential nutrient for man; its sole recognized function in the human organism is its role in the formation of thyroid hormone, of which it is a basic component. Thyroid hormone regulates the metabolic rate of the individual. One of the factors which affect the output of thyroid hormone by the thyroid gland is availability of iodine. In the absence of sufficient iodine, the gland increases its secretory activity in an attempt to compensate for the deficiency; as a result, the gland enlarges and becomes turgid with an iodine-poor secretion. This condition is known as simple, or endemic, goiter.

Once ingested, iodine is absorbed from the small intestine. It is found in the blood both as inorganic iodide and as protein-bound iodine. It is taken up by the thyroid gland as the iodide ion and is selectively concentrated there, oxidized to elemental iodine, and incorporated into the amino acid tyrosine, which, after conversion to diiodotyrosine, thyroxine, and triiodothyronine, becomes part of the thyroglobulin complex—the biologically active hormone.

Synthesis of thyroid hormone may be effectively prevented, even in the presence of sufficient iodine in the diet and the circulation, by certain drugs (thiourea, thiouracil), which block the oxidation of iodide to iodine in the thyroid gland. Cabbage, rutabaga, and other members of the *Brassica* family contain a goitrogenic substance, thiooxazolidone, which acts similarly in interfering with thyroid hormone synthesis. Under ordinary circumstances insufficient quantities of this goitrogen are ingested to be of clinical significance.

Requirements and Deficiency

The iodine requirement for prevention of goiter in adults is 50 to 75 µg per day, or approximately 1 µg/kg body weight. The need for iodine is increased during puberty and pregnancy. Presumably the demand for thyroid hormone increases during these periods, and temporary enlargement of the oversecreting thyroid gland may be observed not infrequently. The need for iodine is increased in pregnancy because the fetus must derive its iodine requirements and stores from the mother. During lactation, maternal iodide is lost through secretion in the milk and the minimal iodine requirement is almost doubled at the time of maximal lactation. The Food and Nutrition Board has set a recommended daily allowance varying from 35 μg of iodine in young infants to 150 μg in lactating women.

Food which is grown on iodine-poor soil contains insufficient iodine to meet human needs. Endemic, or simple, goiter is observed frequently in regions deficient in iodine. A high incidence of simple deficiency goiter has been found in the Alps, the Pyrenees, the Himalaya mountains, the Thames Valley in England, Central America, the Great Lakes basin, and northwestern sections of the United States. Additional areas throughout the world are subject to moderate degrees of iodine deficiency. Though Japan is geologically low in iodine, it represents a remarkable example of a goiter-free population, while Formosa and the interior of China, both similarly depleted in iodine, have a high incidence of goiter in their population. The absence of goiter in Japan results from the Japanese gastronomic predilection for seaweed and fish, which are extensively consumed both in the coastal regions and in the interior of the country and which are unusually rich in iodine content.

Possibly the most pressing reason for preventing simple deficiency goiter is not the attendant mild hypothyroidism itself, but the concomitant cretinism of goitrous populations. The human fetus derives little thyroid hormone from the mother during intrauterine life and must elaborate its own. In the absence of sufficient iodine the fetus fails to develop normally. The physical retardation may be corrected by the administration of thyroid hormone, but the mental retardation in congenital cretinism of long standing is irreversible and the damage irreparable to a great extent.

Sources

Among natural foods, the best sources of iodine are seafoods and vegetables grown on iodine-rich soils. Neither source enjoys universal distribution, and various methods have been proposed to assure an adequate iodine intake, especially for populations in iodine-poor regions. The use of iodized salt has thus far proved the most successful and most widely adopted method. In the United States, commercially iodized salt contains 0.01 percent of potassium iodide. Assuming that the average adult uses 6 to 6.5 g of salt daily, his concurrent iodine intake from this source is 0.48 mg; this amount of iodine represents about twice the normal requirement and provides amply for a sufficient reserve. In Central America iodates are used successfully instead of iodide; they have the advantage of greater stability in salt which is not highly refined. In regions where salt iodization programs cannot presently be undertaken, the intramuscular injection of iodized poppy-seed oil at 2-year intervals is an effective and acceptable prophylactic public health measure. (Each milliliter of oil contains 475 mg of iodine; dosage ranges from 0.2 ml of the oil for children up to 2 years of age to 2.0 ml for individuals 12 years old and up.)

The major source of iodine in the United States is iodized salt. The physician must not overlook this fact when a patient is placed on a low-salt or salt-free diet, especially in the case of pregnant women for whom he may desire a reduced sodium intake because of circulatory or renal disease or a tendency to toxemias of pregnancy. Considering that the iodine requirement in pregnancy is high, an iodine supplement is desirable if rigid salt restriction has been ordered for the patient.

COBALT

Cobalt is a component of the vitamin B_{12} molecule, and this may well be its only biologic function in the human body. Cobalt is found in many common foods; it is readily absorbed from the intestinal tract, and most of the absorbed material is excreted in the urine. Very little of this element is retained; the retained fraction serves no physiologic function since human tissues cannot synthesize vitamin B_{12} and thus do not utilize the available cobalt for this purpose. There is no known human cobalt requirement (except for that contained in vitamin B_{12}), and cobalt deficiency in man is unknown.

ZINC

Physiology

The physiologic importance of zinc is that it is a component of several enzymes which catalyze vital metabolic reactions. Zinc is an integral part of the molecule of carbonic anhydrase (found in red blood cells), without which carbon dioxide exchange could not take place with sufficient dispatch to sustain life. Zinc is also a component of the digestive enzyme carboxypeptidase and of several dehydrogenases active in the liver in animals and, by inference, possibly in man as well. More recently evidence has emerged that zinc, in addition to being a component part of several metalloenzymes, participates in nucleic acid and protein metabolism and is essential for normal maintenance of vitamin A blood levels by facilitating release of vitamin A stores from the liver. Contrary to a widely held belief, zinc is not essential for the physiologic activity of insulin. In experiments in animals and man it has been shown that zinc supplementation may aid the optimal healing of burns and of surgical incisions.

Requirements and Deficiency

The normal daily diet of Western man contains 10 to 15 mg of zinc. How much of it is available for intestinal absorption depends, as in the case of iron, on the precise form of the dietary mineral and the simultaneous presence of substances which make it unavailable (like phytates and other chelating compounds). Excretion occurs primarily through the gastrointestinal tract by way of pancreatic juice and intestinal secretions. On the average, feces contain about 10 mg and urine from 0.4 to 0.5 mg of zinc per day. In tropical climates, sweat excretion may account for a daily loss of as much as 1 to 2 mg. The daily dietary requirement of zinc in adults has been estimated to be about 10 mg. The Food and Nutrition Board recommends a daily allowance varying from 3 mg for young infants to 25 mg for lactating women.

Normal intake and excretion figures appear to indicate that the usual zinc intake of man in cold and temperate climates is generally adequate to maintain a positive balance. Zinc deficiency has been reported to be responsible for growth retardation, hypogonadism, and delayed sexual maturation in selected malnourished teen-age children in the Middle East. In the cases observed to date, factors which make zinc unavailable (unleavened village bread with a high phytate content as the mainstay of the diet, and clay eating) or cause abnormal zinc losses from the body (chronic blood loss from parasitism), or a combination of these, appear to be the underlying causes in addition to a generally inadequate diet deficient in animal protein. Recent evidence suggests that marginal states of zinc nutrition may exist in segments of the population in the United States. Accelerated rates of wound healing and improved rates of growth, appetite, and taste acuity were observed as the result of increased zinc intake in individuals suspected of a deficient zinc nutriture.

Risks of a deficiency in the United States are *generally* slight since zinc appears to be furnished in adequate quantities by a mixed diet, especially one containing sufficient animal protein. The richest dietary sources of zinc are

Table 18   Dietary Sources of Zinc
(Milligrams per 100-g Edible Portion)

Applesauce, canned	1.2–1.4	Liver, pork	3–15
Barley	2.7	Milk, cow's	0.4–3.0
Beef	2–5	Milk, dry skim	4.5
Beets	2.8	Oatmeal	14
Bread, whole wheat	2.4–3.5	Oranges	0.1
Bread, rye	2.2	Oysters	160
Butter	0.3	Peanut butter	2.0
Cabbage	0.2–1.5	Pears, canned	1.5–1.8
Carrots	0.5–3.6	Peas	3–5
Cherries, canned	1.6–2.2	Potatoes	0.2
Clams	2.0	Rice	1.5
Corn, whole	2.5	Rice, cereal	1.9
Eggs, dry whole	5.5	Spinach	0.3–0.9
Egg, yolk	2.6–4	Syrup, maple	5.2–10.5
Herrings	70–120	Wheat	2.5–8.5
Lettuce	0.1–0.7	Wheat bran	14
Liver, beef	3.0–8.5	Yeast, dry	8

oysters and herring, which contain about 100 mg per 100 g. Other high-zinc foods are meats, liver, milk, fish, eggs, nuts, and legumes. Foods and diets high in protein of animal origin supply large amounts of zinc; foods and diets containing mostly carbohydrates and containing only proteins of plant origin provide considerably less zinc.

An excess of zinc may be harmful; enough zinc may be dissolved from galvanized iron containers and cooking utensils by acid foods to produce untoward gastrointestinal symptoms.

MANGANESE

Manganese is part of the molecular structure of arginase, an enzyme necessary for the formation of urea. It also serves as an activator of several enzymes active in the Krebs cycle reactions (Fig. 5 in Chap. 8), particularly in the decarboxylation steps which occur during the metabolism of di- and tricarboxylic acids. Based on its role in enzymatic reactions, it is considered an essential micronutrient.

Manganese is widely distributed in foods of plant and animal origin. The human requirement is unknown, and a deficiency syndrome has yet to be reported.

Table 19   Dietary Sources of Manganese
(Micrograms per 100-g Edible Portion)

Bananas	640	Liver	391
Beans, dry	1,500	Oatmeal	4,945
Beans, snap	325	Peas, dried	1,990
Beets	575	Prunes, dried	436
Corn, whole	680	Rice, white	1,014
Flour, white	710	Rye, whole grain	3,067
Flour, whole wheat	4,300	Spinach	828
Kale	590	Sweet potatoes	407
Lettuce	1,240	Wheat	4,591

MAGNESIUM

Magnesium is a component of soft tissues as well as bone. Cardiac and skeletal muscle and nervous tissue depend on a proper balance between calcium and magnesium ions for normal function. Magnesium is an essential activator for all enzymes which transfer phosphate from adenosine triphosphate (ATP) to adenosine diphosphate (ADP). These reactions are fundamental and widespread and thus influence all basic life processes. Among the many enzymes activated by magnesium are hexokinase, fructokinase, diphosphopyridine nucleotide phosphorylase, pyruvic carboxylase, pyruvic oxidase, and creatine kinase. Physiologically, low magnesium body fluid levels enhance muscular irritability through increased nerve conduction, increased impulse transmission at the myoneural junction, and increased muscular contractility.

A deficiency syndrome resulting from severe renal disease, toxemia of pregnancy, chronic alcoholism with hepatic cirrhosis, sustained losses of gastrointestinal secretions, vigorous, drug-induced diuresis, or the prolonged administration of magnesium-free parenteral fluids has been reported. This syndrome resembles hypocalcemic tetany and is manifested by muscle tremor, choreiform movements, and, in severe cases, convulsions. Delirium may accompany the nervous manifestations. The condition responds to parenteral administration of magnesium.

Since magnesium occurs widely in foods—particularly those of plant origin—a true dietary deficiency of this element seems to be rare and has not been reported in man.

The magnesium content of the average American diet has been estimated at about 120 mg per 1000 cal. The magnesium requirement of man has not yet been determined *precisely*; diets supplying 300 mg for women and 300 to 400 mg for men keep healthy adults in balance. The recommended daily allowances of the Food and Nutrition Board vary from 60 mg for infants to 450 mg for pregnant or lactating women (Table 22).

Table 20   Dietary Sources of Magnesium
(Milligrams per 100-g Edible Portion)

Almonds	252	Oatmeal	145
Barley, entire	171	Oranges, fresh	13
Beans, lima, dry	181	Peaches, fresh	8
Beef, raw	25	Peanuts	167
Brazil nuts	225	Peas, fresh	140
Carrots, raw	12	Pecans	152
Cashew nuts	267	Potatoes, raw	24
Chicken, roast	23	Rice, brown	119
Cocoa	420	Soy flour	223
Cod, cooked	21	Spinach, boiled	59
Corn	121	Tomatoes, raw	11
Flour, whole wheat	122	Walnuts	134
Halibut, cooked	23	Wheat, whole	165
Hazelnuts	140		

MOLYBDENUM

Evidence that molybdenum is an essential trace mineral is based on the fact that it is part of the molecular structure of two enzymes, xanthine oxidase and aldehyde oxidase. Both enzymes are molybdoflavoproteins; the molybdenum is most likely involved in the linkage of flavin nucleotide (the prosthetic group, or coenzyme) to the substrate-specific protein (apoenzyme). A catalytic role in fatty acid oxidation has been ascribed to molybdenum; also, it is an essential component of the enzyme sulfite oxidase. As a component of xanthine oxidase, molybdenum participates in the reduction of cellular ferric to ferrous ferritin.

To date, no characteristic syndrome of molybdenum deficiency has been recognized in man. A positive molybdenum balance (with storage of the element, rather than loss from the body) is obtained when the daily intake approximates 100 µg per day—a condition which is apparently satisfied by average or even marginal diets in the United States.

Claims have been made that molybdenum exerts a stimulatory effect on hemoglobin regeneration when it is used concurrently with iron therapy in hypochromic anemias. These reports still await substantiation.

FLUORINE

Physiology

Fluorine is important inasmuch as it is normally present in bones and teeth and a proper intake is essential to achieve maximum resistance to dental caries. It is discussed here particularly because of the beneficial effects of small amounts of fluorine in the prevention of dental caries in children and adults (Fluoride in trace amounts is essential for normal growth and development in the rat.) Fluorine deficiency in terms of lowered resistance to dental caries is prevalent in large sections of the world. On the other hand, retardation of growth or soft-tissue lesions have not been produced under natural or experimental conditions in man or animal as a result of fluorine deprivation.

Fluorine is widely but unevenly distributed in nature. Water normally contains traces of fluorine; the fluorine content increases, sometimes excessively, when water passes through rocks and soils of special composition. It is found in many foods, seafoods and tea being the most significant dietary source. Information on fluorine metabolism is meager. Its intestinal absorption depends to a large degree on the solubility of the ingested fluorine compound.

The fluorine content of normal human blood is about 0.2 part per million (ppm) and that of saliva, 0.1 ppm. Almost all ingested fluorine, up to 3 mg per day, is quantitatively excreted in the urine (and to a small degree in the feces and sweat). Prolonged, higher intake may result in excessive storage of fluorine in the skeleton and teeth and, in extreme cases, in abnormal hardening of bone (osteosclerosis) and skeletal abnormalities usually beginning with calcification between the radius and the ulna.

An excessive intake of fluorine leads to mottling of the enamel of the teeth. In extreme cases the enamel may become pitted and the teeth appear stained and corroded. This condition of dental fluorosis is endemic in a number of communities, including localities in Colorado and the Texas panhandle where the natural water supply contains from 2 to 6 ppm of fluorine. On the other hand, when the fluorine concentration in the drinking water is about 1 ppm, a

Table 21   Dietary Sources of Fluorine
(Micrograms per 100-g Edible Portion)

Almonds	90	Herring, smoked	350
Apples	5–130	Honey	100
Apricots	2–22	Kale	16–300
Bananas	23	Lamb	120
Beans, string	13	Mackerel	2,700
Beef	29–200	Mackerel, canned	1,200
Round steak	130	Milk	10–55
Beef liver	99	Oats	25
Calf's liver	19	Onions	60
Beets	20	Oranges	7–17
Butter	150	Oysters	65
Cabbage	15	Parsley	80–100
Cantaloupe	20	Peaches	21
Carrots	40	Pears	19
Celery	14	Peas	60
Cheese	160	Pineapple	14
Cherries	25	Plum	21
Chicken	140	Pork	34–98
Chicken, canned	63	Pork, salt	100–3,300
Chocolate	50	Potatoes	7–640
Chocolate milk	50–200	Radish	80
Codfish	700	Rhubarb	40
Corn	62	Rice	10–67
Cornmeal	22	Salmon, canned	450–900
Crab meat, canned	200	Sardines, canned	730–1,600
Cucumber	20	Shrimp, canned	440
Eggs:		Soybeans	130
Whole	120	Spinach	20–180
White	150	Strawberries	18
Yolk	59	Tea infusion	120–6,300
Eggplant	40	Tomatoes	24
Figs	21	Tuna, canned	10
Fish	160	Turnips	30
Frankfurters	170	Veal	90
Gooseberries	11–52	Watercress	100
Grapefruit	36	Wheat	70
Grapes	16	Wheat flour	27–35
Hazelnuts	30	Wheat germ	88–400

marked decrease in dental caries is observed as compared with the national average.

The precise mechanism by which fluorine inhibits the development of dental caries is not known. Fluorine which is incorporated into the tooth enamel during the formative period apparently reduces the solubility of this enamel in the acids which are produced by bacteria in contact with the teeth and which are implicated in tooth decay. It is believed that the ingestion of fluoride results in replacement of hydroxyl ion by fluoride ion, and crystal growth of the apatite phase in bone and teeth, producing a more stable mineral phase. Some workers believe that the fluoride ion is more tightly bound to the apatite structure than the hydroxyl ion is, and thus both solubility and chemical reactivity of the bone mineral are reduced. Other workers have suggested that the incorporation of fluoride into apatite results in a more compact crystal structure with a reduced surface exposed at the interface between bone mineral crystals and the hydrated protein matrix in which they are embedded—thus also reducing the likelihood of ready crystal reactivity and dissolution.

There are strong indications that fluoride reduces mineral loss from the skeleton in general, not only the teeth, and renders bone more resistant to the degenerative demineralization of osteoporosis. In fact, in recent years oral fluoride has been used in the prophylaxis and treatment of osteoporosis.

Fluoridation

At present sodium fluoride is added to the municipal water supply in a large number of communities in an effort to decrease the incidence of dental caries among the young. Such fluoridated water usually contains 1 ppm of fluorine.

An average daily diet provides 0.25 to 0.35 mg of fluorine. In addition, the average adult may ingest daily 1.0 to 1.5 mg from drinking and cooking water which contains 1 ppm of fluorine. This same water contributes from 0.4 to 1.1 mg of fluorine to children 1 to 12 years old. This added quantity of fluorine, if ingested during the childhood years (up to age 16), makes a difference between a high and a low rate of tooth decay.

In every instance where well-controlled studies were made subsequent to the introduction of fluoridation, a marked decrease of carious teeth was noted. Toxic manifestations or other undesirable effects have not been observed as a result of fluoridation at such low levels. All available evidence indicates that consumption of water containing 1 ppm of fluorine is safe and accomplishes a significant reduction of dental decay in children and adolescents. (See Chap. 20 for further discussion.)

This prophylactic action of fluorine should not overshadow the importance of other nutrients which are essential for normal tooth formation. For a maximum of dental well-being, the total diet must be satisfactory and adequate amounts of calcium and phosphorus as well as protein and vitamins A, D, and C must be supplied to the pregnant mother and to her children.

SODIUM

Both sodium and potassium are essential for the normal functioning of the body. Dietary deficiencies, however, are rare under ordinary circumstances; this is probably the reason why little attention is paid to either element in the discussion of dietary requirements.

Practically all the sodium in the body is found in the extracellular fluids. Sodium ions make up 93 percent of the basic ions in the blood. Sodium plays an important role in the regulation of the acid-base balance in the body fluids and determines to a large degree the osmotic pressure of the extracellular fluids (Chap. 3). Under normal conditions, 90 percent of ingested sodium is excreted in the urine, usually in the form of sodium chloride and sodium phosphate. Under conditions of intense perspiration, sweat becomes the main vehicle of excretion. Prolonged, profuse perspiration may lead to sodium chloride depletion, with muscular cramps, weakness, headache, and vascular collapse. The prophylactic use of increased salt in the diet is indicated in occupations where excessive perspiration is a factor. (Under unusual circumstances, such as work in boiler rooms, salt tablets are used to compensate for excessive sodium chloride loss.) A special need for sodium chloride replacement also exists after recurrent vomiting or protracted diarrhea and in adrenal cortical insufficiency.

The normal intake of sodium chloride may range from 2 to 20 g daily. The Food and Nutrition Board states that 5 g is a liberal allowance; one additional gram of salt should be taken for each liter of water in excess of a daily intake of 4 liters. Information regarding the sodium content of foods is found in the Tables of Food Composition in the Appendix. The therapeutic use of sodium restriction is discussed in Chaps. 27, 29, and 30.

POTASSIUM

In contrast to sodium, potassium occurs mainly in the intracellular fluid. The cellular elements of the blood contain about twenty times as much potassium as the plasma; skeletal muscle contains about six times as much potassium as sodium. Potassium influences the contractility of smooth, skeletal, and cardiac muscle and profoundly affects the excitability of nerve tissue. Potassium deficiency can result from protracted diarrhea, abnormal kidney function, diabetic acidosis, and renal disease. Hypopotassemia may also be produced iatrogenically by prolonged maintenance of body fluids with parenteral glucose and sodium chloride infusion. Potassium deficiency is manifested by muscular weakness, increased nervous irritability, mental disorientation, and cardiac irregularities. Excessive concentrations of potassium are toxic. With increasing blood levels of potassium, cardiac irregularities develop; extreme hyperpotassemia (10 millimoles per liter or more) results in serious cardiac arrythmias, progressing to cardiac arrest.

Hyperpotassemia is almost always the result of greatly diminished renal excretion caused by kidney disease or by oliguria accompanying shock and dehydration. It is impossible to produce hyperpotassemia through dietary means in individuals with normal circulation and renal function. Similarly, dietary potassium deficiency does not exist under ordinary circumstances. Potassium depletion with hypokalemia, lassitude, and muscle weakness is frequently found among workers subject to heavy physical exertion and sweating in hot environments or after excessive vomiting and diarrhea. This impairment can be prevented or corrected by an increased potassium intake.

The dietary need for potassium roughly equals that of sodium. Information regarding the potassium content of foods is found in the Tables of Food Composition in the Appendix.

CHROMIUM

In recent years enough experimental evidence has been accumulated to classify chromium as an essential micronutrient for some mammals, concerned with carbohydrate and lipid metabolism. Still lacking are definitive experiments to link the disorders found in chromium-deficient laboratory animals with their human counterparts. There have been observations that abnormal glucose metabolism in some malnourished children with kwashiorkor, and poor glucose tolerance in some nondiabetic elderly men, and in some patients with frank diabetes, can be improved with the aid of supplements of trivalent chromium. A number of workers believe that an organic chromium compound, as yet chemically ill-defined, potentiates the metabolic actions of insulin. Future research in human nutrition will have to establish more fully the precise, and presumably essential, role played by chromium in man.

OTHER TRACE ELEMENTS

There is experimental evidence that certain animals require selenium for normal growth and health. Human requirements or tolerances, however, have not been established. In these animals, the role of selenium as an antioxidant overlaps partially with vitamin E in man.

WATER

A discussion of the inorganic nutrients and their dietary requirements would be incomplete without mention of water. Among the various nutrients, water is second only to oxygen in importance, which is not surprising considering the prompt and dire results which follow the failure of adequate supply. Water is unique because it not only serves as an essential nutrient but also constitutes the major component of the body, its vehicle of chemical transport, and the medium in which practically all metabolic reactions involving ordinary nutrients take place. The fluid compartments of the body and the dynamics of external and internal water exchange have been discussed in Chap. 3.

Both the Food and Nutrition Board and the Canadian Dietary Standards recommend a daily intake of about 2.5 liters, or 1 ml of water for each calorie of food, under conditions of moderate temperature and exercise. Infants should receive 1.5 ml per calorie, particularly when fed high-protein formulas. In hot environments, water consumption must also be increased. The actual intake, in the form of fluid and solid foods and drinking water, varies considerably, but is ordinarily kept within normal bounds without conscious regulation. Infants and sick individuals are exceptions to this rule. Uncontrollable vomiting or copious diarrhea may result in rapid dehydration and even death (due to circulatory failure), especially in infants. Unconscious or comatose patients are also very prone to water deprivation; an adequate fluid supply must be a primary consideration in their care.

Part Three

Nutrition in Health

Chapter 13

Human Nutritional Requirements

A normal diet should conform to the following basic criteria: (1) it should supply all essential nutrients in adequate amounts; (2) it should supply a physiologic quantity of bulk and fluids and should be easily digestible and confer a feeling of satiety; (3) it should be readily available, from the standpoint of both supply and cost; and (4) it should live up to the gustatory expectations of the prospective consumer and conform to the gastronomic customs of his group. Within this framework an infinite variety of foods and menus is possible. There is no single food pattern which must be followed to ensure adequate nutrition.

Dietary Standards

Dietary standards are quantitatively stated summaries of nutritional requirements; they are primarily concerned with the first criterion of the normal diet and are used to formulate, and at times evaluate, food intakes. The first scientific dietary standards, as we know them today, were developed during the 1930s. In 1933 the British Medical Association organized a Committee on Nutrition to determine the minimum food intakes needed to maintain health

Table 22   Food and Nutrition Board, National Academy of Sciences–National Research Council, Recommended Daily Dietary Allowances,[a] **Revised 1974**

(Designed for the Maintenance of Good Nutrition of Practically All Healthy People in the United States)

	Age (yr) from, up to	Weight kg	lb	Height cm	in	Energy kcal[b]	Protein g	Fat-soluble vitamins Vitamin A activity RE[c]	IU	Vitamin D IU	Vitamin E activity[d] IU	Ascorbic acid mg
Infants	0.0–0.5	6	14	60	24	kg×117	kg×2.2	420[g]	1,400	400	4	35
	0.5–1.0	9	20	71	28	kg×108	kg×2.0	400	2,000	400	5	35
Children	1–3	13	28	86	34	1300	23	400	2,000	400	7	40
	4–6	20	44	110	44	1800	30	500	2,500	400	9	40
	7–10	30	66	135	54	2400	36	700	3,300	400	10	40
Males	11–14	44	97	158	63	2800	44	1,000	5,000	400	12	45
	15–18	61	134	172	69	3000	54	1,000	5,000	400	15	45
	19–22	67	147	172	69	3000	54	1,000	5,000	400	15	45
	23–50	70	154	172	69	2700	56	1,000	5,000	...	15	45
	51+	70	154	172	69	2400	56	1,000	5,000	...	15	45
Females	11–14	44	97	155	62	2400	44	800	4,000	400	10	45
	15–18	54	119	162	65	2100	48	800	4,000	400	11	45
	19–22	58	128	162	65	2100	46	800	4,000	400	12	45
	23–50	58	128	162	65	2000	46	800	4,000	...	12	45
	51+	58	128	162	65	1800	46	800	4,000	...	12	45
Pregnant	...	...		...		+300	+30	1,000	5,000	400	15	60
Lactating	...	...		...		+500	+20	1,200	6,000	400	15	60

[a]The allowances are intended to provide for individual variations among most normal persons as they live in the United States under usual environmental stresses. Diets should be based on a variety of common foods in order to provide other nutrients for which human requirements have been less well defined. See text for more detailed discussion of allowances and of nutrients not tabulated.

[b]Kilojoules (kJ) = 4.2 × kcal.

[c]Retinol equivalents.

[d]Total vitamin E activity, estimated to be 80 percent as α-tocopherol and 20 percent other tocopherols.

and working capacity. In 1936, the Health Organization of the League of Nations published a dietary standard based in part on physiologic needs. During World War II dietary standards were formulated in many countries, and since then the World Health Organization and Food and Agriculture Organization, both of the United Nations, have endeavored to formulate universal minimum human dietary standards based on physiologic requirements.

Recommended Dietary Allowances, Food and Nutrition Board

In the United States, nutrition standards have been formulated by the Food and Nutrition Board of the National Research Council under the name "Recommended Dietary Allowances." These dietary allowances are found in

Water-soluble vitamins						Minerals					
Folacin[e] μg	Niacin[f] (B₁) mg	Riboflavin (B₂) mg	Thiamin mg	Vitamin B₆ mg	Vitamin B₁₂ μg	Calcium mg	Phos-phorus mg	Iodine μg	Iron mg	Mag-nesium mg	Zinc mg
50	5	0.4	0.3	0.3	0.3	360	240	35	10	60	3
50	8	0.6	0.5	0.4	0.3	540	400	45	15	70	5
100	9	0.8	0.7	0.6	1.0	800	800	60	15	150	10
200	12	1.1	0.9	0.9	1.5	800	800	80	10	200	10
300	16	1.2	1.2	1.2	2.0	800	800	110	10	250	10
400	18	1.5	1.4	1.6	3.0	1,200	1,200	130	18	350	15
400	20	1.8	1.5	1.8	3.0	1,200	1,200	150	18	400	15
400	20	1.8	1.5	2.0	3.0	800	800	140	10	350	15
400	18	1.6	1.4	2.0	3.0	800	800	130	10	350	15
400	16	1.5	1.2	2.0	3.0	800	800	110	10	350	15
400	16	1.3	1.2	1.6	3.0	1,200	1,200	115	18	300	15
400	14	1.4	1.1	2.0	3.0	1,200	1,200	115	18	300	15
400	14	1.4	1.1	2.0	3.0	800	800	100	18	300	15
400	13	1.2	1.0	2.0	3.0	800	800	100	18	300	15
400	12	1.1	1.0	2.0	3.0	800	800	80	10	300	15
800	+2	+0.3	+0.3	2.5	4.0	1,200	1,200	125	18[h]	450	20
600	+4	+0.5	+0.3	2.5	4.0	1,200	1,200	150	18	450	25

[e]The folacin allowances refer to dietary sources as determined by *Lactobacillus casei* assay. Pure forms of folacin may be effective in doses less than one-fourth of the RDA.

[f]Although allowances are expressed as niacin, it is recognized that on the average 1 mg of niacin is derived from each 60 mg of dietary tryptophan.

[g]Assumed to be all as retinol in milk during the first 6 months of life. All subsequent intakes are assumed to be one-half as retinol and one-half as β-carotene when calculated from international units. As retinol equivalents, three-fourths are as retinol and one-fourth as β-carotene.

[h]This increased requirement cannot be met by ordinary diets; therefore, the use of supplemental iron is recommended.

Table 22. They are designed to maintain good nutrition for healthy persons in the United States under present-day conditions. The nutritive intakes recommended are, in general, higher than average requirements and lower than the amounts needed in illness or in rehabilitation of deficiencies. The allowances are designed to serve as a guide for planning food intakes for population groups, rather than for the evaluation of the nutritional status of such groups.

The latest (1974) Recommended Dietary Allowances (RDA) are defined as levels of intake of essential nutrients considered, on the basis of currently available scientific evidence, to be adequate to meet the known nutritional needs of almost every healthy person. They are recommendations for amounts of nutrients that should be consumed and, therefore, do not allow for amounts lost during processing or preparation of foods. They are appropriate for maintenance of health and do not cóver special needs due to illness. They are estimates of known nutritional needs to ensure a satisfactory rate of growth in children and maintenance of weight and prevention of depletion of nutrients in adults.

The United States allowances have adopted in principle a distinctive feature of the caloric standards of the Food and Agriculture Organization of the United Nations (FAO). The United States recommended calorie allowances for adults are based on a reference man and woman, 23 to 50 years of age, living in a temperate climate at a mean temperature of 20°C, physically only *lightly* active, and weighing 70 and 58 kg, respectively. Adjustments can be made for variations in age, physical activity, or climate, for persons differing from these specifications. Thus it is recommended that energy allowances of persons over 50 years of age be reduced to 90 percent of the amount required by a mature adult. Similarly, the daily energy need of *moderately* active reference persons is increased by about 300 cal, while the allowance for *very active* persons (athletes, miners, heavy-construction workers) should be increased by 600 to 900 cal per day.

Likewise, energy requirements are increased in men performing pre-scribed work and living at high temperatures. While little adjustment appears necessary for rises in temperature between 20 and 30°C, it is desirable, under conditions of *increased* physical activity to increase calorie allowances by 0.5 percent for every degree of temperature rise between 30 and 40°C. Under *resting* conditions no adjustment may be necessary. Average caloric needs for the average individual not engaged in a prescribed or increased physical task at high temperatures may actually be reduced because of a compensatory inclination to lessened activity.

Calorie allowances should be adjusted for variations in energy require-ments which result from differences in body size. Values may be adjusted for men and women who differ from the standard body sizes with the aid of the following formulas:

$$\text{Calories for men} = 725 + 31W \qquad \text{at age 25}$$
$$650 + 28W \qquad \text{at age 45}$$
$$550 + 23.5W \qquad \text{at age 65}$$

$$\text{Calories for women} = 525 + 27W \qquad \text{at age 25}$$
$$475 + 24.5W \qquad \text{at age 45}$$
$$400 + 20.5W \qquad \text{at age 65}$$

where W=desirable body weight, in kilograms. Calorie allowances should always be based on the body weight which is desirable for the individual's height, not on his actual weight, which may be above or below normal. Desirable weights of men and women can be readily obtained from individual height measurements with the aid of Table 35 in Chap. 21. Table 36 gives the recommended calorie allowances for individuals of various body weights and ages.

In Table 22 recommended allowances for infants and children are given in age groups and, after the age of 10, boys and girls separately, since the growth curves and levels of activity differ significantly after this age. Allowances are based on the needs for the middle year in each group and under normal activity at the weight levels indicated in the table. As with adults, adjustments from the standard should be made for children who differ in size and activity.

The recommended allowance values of the table are for nutrients in foods as consumed and do not take into consideration prior losses in storage, cooking, and serving. Provision should therefore be made for these losses in planning practical dietaries. The allowances do provide for possible incomplete availability or absorption of certain nutrients, such as iron and carotene.

The requirements for nutrients not tabulated in the Recommended Daily Dietary Allowances are discussed in the appropriate preceding chapters.

U.S. Recommended Daily Allowances, U.S. Food and Drug Administration

The U.S. Recommended Daily Allowances (U.S. RDA) are a recent innovation formulated by the U.S. Food and Drug Administration to replace the outmoded Minimum Daily Requirements of the past. U.S. RDA values are generally the highest values for each nutrient given in the Recommended Dietary Allowances tables of the Food and Nutrition Board for males and nonpregnant, nonlactating females, 4 or more years of age. The new U.S. RDA were established primarily in connection with legal labeling requirements of foods and vitamin preparation. Table 23 details the U.S. Recommended Daily Allowances which apply to adults and children over 4 years of age.

Canadian Dietary Standards

The Canadian Dietary Standards were formulated by the Canadian Council on Nutrition, a group advising the Department of National Health and Welfare. In Table 24, a summary of the Canadian Dietary Standards, the values are recommended intakes proposed to be adequate for growth and the maintenance of health of the *majority* (presumably over 95 percent) of Canadians; thus they are somewhat higher than *average* requirements.

Recommended intakes were set well above levels below which signs and symptoms of deficiency would appear, to account for biologic variation. These safety factors range in the Canadian Dietary Standards from additions of 50 to 300 percent above minimum values. Values in these standards are intended as a guide in planning diets and food supplies for healthy individuals or groups but not for appraising the nutritional status of individuals. In many cases the Canadian figures are identical with the United States allowances. However, the

Table 23   U.S. Recommended Daily Allowances (U.S. RDA) for Specific Vitamins and Minerals Essential in Human Nutrition

Nutrient	U.S. RDA
Vitamins:	
Vitamin A	5,000 IU
Vitamin D	400 IU
Vitamin E	30 IU
Vitamin C	60 mg
Thiamin (vitamin B_1)	1.5 mg
Riboflavin (vitamin B_2)	1.7 mg
Niacin	20.0 mg
Vitamin B_6	2.0 mg
Vitamin B_{12}	6.0 μg
Folacin (folic acid)	0.4 mg
Biotin	0.3 mg
Pantothenic acid	10.0 mg
Minerals:	
Calcium	1.0 g
Iron	18.0 mg
Phosphorus	1.0 g
Iodine	150 μg
Magnesium	400 mg
Zinc	15 mg
Copper	2.0 mg

allowances for thiamin, vitamin A, and ascorbic acid, as well as for iron in males, are significantly lower than the recommended United States allowances.

British Standards

Table 25 summarizes the Recommended Intakes of Nutrients for the United Kingdom. These recommended intakes are defined as sufficient or more than sufficient for the nutritional needs of practically all healthy persons in the population.

The British standards do not differ appreciably in their requirements from their United States counterparts except for the allowances for iron, thiamin, and vitamin A, which are somewhat lower. Recommendations for ascorbic acid and calcium are significantly lower, in the case of the latter the view being that it is impossible to prevent osteoporosis with dietary calcium.

International Standards

To date, the Food and Agriculture Organization of the United Nations has adopted average minimum standards for calorie and protein requirements.

The FAO calorie standard is based on a hypothetical reference man and

Table 24 Abridged Canadian Dietary Standards (1970)

(Recommended Daily Nutrient Intakes for Canadians)

Sex	Age, yr	Weight, lb	Activity category	Calories	Protein,* g	Calcium, g	Iron, mg	Vitamin A, IU†	Vitamin D, IU	Ascorbic acid, mg	Thiamin, mg	Riboflavin, mg	Niacin, mg
Both	0–1	7–20	Usual	360–900	7–13	0.5	5	1,000	400	20	0.3	0.5	3
Both	1–2	20–26	Usual	900–1200	12–16	0.7	5	1,000	400	20	0.4	0.6	4
Both	2–3	31	Usual	1400	17	0.7	5	1,000	400	20	0.4	0.7	4
Both	4–6	40	Usual	1700	20	0.7	5	1,000	400	20	0.5	0.9	5
Both	7–9	57	Usual	2100	24	1.0	5	1,500	400	30	0.7	1.1	7
Both	10–12	77	Usual	2500	30	1.2	12	2,000	400	30	0.8	1.3	8
Boy	13–15	108	Usual	3100	40	1.2	12	2,700	400	30	0.9	1.6	9
Girl	13–15	108	Usual	2600	39	1.2	12	2,700	400	30	0.8	1.3	8
Boy	16–17	136	B‡	3700	45	1.2	12	3,200	400	30	1.1	1.9	11
Girl	16–17	120	A§	2400	41	1.2	12	3,200	400	30	0.7	1.2	7
Boy	18–19	144	B‡	3800	47	0.9	6	3,200	400	30	1.1	1.9	11
Girl	18–19	124	A§	2450	41	0.9	10	3,200	400	30	0.7	1.2	7
Male	Adult	154	B	3582	47	0.5	6	3,700	…	30	1.1	1.8	11
Female	Adult	124	A	2390	40	0.5	10	3,700	…	30	0.7	1.2	7

*Protein recommendation is based on normal mixed Canadian diet. Vegetarian diets may require a higher protein content.

†Vitamin A is based on the mixed Canadian diet supplying both vitamin A and carotene. As preformed vitamin A, the suggested intake would be about two-thirds of that indicated.

‡B—expenditure assessed as being 113 percent of that of a man of the same weight and engaged in the same degree of activity.

§A—expenditure assessed as being 104 percent of that of a woman of the same weight and engaged in the same degree of activity.

Table 25 Recommended Daily Intakes of Energy and Nutrients for the United Kingdom

Age range[a]	Occupational category	Body weight,[c] kg	Energy[d] kcal	Energy[d] MJ[e]	Protein,[f] g
Boys and girls:					
0 up to 1 year[b]	. . .	7.3	800	3.3	20
1 up to 2 years	. . .	11.4	1200	5.0	30
2 up to 3 years	. . .	13.5	1400	5.9	35
3 up to 5 years	. . .	16.5	1600	6.7	40
5 up to 7 years	. . .	20.5	1800	7.5	45
7 up to 9 years	. . .	25.1	2100	8.8	53
Boys:					
9 up to 12 years	. . .	31.9	2500	10.5	63
12 up to 15 years	. . .	45.5	2800	11.7	70
15 up to 18 years	. . .	61.0	3000	12.6	75
Girls:					
9 up to 12 years	. . .	33.0	2300	9.6	58
12 up to 15 years	. . .	48.6	2300	9.6	58
15 up to 18 years	. . .	56.1	2300	9.6	58
Men:					
18 up to 35 years	Sedentary	65	2700	11.3	68
	Moderately active		3000	12.6	75
	Very active		3600	15.1	90
35 up to 65 years	Sedentary	65	2600	10.9	65
	Moderately active		2900	12.1	73
	Very active		3600	15.1	90
65 up to 75 years	Assuming a	63	2350	9.8	59
75 years and over	sedentary life	63	2100	8.8	53
Women:					
18 up to 55 years	Most occupations	55	2200	9.2	55
	Very active		2500	10.5	63
55 up to 75 years	Assuming a	53	2050	8.6	51
75 years and over	sedentary life	53	1900	8.0	48
Pregnancy, 2d and 3d trimesters	. . .		2400	10.0	60
Lactation	. . .	. . .	2700	11.3	68

[a] The ages are from one birthday to another: e.g., 9 up to 12 is from the 9th up to, but not including, the 12th birthday. The figures in the table in general refer to the midpoint of the ranges, though those for the range 18 up to 35 refer to the age 25 years, and for the range 18 up to 55, to 35 years of age.

[b] Average figures relating to the first year of life.

[c] The body weights of children and adolescents are averages and relate to London in 1965. (Taken from Tanner, Whitehouse & Takaishi, 1966; Tables IV A and IV B, 50th centile.) The body weights of adults do not represent average values; they are those of the FAO (1957) reference man and woman, with a nominal reduction for the elderly.

[d] Average requirements relating to groups of individuals.

[e] Megajoules (10^6 joules). Calculated from the relation 1 kilocalorie = 4.186 kilojoules, and rounded to one decimal place.

[f] Recommended intakes calculated as providing 10 percent of energy requirements.

Thiamin,[g] mg	Ribo-flavin, mg	Nicotinic acid, mg equivalents[h]	Ascorbic acid, mg	Vitamin A, μg retinol equivalents[i]	Vitamin D,[j] μg cholecal-ciferol	Calcium, mg	Iron, mg
0.3	0.4	5	15	450	10	600[l]	6[l]
0.5	0.6	7	20	300	10	500	7
0.6	0.7	8	20	300	10	500	7
0.6	0.8	9	20	300	10	500	8
0.7	0.9	10	20	300	2.5	500	8
0.8	1.0	11	20	400	2.5	500	10
1.0	1.2	14	25	575	2.5	700	13
1.1	1.4	16	25	725	2.5	700	14
1.2	1.7	19	30	750	2.5	600	15
0.9	1.2	13	25	575	2.5	700	13
0.9	1.4	16	25	725	2.5	700	14
0.9	1.4	16	30	750	2.5	600	15
1.1	1.7	18	30	750	2.5	500	10
1.2	1.7	18	30	750	2.5	500	10
1.4	1.7	18	30	750	2.5	500	10
1.0	1.7	18	30	750	2.5	500	10
1.2	1.7	18	30	750	2.5	500	10
1.4	1.7	18	30	750	2.5	500	10
0.9	1.7	18	30	750	2.5	500	10
0.8	1.7	18	30	750	2.5	500	10
0.9	1.3	15	30	750	2.5	500	12
1.0	1.3	15	30	750	2.5	500	12
0.8	1.3	15	30	750	2.5	500	10
0.7	1.3	15	30	750	2.5	500	10
1.0	1.6	18	60	750	10[k]	1,200[m]	15
1.1	1.8	21	60	1,200	10	1,200	15

[g] The figures, calculated from energy requirements and the recommended intake of thiamin of 0.4 mg/1000 kcal, relate to groups of individuals.

[h] 1 nicotinic acid equivalent = 1 mg available nicotinic acid or 60 mg tryptophan.

[i] 1 retinol equivalent = 1 μg retinol or 6 μg β-carotene or 12 μg other biologically active carotenoids.

[j] No dietary source may be necessary for those adequately exposed to sunlight, but the requirement for the housebound may be greater than that recommended.

[k] For all three trimesters.

[l] These figures apply to infants who are not breast-fed. Infants who are entirely breast-fed receive smaller quantities; these are adequate since absorption from breast milk is higher.

[m] For the third trimester only.

Source: Department of Health and Social Security, United Kingdom Reports on Public Health and Medical Subjects No. 120, Her Majesty's Stationary Office, 1969.

woman. The reference man is 25 years of age, weighs 65 kg, and is physically fit. He lives in the Temperate Zone at a mean annual temperature of 10°C and neither gains nor loses weight. He works 8 hours per day at a nonsedentary occupation which requires only occasional periods of hard physical labor. When not at work, he is sedentary for about 4 hours daily, spends about 1½ hours on active recreation or household work, and may walk for up to 1½ hours. This reference man requires, on the average, 3200 cal daily.

The reference woman is 25 years old, weighs 55 kg, is physically fit, and lives in a similar climate. She is either engaged in full-time housework or works in light industry. She walks for about 1 hour each day and engages in active recreation (playing with children, gardening) for about another hour. This reference woman requires, on the average, 2300 cal daily.

Formulas are provided which permit the calculation of caloric needs of actual persons in accordance with their individual physical activity, body size, climate, and physiologic state. The figures obtained are of the same general

Table 26   Essential Amino Acid Pattern in Provisional FAO Reference Protein

Amino acid	FAO reference protein	Human milk	Cow's milk	Whole egg
	Milligrams amino acid per gram protein nitrogen			
Isoleucine	270	411	407	428
Leucine	306	572	630	565
Lysine	270	402	496	396
Phenylalanine	180	297	311	368
Tyrosine	180	355	323	274
Sulfur-containing:				
Total	270	274	211	342
Methionine	144	140	154	196
Threonine	180	290	292	310
Tryptophan	90	106	90	106
Valine	270	420	440	460
	Amino acid per 100 g protein			
Isoleucine	4.2	6.4	6.4	6.8
Leucine	4.8	8.9	9.9	9.0
Lysine	4.2	6.3	7.8	6.3
Phenylalanine	2.8	4.6	4.9	6.0
Tyrosine	2.8	5.5	5.1	4.4
Sulfur-containing:				
Total	4.2	4.3	3.3	5.4
Methionine	2.2	2.2	2.4	3.1
Threonine	2.8	4.6	4.6	5.0
Tryptophan	1.4	1.6	1.4	1.7
Valine	4.2	6.6	6.9	7.4

Table 27   Summary of Average Minimum Requirements for the FAO Reference Protein in Healthy Individuals

	Approximate grams of protein per kilogram body weight
Infants:	
Up to 6 months	2.0
After 6 months	1.5
Up to 2 years	1.2
Children:	
2 to 6	Decreasing from 1.2 to 0.8
6 to 10	0.8
10 to 16 (boys)	0.8–0.9
10 to 13 (girls)	0.8–0.9
Up to 21	0.35–0.4
Adults	0.35
Pregnant women	0.35; add 10 g protein/day
Lactating women	0.35; add 30 g protein/day

Note: Hard physical labor calls for an additional initial temporary protein allowance.

order of magnitude as those set forth by the United States and Canadian standards.

The protein requirements, as provisionally suggested by FAO, are unique in that they are based on a hypothetical reference protein of a provisional, desirable amino acid composition. Table 26 details the specific amino acid pattern of this reference protein, and Table 27 summarizes the average minimum protein requirements through life as set forth by FAO.

Individual Variance in Nutritional Requirements

Individual organisms differ in their genetic makeup and differ also in morphologic and physiologic aspects, including their endocrine activity, metabolic efficiency, and nutritional requirements. The science of human nutrition applies to a genetically heterogeneous group, particularly in the United States, where the population exhibits a very diverse hereditary background. In contrast to inbred strains of laboratory animals, such a human population represents a wide range of physiologic needs. The greater the number of metabolic variants considered, the more heterogeneous the population appears and the smaller is the likelihood that any number of individuals share identical nutritional requirements.

The data on average, normal nutritional needs presented in this chapter should thus be regarded with certain reservations when they are applied to any one individual. Nutritional standards and recommended allowances are working tools to express the nutritional requirements of what is hoped to be the greatest number of healthy individuals in given population groups. Probably no

Table 27A Comparative Dietary Standards for Adults in Selected Countries and FAO with Explanations as to Their Meaning

The purpose for establishing a national dietary standard is not the same in all countries. Therefore, some variation in nutrient allowances from country to country is to be expected. At the same time, it must be recognized that the "reference" individual will vary from country to country. Furthermore, even in instances when there are presumed similar objectives among countries as to the purpose and usefulness of proposed standards, it can be seen that there is by no means uniform agreement as to the nutrient allowances considered desirable as national guides. Standards are also subject to revision as newer knowledge becomes available. Particular attention should be paid to the footnotes, which explain, in brief form, the basis for nutrient allowances in the various countries and those of FAO. The original publications should be consulted for detailed explanations.

Country	Sex	Age, yr	Weight, kg	Activity	kcal	Protein, g	Calcium, g	Iron, mg	Vit. A activity, IU	Thiamin, mg	Riboflavin, mg	Niacin equiv., mg	Ascorbic acid, mg
U.S.A.[1]	M	22	70	Footnote[2]	2800	65	0.8	10	5,000	1.4	1.7	18[3]	60
	F	22	58	Footnote[2]	2000	55	0.8	18	5,000	1.0	1.5	13[3]	55
FAO[1]	M	25	65	Footnote[2]	3200	46[3]	0.4–0.5[4]	...	Footnote[5]	1.3[6]	1.8[7]	21.1[8]	
	F	25	55	Footnote[2]	2300	39[3]	0.4–0.5[4]	...	Footnote[5]	0.9[6]	1.3[7]	15.2[8]	
Australia[1]	M	25	70	Footnote[2]	2900	70[3]	0.4–0.8	10	2,500[4]	1.2	1.5	18[5]	30
	F	25	58	Footnote[2]	2100	58[3]	0.4–0.8	10	2,500[4]	0.8	1.1	14[5]	30
Canada[1]	M	25	72	Footnote[2]	2850	50[3]	0.5	6	3,700[4]	0.9	1.4	9	30
	F	25	57	Footnote[2]	2400	39[3]	0.5	10	3,700[4]	0.7	1.2	7	30
C.A. and Panama[1]	M	25	55	Moderate activity	2700	65[2]	0.45	10	Footnote[3]	1.1	1.6	17.8	60
	F	25	50	activity	2000	60[2]	0.45	10	Footnote[3]	0.8	1.2	13.2	50
Colombia[1]	M	20–29	65	Moderate activity[2]	2850[3]	68	0.5[4]	10[5]	5,000[6]	1.1[7]	1.7[8]	18.8[9]	50
	F	20–29	55	activity[2]	1900[3]	60	0.5[4]	15[5]	5,000[6]	0.8[7]	1.1[8]	12.5[9]	50
France[1]	M	.....	65	Moderate activity[2]	3000[2]	90[3]							
	F	.....	55	activity[2]	2400[2]	75[3]							
India[1]	M	25.4	55	Moderate activity[2]	2800	55[3]							
	F	21.5	45	activity[2]	2300	45[3]							
Japan[1]	M	26–29	56[2]	Moderate	3000	70[4]	0.6	10	2,000[5]	1.5	1.5	15	65
	F	26–29	49[2]	activity[3]	2400	60[4]	0.6	10	2,000[5]	1.2	1.2	12	60
Netherlands[1]	M	20–29	70	Light	3000	70[2]	1.0	10	5,500[3]	1.2	1.8	12	50
	F	20–29	60	activity	2400	60[2]	1.0	12	5,500[3]	1.0	1.5	10	50
Norway[1]	M	25	70	None	3400	70	0.8	12	2,500[2]	1.7	1.8	17	30
	F	25	60	given	2500	60	0.8	12	2,500[2]	1.3	1.5	13	30

Philippines[1]	M	53	None specified	Moderate activity	2400	53	0.5	*	5,000[2]	1.2	1.2	*	70
	F	46			1800	46	0.5	*	5,000[2]	0.9	0.9	*	70
S. Africa[1]	M	73	None specified	Moderate activity	3000	65	0.7	9	4,000[2]	1.0	1.6	15	40
	F	60			2300	55	0.6	12	4,000[2]	0.8	1.4	12	40
U.K.[1]	M	65	20 up	Medium activity[2]	3000	87[3]	0.8	12	5,000[4]	1.2	1.8	12[5]	20
	F	56	20 up		2500	73[3]	0.8	12	5,000[4]	1.0	1.5	10[5]	20
U.S.S.R.[1]	M	:	.....	Moderate activity	.....	:	.....	:	5,000[2]	2.0[3]	2.5	15	70[3]
	F	:			.....	:	.....	:	5,000[2]	2.0[3]	2.5	15	70[3]
E. Germany[1]	M	:	18–35	Light work	2700[2]	85[3]	0.8	10	5,000	1.6[4]	1.5	18	70
	F	:	18–35		2300[2]	75[3]	0.8	15	5,000	1.4[4]	1.3	15	70
W. Germany[1]	M	72	25	Sedentary activity	2550[3]	72	0.8	10	5,000[4]	1.7	1.8	18	75
	F	60	25		2200[3]	60	0.8	12	5,000[4]	1.5	1.8	14	75

Footnotes to Table 27A

U.S.A.

[1]*Sources: Recommended Dietary Allowances*, Revised 1968. NAS Pub. 1694, National Academy of Sciences, Washington, D.C., 1968.

[2]Allowances are intended for persons normally active in a temperate climate.

[3]Niacin equivalents include dietary sources of the preformed vitamin and the precursor tryptophan. 60 mg of tryptophan represents 1 mg of niacin.

FAO/WHO

[1]*Sources:* "Calorie Requirements," *FAO Nutr. Stud. No. 15*, Rome (1957). "Protein Requirements," FAO/WHO. *FAO Nutr. Meetings Rep. Ser. No. 37, WHO Tech. Rep. Ser. No. 301*, Rome (1965). "Calcium Requirements," FAO/WHO. *FAO Nutr. Meet. Rep. Ser. No. 30. WHO Tech. Rep. Ser. No. 230*, Rome (1962). "Requirements of Vitamin A, Thiamine, Riboflavin and Niacin." FAO/WHO. *FAO Nutr. Rep. No. 41. WHO Tech. Rep. Ser. No. 362*, Rome (1967). **Mean** annual temperature, 10°C.

[2]The activity for the reference man is described as "on each working day he is employed 8 hours in an occupation which is not sedentary, but does not involve more than occasional periods of hard physical labor. When not at work, he is sedentary for about 4 hours daily and may walk for up to 1¹/₂ hours. He spends about 1¹/₂ hours on active recreation and household work." The activity of the reference woman is described as "she may be engaged either in general household duties or in light industry. Her daily activities include walking for about 1 hour and 1 hour of active recreation, such as gardening, playing with children, or nonstrenuous sport."

[3]The protein values, stated to be a practical allowance designed to cover the needs of all but a small percent of the population, are based on 0.71 g/kg, representing a level of 20 percent above the requirements for reference protein.

[4]The value is considered a safe practical allowance. A range is given to emphasize that present knowledge does not permit any greater accuracy as to a safe allowance.

[5]750 μg of retinol, both sexes. 1 μg of β-carotene is equivalent to 0.167 μg of retinol.

[6]0.40 mg of thiamin per 1000 kcal.

[7]0.55 mg of riboflavin per 1000 kcal.

[8]6.6 niacin equivalents per 1000 kcal.

Australia

[1]*Sources:* "Dietary Allowances for Australians," 1965 revision, *Med. J. Aust.* (1965) (June, 11th), Vol. 1, p. 1041. The allowances are designed to be used as a basis for planning food supplies for persons or groups.

[2]The activities specified are similar to those of the reference man and woman ("Calorie Requirements," *FAO Nutr. Stud. No. 15*, Rome, 1957). Mean annual external temperature 18°C.

[3]A practical protein allowance may be calculated on the basis of 10 to 12 percent of the calories being derived from protein.

[4]3 IU of carotene equivalent to 1 IU of vitamin A activity.

[5]Preformed niacin plus (g of protein × 0.16).

Canada

[1]*Sources:* "Recommended Daily Intakes of Nutrients Adequate for the Maintenance of Health Among the Majority of Canadians." *Can. Bull. Nutr., 6,* 1 (1964).

[2]Five categories of activity are listed and described. The values for calories and nutrients given here apply to "most household chores," "office work," "laboratory work," "shop and mill work," "mechanical trades or crafts," and various sports.

[3]Based on normal mixed Canadian diets.

[4]Based on mixed Canadian diet supplying both vitamin A and carotene. As preformed vitamin A, the suggested intake would be two-thirds of amounts indicated.

Central America and Panama

[1]*Sources: Publicaciones Cientificas del Instituto de Nutricion de Centro America y Panama, Recopilacion No. 5*, pp. 75–76 (1966). The figures for nutrients are designed to meet the needs of nearly all individuals. Average annual temperature, 20°C.

[2]Protein. 30 percent as protein of high biological value.

[3]The table lists 1.3 mg of vitamin A alcohol for both sexes and assumes that one-fifth of the ingested total is preformed vitamin A and four-fifths is β-carotene. Based on the relationship: 1 IU = 0.3 μg of vitamin A alcohol.

Colombia

[1]*Sources: Archivos Latinoamericanos de Nutricion, XVII, 255,* September (1967). Values are tabulated separately at 10°C, 20°C, and 30°C. Those used here are at 20°C.

[2]Activities for reference man are described as farming and day laborer, for example; activities for reference woman include housework, factory work, office work, and minding children.

[3]To be reduced by 3 percent between ages 30 and 39; by 5 percent between ages 40 and 49; by 5 percent between ages 50 and 59; by 8 percent between ages 60 and 69; by 8 percent between ages 70 and 79; and by 10 percent after age 79.

[4]Based on FAO/WHO Expert Group report, "Calcium Requirements" (1962).

[5]Based on NRC recommendations with allowances for difference in weights.

[6]Based on NRC recommendations.

Footnotes to Table 27A

[7]0.4 mg of thiamin per 1000 kcal.
[8]0.6 mg of riboflavin per 1000 kcal.
[9]Niacin equivalent of 6.6/1000 kcal.

France
[1]*Sources:* "Rations—Types et Precóniser pour le Francais." *Inst. Nat. Hyg., Nutr. Sect., Bull. Inst. Nat. Hyg. 7*:761, 825 (1952). (Based on surveys, see *Nutritio et Dieta, 1,* 1959.)
[2]Include up to 10 percent of alcohol.
[3]More than 25 percent as animal protein.

India
[1]*Sources:* Patwardhan, V. N., "Dietary Allowances for India. Calories and Protein." *Indian Counc. Med. Res., Spec. Rep. Ser. No. 35,* New Delhi (1960). The data are 1958 revisions of earlier figures.
[2]The activities corresponding to the calorie recommendations are detailed in the above publication. "Moderate" refers to activity in a "light industrial occupation."
[3]An allowance of 1 g of protein per kilogram of body weight of vegetable proteins in properly balanced diets.

Japan
[1]*Sources: Nutrition in Japan, 1964,* Ministry of Health and Welfare, Tokyo (1965). Data adopted by the Council on Nutrition in 1960. The allowances are believed to be sufficient to establish and maintain a good nutritional state in typical individuals.
[2]1961 averages.
[3]Five categories of activity are specified for men and four for women, with corresponding intakes for calories and B vitamins.
[4]Higher intakes are specified for heavy and very hard work.
[5]Requirement for both sexes specified as 2,000 IU of preformed vitamin A or 6,000 IU of carotene.

Netherlands
[1]*Sources:* Recommended quantities of nutrients, Committee on Nutritional Standards of the Netherlands Nutrition Council. The figures for nutrients are set to cover individuals having high requirements. The figures for calories are average requirements.
[2]Assumes one-third is from animal sources. Figures are increased for heavy and very heavy work.
[3]Assumes 1,500 IU as preformed vitamin A and 4,000 IU of activity as carotene.

Norway
[1]*Sources:* Evaluation of nutrition requirements, State Nutrition Council, 1958. Figures are "somewhat higher than average requirements."
[2]Vitamin A as present in animal foods.

The Philippines
[1]*Sources:* Recommended daily allowances for specific nutrients, Food and Nutrition Research Center, 1960 (revisions based on a letter from Conrado R. Pascual, January 10, 1967. No new publication cited). "Objectives toward which to aim in planning practical diets."
[2]Assumes 90 percent contributed by carotene.
*No definite recommendations at present for iron and niacin.

South Africa
[1]*Sources:* "Recommended Minimum Daily Dietary Standards," National Research Council, *S. A., Med. J., 30,* 108 (1956).
[2]Assumes two-thirds contributed by carotene.

United Kingdom
[1]*Sources:* Report of the Committee on Nutrition, British Medical Association, 1950. The levels of nutrients recommended are believed to be sufficient to establish and maintain a good nutritional state in representative individuals of the groups concerned.
[2]Values are given for six levels of activity for males and five for females. Medium work is described as 8 hours at 100 kcal/h and traveling (130 kcal for men, 100 kcal for women).
[3]The protein allowance is increased with calories on the basis that the protein in the diet should provide not less than 11 percent of the energy for adults not engaged in hard work.
[4]A mixed diet containing one-third vitamin A and two-thirds carotene.
[5]Allowances are for preformed vitamin only.

U.S.S.R.
[1]"New Daily Vitamin Supply Standards in Man, 1961," Yarasova, N. S., *Vop. Pitan., 20,* 3 (1961).
[2]IU is equivalent to 0.3 μg of natural vitamin.
[3]To be increased up to 50 percent in far north.

Footnotes to Table 27A

E. Germany

[1]*Source:* Deutsche Akademie der Wissenschaften zu Berlin, Institut für Ernährung, Potsdam-Rehbrücke.

[2]For practical calculations for group feeding, recommended values are developed for the age category of 35 to 55 years for lightly working persons.

[3]Protein requirements are 12 percent of kcal.

[4]0.6 mg/1000 kcal.

W. Germany

[1]*Sources:* Die wünschenswerte Höhe der Nahrungszufuhr; Empfehlungen des Ausschusses für Nährungsbedarf der Deutschen Gesellschaft für Ernährung e.V., Frankfurt/M., 2. überarb, Ausg., Umschau-Verlag (Frankfurt/M. 1962).

[2]Activity for the reference man or woman: On each working day he or she is employed 8 hours. For stronger activities, in addition for man: 75 to 150 kcal/h at moderate work, 150 to 225 kcal/h at heavy work, 225 kcal/h and more at very heavy work; for women: 60 to 120 kcal/h at moderate work, 120 kcal/h and more at heavy work.

[3]At age 45, men 150 kcal less; 65 years, 300 kcal less; women 45 years, 100 kcal less; 65 years, 200 kcal less.

[4]Assumes four-fifths contributed by carotene.

Source: Food and Nutrition Board, National Research Council (1968).

one is more aware of the wide variation in individual nutritional requirements than the workers who have set these standards. The danger lies in too strict an interpretation of such working formulas by physicians and nutritionists who apply them to the individual in their daily work.

It is often taken for granted that the human population is made up of individuals who exhibit average physiologic requirements and that a minor proportion of this population is composed of those whose requirements may be considered to deviate excessively. Actually there is little justification in nutritional thinking for the concept that a representative prototype of *Homo sapiens* is one who has average requirements with respect to all essential nutrients and thus exhibits no unusually high or low needs. In the light of today's genetic and physiologic knowledge and the statistical interpretations thereof, the typical individual is more likely to be one who has average needs with respect to many nutrients and also exhibits some nutritional requirements for a few essential nutrients which are far from average.

If the range in individual nutritional requirements were relatively small (e.g., 20 to 50 percent), the individual biologic variation could be adequately compensated for by setting uniformly higher standards—the average plus 50 percent for good measure. However, the range may be about threefold with respect to some nutrients, and even greater ranges have been reported. In the case of ascorbic acid, daily intakes varying anywhere from 0.6 to 2.85 mg/kg body weight may be needed to produce tissue saturation (this does not imply that protection from scurvy is related in the same manner). Synthesis of thiamin and vitamin B_{12} by intestinal organisms varies considerably from individual to individual and may influence the respective individual dietary requirements. Thus some subjects may develop clinical thiamin deficiency on an experimental diet after a few weeks, while others will remain asymptomatic and excrete thiamin in their feces.

After a test dose of tryptophan, some infants require three to four times as much pyridoxine as others to prevent excessive excretion of xanthurenic acid.

That these infants develop clinical pyridoxine deficiency on a restricted vitamin B_6 intake while others do not was inadvertently demonstrated in the not-so-distant past. In 1951 there was a widespread occurrence of convulsions of unknown origin among infants in the United States. The etiology was eventually traced to a widely used proprietary milk formula which had become deficient in pyridoxine as the result of changes in the sterilization process. There is no doubt that at the time literally tens of thousands of infants subsisted on this formula exclusively. Nevertheless, not all these babies reacted to this vitamin B_6 deprivation. A large proportion of this group undoubtedly exhibited subclinical symptoms which never came to medical attention, such as restlessness and irritability and excessive crying, which were being blamed on "colic" and passing unhappiness. A smaller percentage showed clinical symptoms, and a still smaller group became very acutely ill. Subsequent follow-up studies showed that some of the infants who had gotten into acute trouble had unusually high, genetically conditioned pyridoxine requirements.

Large numbers of individuals are not required to demonstrate biologic variance; the same long-term experimental diet administered to three volunteers may induce niacin deficiency symptoms in one subject and equivocal symptomatology in another, while leaving the third subject asymptomatic. Because of a variety of factors, including such variability, some individuals reach a healthy old age while disregarding the maxims of good nutrition which apply to the majority of the population. Such individuals may have unusually low requirements for some essential nutrients, coupled with a high demand for other crucial nutrients which abound in the foods of their preference. Other individuals constitute the antithesis of this group, and it is they who require special attention. The physician and the nutritionist must be on the lookout for mute cases of malnutrition of a type based on the individual's genetically and/or physiologically induced specific high nutritional demands, even though the particular patient may consume what appears to be an average diet supplying average nutritional needs.

Chapter 14

The Nutritional Characteristics of Major Food Groups

Knowledge of the nutritive value of foods is essential if scientifically established dietary standards are to be translated into applicable, practical information for the qualitative and quantitative selection of the diet. In discussing the nutritive composition of specific foods or food groups, it is necessary to talk in terms of representative average values. Foods, being of biologic origin, are subject to considerable variations in composition as the result of genetic and climatic factors; before being consumed, they are exposed to storage, cooking, and processing conditions which may have a bearing on their nutritional contribution. The modifying influence of technological practices is discussed separately in Chap. 42. The present discussion will deal primarily with the inherent basic nutritive characteristics of specific common foods and food groups.

Detailed information concerning the composition of individual foods—raw, cooked, canned, or frozen—is assembled in convenient form in the tables in the Appendix. To obtain a maximum of benefit, the reader is urged to acquaint himself with the entire contents of the Appendix, including the introduction to and a commentary on these tables.

Meat, Poultry, and Fish

Meat Probably the most important contribution of meat to the human diet is protein, practically all of which is of high biologic quality. The proteins of meat are surpassed in quality only by those provided by eggs. In general, meat contains about 20 to 23 percent protein, a variable amount of fat and lesser constituents, and about 60 percent water. Muscle meats are consumed in much larger quantities than organ meats, though, on the whole, the latter are nutritionally superior. The amount of fat in meats varies with the nutritional state of the animal and the extent of trimming and method of preparation of the meat. In most meats, the fat occurs in distinct tissue layers and can be easily trimmed off; on the other hand, pork fat is interspersed throughout the muscle fibers in minute amounts, making it difficult to separate. On the basis of its higher fat content, pork is more slowly digested.

In addition to protein, muscle meat contributes moderate amounts of thiamin and riboflavin, moderate amounts of iron, and generous quantities of niacin and phosphorus. The organ meats, particularly liver and kidney, furnish proteins of a very high quality, generous quantities of practically all the B complex vitamins, iron, phosphorus, copper, and other trace minerals, and even moderate amounts of ascorbic acid; and in addition, liver contains very large quantities of vitamin A. Organ meats combine comparatively low cost with a highly desirable nutritive composition; it is unfortunate that they are not accorded more dietary recognition in the United States.

Except for pork, which is characterized by a higher fat content and by a high level of thiamin, the nutritive value of most edible meats is similar. Beef, veal, pork, mutton, lamb, goat, and game are equally desirable from the standpoint of their nutritional contribution.

Poultry Poultry meat does not differ materially from other meats. Chickens, turkeys, ducks, geese, and game birds make approximately similar nutritive contributions to the diet. Goose and duck meat contain more fat than other poultry and are, on this basis, somewhat less readily digested by some individuals. The white meat and dark meat of poultry are similar in composition; on the average, white meat contains somewhat more niacin and less fat.

Fish and Other Seafoods From the standpoint of nutrition, fish does not differ markedly from other meats. On the whole, it contains more water and less fat, but the desirable quality of its proteins is similar to that of other animals. Oysters and other seafoods—crabs, lobsters, and shrimp—fall into the same category. Seafoods are as readily digested as other meats. Crabs and fat fish (salmon, herring, shad) rank in digestibility with fat meat and poultry (pork, goose), and lean seafood (cod, clams) is as easily and quickly utilized as lean beef.

Milk and Milk Products

Milk is distinguished by the high quality of its proteins and its high content of calcium and phosphorus. It is also a good source of riboflavin and vitamin A and supplies generous quantities of lactose and readily digested milk fat. The fact that it contains most essential nutrients (especially proteins, calcium, and riboflavin) makes it indispensable to the infant and highly desirable to the growing child and the pregnant and lactating woman.

The major protein of milk is casein; smaller amounts of lactalbumin and lactoglobulin are also present. The casein found in the milk of most warm-blooded animals is similar, if not identical; the lactalbumin and lactoglobulin are, however, species-specific and differ in the composition and immunologic properties. Cow's milk is poor in iron and vitamin C and cannot be relied upon to supply these essentials. The vitamin A content of milk varies with the feed of the cow; the vitamin D content of nonenriched milk varies with the availability of sunlight and is greater in the summer months.

Much of the nutritional excellence of fresh, whole fluid milk is also found in evaporated and powdered milk. Fat-free skim milk is practically as desirable (especially if the vitamin A and D content is restored), and skim milk powder is the most economical source of good protein, calcium, and phosphorus.

Cheese contains all the casein and some of the albumin and minerals of the milk from which it is derived. When made from whole milk, it also contains the original butterfat. It is a highly nutritious, economical food and a desirable form of milk protein, calcium, and phosphorus for those who do not care to drink fluid milk. (About $1\frac{1}{2}$ ounces of cured cheese—not cottage cheese—may be substituted for 8 ounces of fluid milk in diets calling for a relatively high consumption of the latter.)

Eggs

The average hen's egg contains roughly 13 percent protein and 12 percent fat. Eggs contain very little carbohydrate, which is no detraction since this is supplied by almost any other food. Egg proteins, both the albumin of the white and vitellin of the yolk, are of the highest quality. The fat of the egg is finely emulsified and easily assimilated. The egg yolk is more nutritious than the white; it contains most of the vitamins, minerals, and fat. Egg yolk is very rich in vitamin A, phosphorus, and iron; it also contains liberal amounts of thiamin and vitamin D, while the egg white is a rich source of riboflavin.

Eggs, like milk, are easily digested; the proteins are about 98 percent absorbed, and the figure for the utilization of the fatty fraction is about the same.

Cereals and Cereal Products

Cereal grains are the backbone of man's food supply, be it in their original form or in the form of flour, bread, or noodles. Quantitatively, on a worldwide scale, rice is probably the most important grain; wheat and corn also figure very largely as mainstays of national diets, followed by rye, barley, millet, and oats. The common grains have a roughly similar composition. They contain from 7 to 14 percent protein and 75 percent carbohydrate. The proteins are of low biologic value; however, when supplemented with simultaneously consumed proteins of a better quality, they are capable of supplying man's protein requirement (Chap. 7).

The vitamin and mineral constituents of grains are held mostly in the outer layers of the kernel or in the embryo ("germ"). Since much of this is lost in the process of milling, phosphorus remains the major mineral contribution of most grains. Enrichment of flour as practiced today restores thiamin, riboflavin, niacin, and iron to the grain and is a laudable procedure which should be extended to every corner of the world. There is no doubt that the mandatory enrichment of flour in the states and countries where it is practiced has contributed materially to higher standards of nutrition and health.

The enrichment of many breakfast cereals and of precooked infant cereals has become a standard procedure in the food industry. In the United States, these precooked infant cereals supply the bulk of the highly needed dietary iron of infants, as well as much of their thiamin and niacin intake. Enrichment of wheat flour, corn meal, and grits with niacin (as well as thiamin, riboflavin, and iron) has aided considerably in reducing the incidence of pellagra in the Southern states. Recently, a program of rice enrichment was started, both in the United States and abroad. This is an important factor in the eradication of beriberi, still a significant problem in many parts of the world. In food planning and preparation, whole-grain or enriched cereals and cereal products should always be given preference.

Vegetables

Roots and Tubers The white potato makes up an important part of the diet of man in both Europe and North America, and its nutritive value is consequently of importance. It contains about 20 percent carbohydrate—mostly starch—and 2 percent protein. The protein, though relatively scanty, is of high biologic value. The white potato is primarily an energy-yielding food; it is low in fiber and highly digestible. It contains a fair amount of vitamin C, which is preserved best in whole potatoes, cooked or baked in their skins. White potatoes also supply generous amounts of potassium and small quantities of thiamin and iron.

Sweet potatoes, though actually unrelated, have a composition similar to the common white potato. They are richer in carbohydrates and are noteworthy for their high carotene (provitamin A) content.

Carrots are of value primarily because of the large quantity of carotene which they contain. Beets and turnips are carbohydrate-rich foods; their leaves, however, contribute generous amounts of minerals and vitamins, including ascorbic acid.

Leafy Vegetables   In the amounts commonly consumed, leafy vegetables are not important energy-yielding foods; however, their less digestible carbohydrates (hemicelluloses and cellulose fiber) provide an abundance of roughage, which is an important component of a normal diet. Their protein is generally of high quality, though not abundant in quantity. The value of leafy vegetables lies primarily in their vitamin and mineral content. Most vegetable leaves are rich sources of provitamin A and good sources of iron, calcium, riboflavin, and folic acid. The greener the leaf, the higher the carotene content. Carotene from leafy vegetables is more readily absorbed and utilized than that from yellow ones. Fresh vegetable leaves are also good sources of vitamin C; unfortunately much of this ascorbic acid is often lost before consumption through oxidation and leaching during preparation. Though little carotene is lost in cooking, portions of the water-soluble vitamins and appreciable quantities of iron, magnesium, and phosphorus may be lost if the cooking water of leafy vegetables is discarded.

Tomatoes   Though generally regarded as a vegetable, the tomato is really a fruit; it is outstanding because of its generous provitamin A and vitamin C content. When canned, tomatoes and tomato products tend to retain their vitamin C better than other vegetables, which makes them particularly useful.

Legumes   Dry legume seeds, such as beans, peas, and lentils, contain approximately twice as much protein as the cereals and almost as much carbohydrate. Though of a somewhat higher quality than cereal proteins, most legume proteins are still incomplete proteins which are best supplemented with concurrently consumed higher-quality proteins (such as those found in cheese or meat). Beans are noteworthy as an inexpensive protein food. As a rule, most legumes are good sources of thiamin and contribute moderate amounts of riboflavin and niacin. They also contain significant quantities of phosphorus and iron and smaller amounts of calcium.

Soybeans (and soybean flour) are outstanding because of their very high protein content and the high biologic quality of this protein. They are also a good source of calcium and iron and contain more fat than most other legumes.

The digestibility of legume proteins is somewhat less than that of animal proteins; on the average, about 90 percent is utilized—still a highly respectable figure.

Peanuts resemble other legumes in composition, except for their high fat content. They are also characterized by high niacin values.

Nuts

As a rule, most edible nuts contain less carbohydrate than legumes and are rich in protein and very rich in fat. They contain fair to generous amounts of thiamin, riboflavin, and niacin and represent good sources of iron and phosphorus. The proteins of nuts have a biologic value similar to the legumes (soybeans excepted). The digestibility of nuts is rather low, primarily because of their compact physical state. Thorough mastication (or grinding, as in the case of peanut butter) considerably increases the utilization of the nutrients which they contain.

Fruits

Ordinarily, fruits do not contribute important quantities of calories or proteins to the diet. They are valuable because of the vitamins and minerals which they contain, as well as for their bulkiness and laxative properties.

The citrus fruits are distinguished by their high ascorbic acid content. Orange juice, for example, is given routinely to infants for the prevention of scurvy. Fresh berries are also valuable for their vitamin C content. Bananas, apricots, and peaches contribute varying amounts of provitamin A and vitamin C. Apples are primarily beneficial because of the roughage and bulk which they impart to the diet. In addition to bulk, figs and prunes contribute their specific water-soluble laxative factors; they are helpful adjuncts in geriatric and pregnancy diets. Practically all dried fruits are rich in minerals (and some in vitamin A and riboflavin); this nutritive wealth is best judged in the light of the individual's capacity to consume these highly concentrated fruits. Reconstituted, stewed dried fruits have, on the average, somewhat less nutritive value than their fresh counterparts.

Fats and Oils

The fats and oils are primarily sources of energy and, to a varying degree, of the essential fatty acids and fat-soluble vitamins (Chap. 9). The fish oils, butter, and fortified margarine contribute vitamins A and D. Corn oil, cottonseed oil, safflower oil, and soybean oil are significant sources of linoleic acid, the main essential fatty acid. With the exception of the fish oils, most of the common animal fats serve largely to bolster the caloric value, flavor, and satiety value of the diet.

Sugars and Sweets

In the quantities usually consumed, sugars, syrups, honey, molasses, and most jams and jellies contribute calories to the diet and very few other incidental nutrients. Unrefined dark cane molasses is a rich source of calcium and iron. However, today this product has little dietary significance since it is used very little and since primarily refined molasses is marketed in the modern grocery store or the supermarket.

As in the case of many fats, excessive consumption of sugars is disadvantageous inasmuch as it leads to a smaller consumption of nutritionally more desirable foods.

Miscellaneous Food Items

Salt   Sodium chloride is not merely a condiment; it is a dietary necessity since natural foods do not supply enough chloride and sodium to meet the body's requirements under all conditions. Excessive consumption of salt is inadvisable, especially in cardiovascular or renal disease where there is inadequate excretion of salt in the urine; in these cases incomplete sodium clearance leads to water retention in the tissues. For reasons outlined in Chap. 12, iodized salt is the preferred variety.

Coffee and Tea   When consumed without the addition of sugar, milk, or cream, neither beverage contributes nutrients to the dietary, except for coffee, which contains varying amounts of niacin, depending on the degree of roasting which the coffee bean has undergone. One 8-ounce cup of coffee (medium roast) contributes about one-tenth of the daily requirement of niacin.

Alcoholic Beverages   Ethyl alcohol is readily oxidized in the body to yield calories. In contrast to carbohydrates or fats, alcohol yields 7 cal per oxidized gram; it is metabolized at a steady rate which is not accelerated by exercise. Not all ingested alcohol is oxidized; a portion is excreted as such by the lung and kidney.

Aside from the more obvious considerations, a large consumption of alcohol is undesirable inasmuch as in some individuals it leads to an excessive caloric intake from the alcohol and associated calorie-yielding ingredients (carbohydrates of beer or sweet wines); in others it may lead to a smaller consumption of nutritionally more desirable foods, either indirectly because the caloric requirement is already met by the alcoholic beverage or directly, in the problem drinker, through deterioration of habits and outright neglect. In the feeding of the elderly and of debilitated patients, small amounts of alcoholic beverages before a major meal serve to stimulate the appetite and to relax the anxious. They are also said to exert a desirable, vasodilating effect in the elderly borderline cardiac patient before the additional circulatory burden, associated with the digestion of a large meal, is placed on his heart.

Chapter 15

The Normal Adult Diet

Given the freedom of choice and left to his own devices, the average, normal adult can be relied upon to consume sufficient food and drink to meet his energy and fluid requirements. He may, indeed, choose a well-balanced diet which satisfies all needs for essential nutrients. On the other hand, influenced by custom and dietary prejudices (and at times fad diets), beset by economic limitations, and guided largely by his taste buds and his olfactory sense, he may not arrive at a satisfactory choice of diet. Foods which are good sources of essential nutrients (*protective foods*) are not always the easiest to prepare, the least expensive, or the most appealing to the sense of taste; many of them might be neglected were it not for educational efforts designed to influence the food choice of the population with a view to ensure a maximal level of health, insofar as that can be done through good nutrition.

Food Selection through Food Groups

In the United States, a widely accepted pattern of food selection is based on a system whereby the desirable foods are grouped together on the basis of similar nutritive composition. It is then quite easy and practical to formulate a diet by specifying the number of servings from each group which should be eaten each day. In the late 1940s, the system of the "seven basic food groups" was used by most workers in the field of public health and nutrition. Under this system, seven basic food groups were recognized: (1) green leafy and yellow vegetables; (2) citrus fruits, tomatoes, raw cabbage; (3) potatoes, other vegetables, other fruits; (4) dairy foods; (5) meats; (6) breads and cereals; and (7) butter and margarine. A number of daily servings of each group were specified to provide a nutritionally adequate diet.

Later, the Agricultural Research Service of the U.S. Department of Agriculture developed and published a food plan which is organized around four basic food groups. The following are the suggested food intakes:

Daily Meal Plan

MILK GROUP
Children	3 cups
Teen-agers	4 or more cups
Adults	2 or more cups
Pregnant women	3 or more cups
Nursing mothers	4 or more cups

Cheese and ice cream can replace part of the milk.

MEAT GROUP: 2 or more servings
Beef, veal, pork, lamb, poultry, fish, eggs, with dry beans, peas, and nuts as
    alternatives.

VEGETABLE-FRUIT GROUP: 4 or more servings, including
A dark green or deep yellow vegetable (important for vitamin A) at least every
    other day.
A citrus fruit or other fruit or vegetable (important for vitamin C) daily.
Other fruits and vegetables including potatoes.

BREAD-CEREAL GROUP: 4 or more servings
Bread or cereals—whole-grain, enriched, restored.

The milk group is relied on to provide most of the calcium requirement, as well as a good contribution of high-quality protein, riboflavin, and other nutrients. The meat group provides protein, iron, thiamin, riboflavin, and niacin. The alternative protein-rich foods listed supply proteins of lower quality which should be supplemented with animal proteins consumed at the same meal. The vegetable-fruit group is an important source of vitamins and minerals (particularly vitamins A and C). The enriched bread–cereal group is counted on to provide thiamin, niacin, iron, and protein (the latter is of low quality, to be improved by simultaneous supplementation with animal proteins).

In any ordinary diet, fats, oils, sugars, and unenriched cereal derivatives are usually combined with the specific foods mentioned. They will be eaten to satisfy the appetite and will round out the caloric requirements. It should be noted that these recommendations make no expressed provision for an adequate supply of iodine or vitamin D.

Another easy-to-follow (and more specific) dietary pattern on which to base the daily food intake is a slight modification of Canada's food rules:

Daily Meal Plan

MILK
Children (up to about 12 years)	At least 1 pt
Adolescents	At least 1½ pt
Adults	At least 1 pt
Expectant or nursing mothers	1 qt or more

Other milk products may be substituted at times; 1½ oz cured cheese or 2–3 large scoops of ice cream may be counted as 1 cup of milk.

MEAT, FISH, AND POULTRY
1 large serving. This may be alternated with eggs or cheese, and dried peas, beans, or lentils. Use liver frequently.
EGGS, in addition, at least three times a week.

FRUITS
1 serving of citrus fruit or tomatoes (or their juices) and 1 serving of other fruit.

VEGETABLES
At least 2 servings of vegetables, preferably dark green leafy or deep yellow; and 1 serving of potatoes at times.

CEREALS AND BREAD
1 serving of enriched or whole-grain cereal, and 2 to 4 slices of enriched or whole-grain bread. Noodles and rice may be used as alternatives to the above.

FLUIDS
For most people, 4–8 cups (1–2 qt) total fluids each day.

ADDITIONAL FOODS
As needed to supply caloric value and to make meals palatable.
(*Note:* Use iodized salt exclusively. All growing persons and expectant and nursing mothers require 400 IU vitamin D daily.)

Ordinarily, at least three meals should be eaten each day. More frequent feedings may be adopted if desired. The division of food among the various meals is immaterial, except that the principle of mutual supplementation of incomplete and complete proteins should be upheld, so that foods supplying low-quality proteins should always be consumed concurrently with some source of proteins of high quality. Breakfast should be a substantial meal; it should never be skimpy since it follows a prolonged period of fasting. Experience has shown that a mere coffee-and-doughnut breakfast, or outright abstention from breakfast, leads to a decreased attention span and working efficiency in the late morning hours.

Both meal plans are basically similar inasmuch as they concentrate their attention on the protective foods, and when followed, both will ensure an adequate intake of all essential nutrients. The total caloric value of either plan is actually low for a physically moderately active adult, unless additional foods are included of the types which conventionally serve to make meals palatable—such as butter, margarine, jams, sweetening for beverages, and the like. Individuals can make an upward adjustment of their total caloric intake to meet higher energy requirements by consuming larger portions and by the inclusion of additional food items.

Sample Menus

Inexpensive and light

BREAKFAST
Enriched breakfast cereal with glass of milk and sugar
Oranges (or orange juice)
Toast, enriched margarine, jelly
Coffee or tea optional

LUNCH
Chicken soup
Macaroni and cheese (or egg or cheese sandwich)
Sliced tomatoes
Fruit
Beverage

DINNER
Hamburger steak and
Baked potato
        (or a large serving of beef stew)
Mixed green salad or green vegetable
Bread, margarine
Ice cream or pudding
Beverage

BEDTIME SNACK
Fruit and cookies or cheese and crackers

Elaborate and hearty

BREAKFAST
Eggs (2)
Ham or sausage
Grapefruit sections
Toast, butter, marmalade
Enriched breakfast cereal with milk and sugar
Coffee or tea

LUNCH
Tomato soup and crackers
Grated carrot and raisin salad
Chicken stew with dumplings
Hot biscuits, butter
Honeydew melon with lime
Beverage

DINNER
Consommé
Pineapple, avocado, and cottage cheese salad
Lamb chops
Baked potato
Broccoli spears, mustard sauce
Hot breads, butter
Ice cream
Beverage

BEDTIME SNACK
Chocolate milk and graham crackers or cheese and crackers

Flexibility and Adaptability

It is important to recognize that adequate nutrition may be achieved by a variety of dietary patterns and that no one formula is correct to the exclusion of others. The meal patterns mentioned above are easily adapted to most North American and western European palates, living standards, and religious customs. These patterns may even be adapted for use by vegetarians, provided eggs, milk, and cheese are substituted for the meat items.

Nevertheless, a word of caution is indicated lest these patterns be used to abet rigid thinking on the part of the nutritionist. Dietary recommendations must be flexible enough to accommodate regional and social gastronomic customs and still provide the nutritional essentials. In Iceland the American's beef may have to yield to mutton, while in Japan smoked fish may take its place; a fisherman on the coast of Norway may think that herrings and potatoes make the best staple diet, while the Iowa farmer might like potatoes well enough but would draw the line at the herring. The economics of food selection are equally powerful: where citrus fruit is economically unfeasible as a source of vitamin C, an adequate supply of ascorbic acid may have to be sought in more available foods, be it potatoes, tomatoes, brussels sprouts, or turnip greens. Thus the diet selected is likely to vary from family to family and region to region, and the major valid criterion of judgment should be the completeness with which it satisfies the nutritive requirements.

Chapter 16

Nutrition in Pregnancy and Lactation

Pregnancy is probably the greatest physiologic stress and the most common major alteration of the normal biologic life processes to which the human female is subjected during her lifetime. Because of the demands of the growing fetus and physiologic and metabolic changes which take place in the mother, different nutritional requirements apply to this period and to the subsequent period of lactation. However, contrary to often-repeated fallacies, these changed requirements do not call for "eating for two" or for an automatic loss of one's figure or of a "tooth for each baby," nor are pernicious vomiting and bizarre appetites an essential part of the clinical or nutritional picture.

Nutritional Status and Pregnancy

The relation of the nutritional status of the mother to the course of the pregnancy and to the health of the infant has been the subject of much study. According to numerous studies, there are fewer stillbirths, premature births, toxemias of pregnancy, and illnesses in the newborn infant if the mother has consumed an optimal diet before her pregnancy and during gestation. Famine conditions during World War II in Holland and the siege of Leningrad led to the well-documented observation that severe undernutrition in terms of total calories also significantly reduces the birth weight of the full-term infant and decreases its length markedly, though not to an equal degree. Poor prenatal maternal nutrition is also reflected in low vitamin and mineral stores in the newborn. Infants of anemic mothers are frequently born with a subnormal iron endowment, while infants born to mothers treated with oral iron during pregnancy exhibit higher serum iron values than control groups.

Probably the most common harmful nutritional aberration seen in pregnant women in the United States is weight abnormalities. Markedly overweight women are more likely than nonobese women to develop preeclampsia or eclampsia. It is an interesting circumstance that the incidence of preeclampsia in markedly underweight mothers is also significantly higher than among the average-weight group. The role of the diet in these toxemias of pregnancy has been much debated. Frequently prenatal diets have been prescribed which limit calories or salt intake as a toxemia-preventive measure. There is no justification for such routine limitation of calories or salt in pregnancy (or for the use of diuretics to limit weight increase and to avoid edema). Any limitation must be specifically indicated.

Weight Gain in Pregnancy

Normally the majority of women experience a marked increase in appetite and thirst during the first trimester. Although at first morning nausea may temporarily counteract the increased desire for food, a notable appetite is soon the order of the day. A significant number of women may also develop temporary cravings for some foods and aversions to others. A small minority of women may even develop pica, a bizarre appetite for starch, chalk, clay, or coal. The sudden craving for particular foods—pickled onions or a specific brand of sardines—is unexplainable on physiologic ground and is looked upon by some psychiatrists as an attention-getting mechanism. The culinary cravings of pregnancy are self-limited and invariably disappear after delivery.

Normal pregnancy is associated with a weight gain of from 15 to 25 pounds. This increase in weight is due to (1) the weight of the fetus, (2) the weight of the placenta, (3) the increase in maternal uterine and mammary tissues, and (4) water retention in the mother's body, which may occur during the latter part of pregnancy.

Normally there is only a slight weight gain during the first trimester; about 21 pounds out of a total average increment of 24 is usually gained during the second and third trimesters. Once the patient has been seen and has received definite instructions as to her diet, an almost uniform, gradual gain should take place. In selected cases, if the prospective mother is conspicuously overweight when she presents herself during the first trimester and if she is well supervised and cooperates intelligently, a somewhat decelerated weight gain may be achieved; this must be accomplished on an adequate intake of all essential nutrients except for too generous a complement of calories. However, as a rule the period of gestation should not be chosen to reduce an overweight individual, and major weight adjustments should be made either before or after pregnancy.

The patient who is definitely underweight when she becomes pregnant and who fails to gain acceptably during the first (and later, second) trimester requires strict dietary attention. A subsequent excessive weight gain during the late second trimester or third trimester is undesirable since experience has shown it to be associated with a greater incidence of preeclampsia. It is also believed that in the case of the excessively underweight patient the pattern for premature labor is established early in pregnancy and that such patients can be significantly protected by an early metabolic and physiologic stabilization which should be reflected by a steady increase in weight beginning in the first trimester.

Pregnancy in Adolescence

In recent years, pregnancy in adolescence has become more frequent in the United States than in any other Western nation. The nutritional demands of pregnancy in adolescence are particularly critical since the growing youngster who becomes pregnant has the task of developing another human being before her body has completed its own growth. Because they are still growing, most girls under 17 have greater nutritional requirements than adult women of equal size, and pregnancy may compromise their growth potential and increase the risks in pregnancy of complications such as iron-deficiency anemia, fetopelvic disproportion, prolonged labor, toxemia, or premature labor. The average birth weight of infants born to adolescent mothers is substantially lower, the proportion of infants with abnormally low birth weight (an index of risk) is greater, and infant mortality rates are higher. Thus special attention must be paid to fulfillment of the nutritional requirements of the adolescent mother and fetus with particular emphasis on an adequate intake of calories, protein, calcium, iron, and folic acid, with resort to supplementation with the latter three where needed.

Maternal and Fetal Nutritional Requirements

Protein Normal pregnancy is associated with endocrine and metabolic changes which, among other phenomena, result in altered nutritional requirements. There is an increased secretion of the pituitary growth hormone and of the two sex hormones, estrogen and progesterone. In response, protein catabolism is curtailed, protein is spared, and the nitrogen balance becomes positive. This is principally a mechanism to provide a continuous supply of extra protein which the growing fetus requires for the synthesis of its tissues. Actually, the mother retains more protein than is required for the fetus or the enlarging placenta, uterus, or breasts. The accumulation of excess protein in the maternal tissues may be regarded as an emergency reserve for use of the fetus in case of any possible future deprivation before delivery; it may also satisfy future protein needs during lactation. In view of the higher protein requirement, the amount of protein in the pregnancy diet should be increased above normal adult levels. The Food and Nutrition Board (Table 22 in Chap. 13) recommends a daily intake of 76 g of protein during the second half of pregnancy, an increase of 30 g over the recommended normal intake. The Canadian Dietary Standards call for a similar increment.

A liberal protein intake is desirable throughout the entire period of pregnancy to compensate for any possible inadequate protein intake before conception and during the early weeks of pregnancy. The recommended daily protein intake during the subsequent period of lactation is 66 g, in keeping with the extra requirements imposed on the mother by the production of protein-containing breast milk and its continuous withdrawal by the infant.

Calcium   As in the case of protein, an increased retention of calcium is required both for fetal bones and teeth and for storage in the maternal skeleton to satisfy future demands during lactation. Concurrent with the increased requirement for calcium, there is a hormonally mediated increase in the efficiency of absorption of dietary calcium. The Food and Nutrition Board's recommendation of 1.2 g of calcium per day satisfies the higher requirement during pregnancy.

The allowance is also increased to 1.2 g during the period of active lactation when the mother loses substantial amounts of calcium in the breast milk.

Iron   As in the case of calcium, iron storage takes place during pregnancy and the absorption of dietary iron from the intestine becomes more efficient. Fetal demand alone does not account for all the stored iron; the iron reserves accumulated during pregnancy (over and above the iron utilized by the fetus for the synthesis of its own tissues) approximate the quantity of iron required for the elaboration of breast milk during 9 months of lactation. The recommended intake of 18 mg of dietary iron per day is adequate to supply the additional needs associated with pregnancy and lactation, but this goal is not easily attainable with today's diet pattern without resort to some supplementation—usually in the form of oral ferrous salts (sulfate, gluconate, or fumarate). Adequacy of the diet with respect to all nutrients is essential for good utilization of the increased supply of iron.

Dilution of the maternal blood during pregnancy is part of the general retention of water in the body during the latter months of pregnancy. This hydremia is a normal and universal occurrence. The increase in plasma volume (an average of 10 to 15 percent) is reflected in an "apparent anemia" since the hemoglobin concentration decreases in relation to the total blood volume, though there may not have been any change in total maternal hemoglobin. Thus anemia should not be suspected unless the hemoglobin values have dropped below 80 percent of normal. On the other hand, a microcytic, hypochromic anemia (Chap. 33) may occur during pregnancy in women who had deficient iron stores before pregnancy and in whom the increased demands of this period have aggravated the severity of their deficiency. Indeed the most commonly found complication of pregnancy and the puerperium in the United States is mutually reinforced dietary iron-deficiency anemia and anemia due to blood loss. Pregnant women who have received iron supplementation usually have an average hemoglobin concentration of 12 g per 100 ml. Hemoglobin concentrations below 11 or 10 g/ml are found frequently and are indicative of iron-deficiency anemia. Since the usual American diet is not likely to supply sufficient iron to meet the increased needs of pregnancy, a daily supplement of 30 to 60 mg of iron is recommended for all pregnant women during the second and third trimesters.

Folic Acid   Another anemia of pregnancy with macrocytic megaloblastic characteristics is discussed in Chap. 33. This disease is not as rare as previously thought. It is more frequently associated with a lifelong marginal diet and presumably more prevalent among less affluent population strata; nevertheless, it is also found among private obstetrical patients with adequate means. —he condition responds readily to folic acid therapy. Supplementation with folic acid is warranted in cases of multiple pregnancy and where the blood picture is marginal. A daily supplement of 400 mg of folic acid suffices to prevent a deficiency in pregnant women.

Iodine   During the second half of pregnancy, the basal metabolic rate may increase up to 23 percent. This enhanced metabolism, associated with increased activity of the thyroid gland and secretion of thyroid hormone, augments the need for iodine throughout pregnancy. It is widely recognized that goiter is more likely to develop during pregnancy. Consequently, the use of iodized salt, advisable during normal periods, must be strongly recommended throughout pregnancy, since few foods, except seafoods, can serve as adequate sources of iodine. If iodized salt is the only source of iodine and the physician restricts the intake of salt as a prophylaxis against the toxemias of pregnancy, a supplementary source of iodine is indicated.

Calories   It is commonly agreed that the energy allowance should be increased during the latter part of pregnancy unless physical activity is severely curtailed. This is consistent with the increase in metabolism during this period and helps spare protein for use of the fetus and storage by the mother. This small increase in caloric intake is justified even in the case of the overweight pregnant woman. An extra allowance of 300 cal per day is recommended by the

Food and Nutrition Board late in pregnancy; the Canadian Dietary Standards call for an increment of 500 cal during the second half of the term.

The extra allowance during the period of lactation is 500 cal, which is ample to cover the increased requirements attendant on the active elaboration of milk.

Vitamin Requirements   As yet, there is little precise information as to vitamin requirements during pregnancy and lactation. It is generally agreed, however, that hand in hand with an increased need for calories and for the specific nutrients mentioned, the vitamin requirements are increased. This increase is roughly proportionate to the caloric intake; hence the diet pattern need not change, nor is special supplementation required to meet the body's needs. This normal adjustment is reflected in the recommended intakes in Table 22.

Vitamin D is necessary for the utilization of calcium and phosphorus by both the fetus and the pregnant or lactating mother; thus a daily intake of 400 IU of the vitamin should be supplied, preferably by the diet ("vitamin D milk"). The possibility of vitamin K deficiency in the mother is normally not very likely. However, many newborn infants have low vitamin K stores and exhibit low prothrombin levels. The prophylactic administration of vitamin K to the mother in the last weeks of pregnancy or just prior to the onset of labor is practiced to some extent, in an effort to improve the infant's blood clotting performance.

Dietary Recommendations in Pregnancy

Except, perhaps, for vitamin D, the nutrient intakes discussed above and recommended by the United States and Canadian dietary standards can be achieved through the proper selection of foods and without the addition of special supplements. For maximal results, such an improvement in food intake should be instituted at the beginning of pregnancy. In women of known poor nutritional status or patients with a history of catastrophes during earlier pregnancies, this special dietary regimen is best begun well in advance of the onset of pregnancy. A well-chosen prenatal diet is a good means of educating the mother with respect to good general dietary practices and provides an excellent opportunity to change poor food habits.

The pregnancy diet is basically a well-balanced ordinary diet, modified through an emphasis on a higher animal protein intake and a decrease in fat and carbohydrate foods. Each day the expectant mother should have about 1 quart of milk (this may be skim milk), one egg, and an ample serving of lean meat, fish, or poultry. Occasionally, less expensive protein foods like evaporated or dried skim milk, soybean flour, and beans or peas may be partially substituted to meet a tight family budget. Generous amounts of citrus fruits, tomatoes, and deep yellow and dark green leafy vegetables should be eaten daily; in addition to filling nutritional needs, the higher intake of fruits and vegetables tends to maintain normal bowel function and counteracts the tendency to constipation during pregnancy. (If needed, small amounts of stewed prunes or prune juice will promote easier elimination; laxatives should not be used except by the physician's current advice.) The intake of butter, cream, margarine, or other fats, and noodles, pies, pastries, rich desserts, soft drinks, and sweets may be decreased.

Foods known to cause digestive distress or gaseousness, alcoholic beverages, highly spiced foods, fried foods, "rich" gravies, and "heavy" desserts are best avoided. Excessive amounts of salt or salted foods are ill-advised, especially during the last 2 months of pregnancy.

The fluid intake should be adequate. About 2 quarts of fluids (including the daily milk ration) or more is indicated; this may take the form of water, fruit juices, soups, and coffee and tea in moderation.

In an effort to avoid excessive weight gain, the total amount of food eaten during the first 4 months should be unchanged if the expectant mother has a normal body weight; however, it should be judiciously checked for adequate representation of protective foods in the dietary pattern. During the latter half of pregnancy the total intake may be increased to permit a gradual weight gain of about 2 pounds per week. If a well-controlled caloric intake is advisable, skim milk may be used instead of whole milk, and at this point the use of a vitamin D supplement should be considered, unless the skim milk is fortified with this vitamin.

Five to six small meals are preferable to three large ones. As the enlarging uterine mass begins to affect gastrointestinal capacity, gaseousness, indigestion, and "heartburn" are more effectively controlled by small frequent feedings. This is particularly indicated for the mother's comfort during the last trimester.

Frequent small meals also have a salutary effect on the tendency to morning nausea in early pregnancy. A morning snack of dry toast or crackers, well chewed and taken in bed 10 to 15 minutes before rising, is also often helpful.

Meal Plan for Pregnancy

MILK
1 qt/day, as a beverage or in foods (puddings, custards). 1¹/₂ oz hard cheese may be substituted for 1 cup milk. If caloric restriction is indicated, skim milk should be used.

LEAN MEAT, SEAFOOD, OR POULTRY
1 to 2 servings per day. Liver or organ meats are recommended once a week.

EGGS
1 per day.

VEGETABLES
2 or more servings of dark green leafy vegetables and deep yellow ones (or
    tomatoes); potatoes to be used in moderation.

FRUITS
2 or more servings per day, one or more of citrus fruits and one or more of
    other fruits, with emphasis on vitamin C.

WHOLE-GRAIN OR ENRICHED CEREAL AND BREAD
1 small serving of cereal and 2 slices of bread suffice. Enriched noodles and rice
    to be used occasionally as alternatives to the above.

BUTTER OR MARGARINE
In moderation; 2 to 3 pats suffice.

A vitamin D supplement is desirable during the second half of pregnancy,
    especially in the fall and winter. Iodized salt should be used.

Sample Menu

BREAKFAST
Grapefruit or orange
Whole-grain cereal with milk
Egg
Buttered toast (1 slice)
Beverage

MIDMORNING SNACK
Milk
Graham crackers (2)

LUNCH
Tomato soup
Liver sausage sandwich
Cottage cheese and lettuce salad
Fresh fruit (preferably citrus)
Beverage

MIDAFTERNOON
Chocolate milk

DINNER
Beef pot roast
String beans
Small baked potato
Raw carrot sticks
Puddings or ice cream (small serving)
Beverage

BEDTIME SNACK
Milk
Cookie (1)

Dietary Recommendations during Lactation

The composition of human milk is more variable than is commonly appreciated, and the maternal diet is the principle determinant of its qualitative and quantitative constitution. The nutritional requirements during lactation are shown in Table 22. Except for two principal modifications, the pregnancy diet lends itself well to supplying the needs during the months of lactation since it emphasizes essential, protective foods.

During lactation, the energy requirement increases considerably over the normal requirements, consistent with the caloric value of the milk secreted and the energy expenditure required for its elaboration. Thus additional cereals, bread, noodles, potatoes, and fats of the lactating mother's choice should be included in the diet; the quantities used will vary in accordance with individual needs. There should be a reasonable intake of the essential fatty acids since their content in breast milk appears to be dependent on dietary sources; hence the diet should include some unsaturated fats in addition to saturated fats (Chap. 9).

An additional pint of milk, bringing the daily milk ration to 1½ quarts, is often recommended and will satisfy the additional protein, calcium, phosphorus, and riboflavin needs, especially since the mother normally accumulates protein and calcium reserves during pregnancy which are utilized during the period of lactation. Liberal amounts of vegetables and fruits, especially citrus fruits, will take care of the increased vitamin A and ascorbic acid requirements. An increased fluid intake is also recommended because of its salutary effect on successful lactation.

Chapter 17

Nutrition in Infancy

In contrast with young animals, the human young take a seemingly infinite time to learn to feed themselves without outside help. For almost 3 years, the infant is at the mercy of its mother's ability to provide and select its food. The first 9 months of this period are spent in utero abstracting from the mother's bloodstream whatever nutrients are required. If the mother's diet is insufficient, her tissues may have to yield some of the missing nutrients, as in the case of calcium and phosphorus derived from the maternal skeleton. A number of neonatal defects may be attributed to defective prenatal maternal nutrition, such as a low fetal prothrombin level due to deficient maternal intake of vitamin K, or low iron stores and anemia due to iron deficit in the mother. Thus maternal nutrition affects the fetus long before it first encounters the perils of extrauterine life.

Nutritional Needs in Infancy

The recommended daily dietary allowances for infants 0 to 6 and 7 to 12 months old are shown in Table 22 in Chap. 13. It may be useful, however, to elaborate on certain aspects of the infant's nutritional needs here.

Calories The normal infant requires about 50 cal per pound per day. It will consume more during the first 6 months of life and somewhat less toward the end of the first year. It will determine its own caloric intake by accepting or rejecting the breast, bottle, and its solid foods.

Protein A high protein intake is essential because of the rapid growth of the infant. During the first year a normal baby approximately triples its birth weight. Protein needs in early infancy are fully met by breast milk when its supply is adequate. Usual quantities consumed by nursing infants afford an intake of about 1.5 to 2.5 g of protein per kilogram of body weight during the first 6 months of life. Allowances for the artificially fed infant may lie in the range of 2.2 g of protein per kilogram from 0 to 6 months and 2.0 g per kilogram during the remainder of the year. In current practice, diets furnishing 3 g of protein and more per kilogram are in common use.

Fat The infant appears to require small amounts of fat as a source of the essential fatty acids (Chap. 9). The amount of fat in the usual intake of breast milk or cow's milk formula fulfills this requirement. Quantities of fat greatly in excess of this are not well tolerated.

Carbohydrate The daily requirement depends on the caloric needs. Formulas should not be overenriched with carbohydrates, in order to avoid satiating the infant before it has satisfied its other, more essential, basic nutritional needs.

Water (in terms of total fluid intake) The infant has a relatively high fluid requirement. Its obligatory water loss through the kidney and skin is great, and it is subject, far more than the adult, to pathologic water loss by way of vomiting and diarrhea. In infants symptoms of dehydration appear rapidly and may have quite serious consequences. Two and a half ounces of fluid per pound of bodyweight per day is adequate for the normal infant in a temperate climate. This may have to be increased in a hot climate or during the summer months.

Calcium About 35 mg per pound per day appears sufficient for adequate mineralization of teeth and bones. The brest-fed infant may receive less, while the bottle-fed baby may receive more (but mineralization is good in either case).

Phosphorus A deficiency of this mineral is unlikely as long as sufficient breast milk is consumed to satisfy the infant's other nutritional requirements. An excess is actually ingested with a similar quantity of undiluted cow's milk.

Iron The need for iron in proportion to body size and food intake is greater during infancy than at any other period of life. The iron requirement is based on the amount of iron available at birth and that needed for growth and hemoglobin production. The recommended daily dietary allowance is 1 mg/kg/day for infants in the United States, which takes into account normal individual variability in maternal iron endowment and intestinal absorption. Infants with a low initial hemoglobin endowment—premature infants, those of low birth weight (less than 2.5 kg), those of multiple births (twins), and possibly those born to mothers with several recent consecutive pregnancies—require 2 mg/kg/day for many months.

Neither breast milk nor cow's milk satisfies the infant's requirement of 6 to 15 mg per day. If the mother's prenatal diet was adequate with respect to iron, the infant will have been born with sufficient iron (chiefly in the form of circulating hemoglobin in its erythrocytes) to last about 3 months. Since this is not always the case and since many infants walk a tightrope with regard to their iron requirement, present-day pediatric custom adds a safe quantity of dietary iron in the form of iron-enriched special infant cereals, or iron-enriched proprietary milk formulas (which should be given after the first 3 months), and, subsequently, in the form of foods naturally rich in iron, such as egg yolks and meats. The reader is referred to Chap. 33, Nutrition and the Anemias, for a more detailed discussion of iron requirements and iron-deficiency anemia in infancy.

Vitamin D   Neither cow's milk nor breast milk contains sufficient vitamin D to meet the daily requirement of 400 IU. Practically all canned evaporated milk is fortified with vitamin D and supplies a minimum of this nutrient with the quantity of formula normally consumed. The daily allowance of vitamin D is best supplied by a special supplement, either in the form of cod-liver oil or by the multivitamin supplement which many pediatricians prescribe for their charges.

Vitamin A   The recommended 1,400 IU is usually found in the daily quota of breast milk or formula. However, human and cow's milk may fluctuate considerably in their vitamin A content, and it is helpful that most vitamin D supplements also contain a supplement of vitamin A. Once strained vegetables are fed, the infant will receive enough vitamin A from this source; the initial supplementation may be a wise precaution for the very young infant (1 to 6 months of age) who may be exclusively milk-fed because of maternal preference or habit.

Ascorbic Acid   The recommended 35 mg may be obtained in the milk of a mother whose own diet is adequate with respect to vitamin C. Cow's milk formula is deficient in vitamin C. It is safest to complement the diet of the milk-fed infant with orange juice or a similar source of ascorbic acid.

Thiamin   Breast milk and cow's milk formula supply somewhat less than the recommended allowance of 0.3 to 0.5 mg daily. Nevertheless, the infant's thiamin requirements appear to be adequately met, especially after early introduction of enriched cereals. Where thiamin deprivation is a factor in the nutrition of the mother, as in the rice-eating regions of Southeast Asia, breast milk provides insufficient thiamin and a clinical deficiency in infants is not uncommon.

Riboflavin and Niacin The usual quota of breast milk and cow's milk supplies the recommended allowance of 0.4 to 0.6 mg of riboflavin. What both sources lack in niacin is compensated for by the tryptophan which is contained in milk protein. The normal human organism constantly converts small amounts of this amino acid into niacin (Chap. 11).

Linoleic Acid The *minimal* essential fatty acid requirement of infants, in the form of linoleic acid, is 1 percent of total calories consumed. It has been demonstrated that maximal growth and freedom from the dermatologic manifestations related to essential fatty acid deficiency in infants 2 to 4 months old is obtained when 1.4 percent of the caloric intake is derived from linoleic acid.

But for the exceptions noted above, the quantity of breast milk or cow's milk formula which satisfies the infant's protein and caloric requirements will ordinarily also meet all its other nutritional needs.

Breast Feeding

Breast feeding is generally the safest and most desirable method of nourishing a baby, and human breast milk may be considered the ideal starting food. With an adequate supply of human milk most of the nutritional requirements of the newborn are met, except for iron and vitamin D. Breast feeding should not, however, be relied on exclusively for optimal nutrition beyond the first semester of life.

The prospective mother should be mentally prepared for her breast feeding task. Anticipation of her role as provider of her baby's food will aid in making this undertaking successful. Beginning with the day after delivery, the infant is put to each breast for about 5 minutes every 6 hours. At this point only small quantities of watery colostrum are available, and the infant should receive supplementary feedings of 5 to 10 percent sugar solution. This preliminary nursing stimulates milk production, and by the third day (or, in the case of a nervous mother, by the time she is in the privacy of her home and unharried by hospital schedules and attendants), a full supply of milk is ordinarily available. Once the secretion of milk has been established, the baby should be fed about every 4 hours—granted that sufficient milk is available at such intervals. The average nursing time is about 15 minutes; longer nursing sessions will usually not produce additional milk, but may predispose to injury of the nipples. If possible, only one breast should be offered at each nursing; this facilitates complete emptying and stimulates lactation.

Weighing the baby before and after nursing will establish the amount of milk consumed. Each ounce supplies about 22 cal, and the total amount should suffice to meet the infant's daily caloric requirement.

There are few contraindications to breast feeding. Nursing should not be attempted if the mother is not in good health. A past history of tuberculosis also precludes breast feeding. The mother's diet must be adequate, as described in Chap. 16. Freedom from emotional stress is another essential for successful nursing since psychologic upsets interfere with a normal "letting down" of the milk. Regularity of nursing and the complete emptying of the breast after each feeding help to maintain lactation on the desired level. If the maternal diet is adequate and the quantity of milk is sufficient, its composition may be assumed to be satisfactory as well.

A normal weight gain of the infant and freedom from digestive upsets indicate that the breast feeding is successful. Poor nursing technique or insufficient elaboration of milk is indicated by a constantly hungry infant who fails to thrive. In the case of prolonged insufficient lactation, the maternal milk supply must be supplemented with bottle feeding and a gradual changeover to the bottle is indicated. The most frequent cause for early weaning from the breast is an inadequate milk supply—in many cases the result of inadequate emptying of the breasts several times daily.

In the Western world, breast feeding past the first year is uncommon and most infants are nursed from 6 to 9 months. In the United States, few infants are nursed beyond the fourth month since solid foods are usually introduced before this time and weaning becomes desirable (in the United States, over half the infants are not nursed at all). Weaning is best done gradually, for the mother's own comfort. Over a period of 2 to 3 weeks gradually one and then more breast feedings are replaced by a bottle until the infant is completely weaned.

Beginning with the first month, breast-fed infants should receive 400 units of vitamin D daily and, if not breast-fed, orange juice or a similar source of vitamin C, supplying 35 mg or more. Selected solid foods are usually started by the second or third month, and the precooked infant cereals which are usually the first solids will supplement the infant's iron and B vitamin intake.

Artifical Feeding

Breast feeding is less expensive than bottle feeding. It also entails less bother with equipment for preparation and feeding of a cow's milk formula and concern about the temperature of the milk. More important, breast feeding is a gratifying emotional experience for the mother and a source of desirable emotional gratification for the infant. It is also a rather safe method and entails less risk to the infant than artificial feeding at the hands of a mother whose comprehension is limited and whose sanitary standards (as applied to preparation of a sterile infant formula) may not be adequate. In these two respects breast feeding is indeed the preferable method. However, given an understanding and willing mother, adequate initial guidance, and an acceptable supply of

Table 28   Average Composition of Human and Cow's Milk

	Breast milk, %	Cow's milk, %
Water	87.6	87.2
Total solids	12.4	12.8
Casein	0.4	2.7
Lactalbumin	0.4	0.4
Lactoglobulin	0.2	0.2
Total protein	1.1	3.3
Fat	3.8	3.8
Lactose	7.0	4.8
Ash	0.21	0.71
Sodium	0.015	0.058
Potassium	0.055	0.138
Calcium	0.034	0.126
Magnesium	0.004	0.013
Iron	0.00021	0.00015
Chlorine	0.043	0.100
Phosphorus	0.016	0.099
Sulfur	0.014	0.030
Calories per ounce	22	21
Calories per 100 ml	71	69
Vitamins per 100 ml:		
Vitamin A	53 μg	34 μg
Carotinoids	27 μg	38 μg
Thiamin	16 μg	42 μg
Riboflavin	43 μg	157 μg
Niacin	172 μg	85 μg
Pyridoxine	11 μg	48 μg
Folic acid	0.18 μg	0.23 μg
Vitamin B_{12}	0.18 μg	0.56 μg
Vitamin C	4.30 mg	1.80 mg
Vitamin D	0.4–10.0 IU	0.3–4.0 IU

Source: Modified from *National Research Council Bulletin 254.*

cow's milk, the results of artificial feeding apparently equal those of breast feeding in most instances.

A great simplification has taken place in bottle feeding in recent years. The introduction and gradual common acceptance of the terminal sterilization method—in which the filled bottle is subjected to boiling temperatures within a closed, covered vessel—not only assures adequate pasteurization and freedom from potential pathogenic bacteria, but also improves the digestibility of the cow's milk by decreasing its curd tension. (The curd of raw milk in an infant's stomach is quite dense and plastic, whereas that of pasteurized milk is less so; boiled milk has a friable, soft curd, and canned evaporated milk, an even softer one. The softer the curd, the more easily it is digested.)

Table 28 outlines the respective composition of breast milk and cow's milk. As is readily seen, they are alike in total fat content (not in fatty acid composition), but cow's milk contains considerably more protein and ash and less carbohydrate than human milk. The concentration of protein in breast milk is sufficient to meet the infant's protein requirements. In the case of cow's milk, the excess protein is metabolized for energy purposes. The higher protein content of cow's milk may put a rather high excretory load on the infant's kidney, as it increases the water requirements for renal clearance of the relatively large amounts of resulting urea and of other solutes which are present in cow's milk formulas in greater concentrations than in breast milk. In fact, it has been shown that there is a direct relationship between the dietary solute load of too-concentrated cow's milk formulas and the appearance, in urine of premature and very young infants, of casts and albumin. There also seem to be greater incidence and severity of diaper rash among infants fed undiluted cow's milk than among breast-fed babies (presumably since the urine of the former contains more urea and thus supports greater ammonia production by urea-forming bacteria in the diaper). Another advantage of breast milk is its higher concentration of amino polysaccharides, which play a significant role in stimulating a rapid development of a favorable microflora in the intestinal tract of infants. Such a flora is characterized by the prevalence of lactobacilli (especially *Lactobacillus bifidus*) which seem to exert a protective action against the growth of undesirable pathogenic enteric organisms. In contrast to cow's milk, breast milk also provides protective antibodies against a number of human pathogenic bacteria and viruses and has a much higher protective lysozyme content.

In general, in order to obtain a formula which resembles breast milk, it is the commonly accepted practice to dilute the cow's milk used for the bottle formula of the very young infant in order to reduce its protein content and to make up the caloric deficit with a carbohydrate supplement.

The Bottle Formula and Its Use

The usual daily cow's milk formula contains the following:

$1^1/_2$ to 2 fl oz whole milk/lb body weight
1 oz sugar (as such, or in the form of syrups or dextrins) for each 10 oz milk used
The total fluid requirement is $2^1/_2$ oz/lb body weight, and the formula is diluted with water accordingly

Evaporated milk is widely used in the preparation of formulas. It combines the advantage of constancy in composition, sterility, a readily digested fine curd, good keeping quality, and almost universal availability. It can be used in the above formula as "whole milk" by reconstitution with an equal amount of water. Sweetened condensed milk contains a disproportionately high amount of sugar and should not be used.

Different carbohydrates are used in the formula. The choice is usually made by the pediatrician. They have varying laxative effects, from lactose on down through corn syrup, plain sugar, Dextri-Maltose, starch, and rice or barley flour.

It is customary to prepare a 24-hour supply of formula at one time and to divide it into bottles according to the number of feedings. To assure freedom from pathogenic microorganisms, two methods of sterilization may be used. In one method the fluid mixture is boiled for 3 minutes and then poured into presterilized bottles which are capped and refrigerated. In the simpler and more foolproof terminal sterilization method the formula is divided into clean bottles which are capped and then placed in a closed vessel, half-filled with boiling water. Boiling is continued for 25 minutes and the pasturized bottles are then refrigerated.

The number of feedings per day varies with the age of the infant. Initially, newborn babies are fed at 4-hour intervals. As soon as possible, the midnight feeding is discontinued; eventually the number of feedings decreases as the amount taken at each feeding increases and as solid foods are subsequently introduced. A fixed schedule is not essential, and though a measure of regularity is convenient for all concerned, spontaneous "demand feeding" is popular and frequently used. A baby's appetite varies from time to time, and there is no imperative rule that each prescribed bottle must be finished at each feeding. Conversely, there is no reason to withhold from a hungry infant quantities larger than those scheduled.

Beginning with the second or third week, formula-fed infants should receive 400 units of vitamin D daily, as well as orange juice or a similar source of vitamin C, supplying 35 mg or more.

The formula-fed infant may receive undiluted, boiled cow's milk when the amount of milk in its formula reaches 1 quart. The amount of added carbohydrate and water is lessened gradually for several days before the changeover to straight milk takes place. It is important that the milk be boiled, both for digestibility and freedom from pathogenic organisms, until the infant is at least 6 months old; thereafter pasteurized milk may be used. Weaning to the cup should take place sometime before the end of the first year.

Proprietary Preparations

A number of premixed, concentrated proprietary formulas in liquid or powder form are available. Some of them simulate the composition of human milk; others are modified or unmodified mixtures of milk, sugars, and fats, with or without added minerals and vitamins. They are primarily characterized by convenience at an appropriate cost. A number of these proprietary formulas are specifically formulated to serve the infant who is allergic to cow's milk. There is a definite need and use for *this* type of preparation. The problem of food allergy in infants and adults is discussed in detail in Chap. 39.

Feeding the Premature Infant

The premature infant presents a series of special problems. Its reflexes are imperfectly developed, it has difficulty sucking or swallowing, and it often regurgitates and aspirates its food with dire consequences. Its caloric and ascorbic acid requirements are quite high, and it absorbs fats and the fat-soluble vitamins poorly. It possesses few nutritional reserves despite its higher basal metabolic requirements. Almost invariably, the premature infant suffers some degree of anemia. This deficiency in iron stores combined with a relatively inactive bone marrow and concurrent rapid growth may be reflected in a further decline in hemoglobin levels after birth. In view of the infant's increased nutritive requirements, human milk is not the food of choice for the premature infant.

Though in some places a medicine dropper is used, premature infants are preferably fed with the aid of a small rubber stomach tube or a polyethylene catheter which may be left in place between feedings. The nutritional program is the same as in the case of a full-term infant except for the following: the caloric intake should be increased to 55 to 60 cal per pound body weight; the daily dose of ascorbic acid is increased to 70 mg; the daily vitamin D intake may be increased to 800 IU though 400 IU appears sufficient. The milk protein, calcium, and phosphorus intakes should be adjusted to a higher level than is found in artificial formulas for full-term infants. (From 4 to 6 g protein and 100 to 120 cal per kg body weight have been suggested.)

Introduction of Solid Foods

There have been divergent trends with regard to the appropriate time at which solid foods should be introduced into an infant's diet. It is generally agreed that they should not be given later than the third or fourth month to either breast-fed or formula-fed babies, since a prolonged, exclusive milk diet does not supply all the essential nutrients, particularly iron and thiamin. The conservative upper time limit of 3 to 4 months is in great contrast to the present trend of introducing selected solid infant foods between the sixth and eigth week. (As far back as 1954 it was ascertained in a survey conducted by the *Quarterly Review of Pediatrics* that 66 percent of some 2,000 responding pediatricians routinely began feeding solid foods before 8 weeks of age.)

Digestion, absorption, and utilization of solid foods appear to be adequate even during the first days of life. Strained meat has been shown to be the equivalent of milk as a source of protein and is well tolerated by full-term and premature infants alike. An increased incidence of allergy has not been demonstrated in connection with the introduction of solid foods in the early weeks of life. If a psychologic advantage is present in early feeding of solids, as has been claimed by some, it accrues primarily to the mother. Weakened by her recent delivery, harried by an older child, and beset with a demanding infant who is clamoring for its milk at 4-hour intervals throughout the night, she welcomes the wider spacing of feedings and the earlier cessation of midnight hunger which accompany the introduction of solids to the baby's diet. The extreme point of view is represented by a group of physicians who begin the feeding of solid foods on the second or third day on a 6-hour schedule. According to this system, the first food offered is cereal, morning and night, followed by strained vegetables at 10 days of age. Strained meats are introduced at 14 days, and strained fruits at 17 days. Dropping the midnight feeding is advised at this point, and the infants continue henceforth on a three-meal schedule.

Thus within the last three to four decades, the pendulum has swung from late introduction of solid food supplementation to its introduction in the first weeks and even days of life. The fact that infants seem to do equally well whether solids are introduced at once or at the end of 2 to 3 months attests to the high adaptability of the baby to the whims of its caretakers, provided its nutritional requirements are met.

There should be no time schedules for the feeding of certain foods at particular ages since it only seems to upset the mother if her baby does not follow them. The initial solid food is usually one of the precooked infant cereals. Most infant cereals are enriched with iron and the major B vitamins, which is important since at this point the infant requires a generous allowance of iron (see Chap. 33) and since milk supplies only a minimum of thiamin.

It is easiest to adapt the infant to its first solids by offering it a semiliquid mixture of formula, or milk, and precooked cereal. After several feedings the consistency may be adjusted to a porridgelike quality. Once the baby has accepted one food, a second one may be conveniently added before the regular mealtime bottle. If a particular food is refused, another one should be substituted, and mothers should not persist in forcing a rejected food since this is one way in which feeding problems are started. Gradually a variety of foods is introduced, one at a time, and the infant becomes accustomed to different textures and flavors. Eventually the infant will receive solid foods before all mealtime bottles, and the number of feedings is reduced to three, with milk snacks between meals as demanded by its individual requirements.

The Widening Diet

Next, after infant cereals, strained fruits and vegetables, strained egg yolks, and meats are usually added. (Egg white is commonly postponed until the end of the first year as a precaution against sensitization of an infant who has a latent predisposition to allergies.) As this variety of foods is introduced, feeding by appetite becomes the rule. Meat, eggs, vegetables, and fruits are essential foods for any age. A high intake of meat, eggs, vegetables, and fruit, in contrast to bread, noodles, potatoes, and desserts, should continue in order to encourage the development of desirable food habits as well as to supply needed nutrients.

As teeth come in, the baby may be given crackers and toast to train it to chew its food. Once the infant is capable of chewing, minced or chopped foods ("junior foods") serve as a mechanical transition form; their nutritive makeup is essentially the same as the previously eaten, mixed strained diet. By the eighteenth to twenty-fourth month, most infants are considered ready for a well-balanced "adult" diet (Chap. 15).

Plotting a progressive growth record of the infant in terms of weight and height is an excellent means of determining the adequacy of its dietary intake as well as an aid in the clinical appraisal of its health. Tables 29 and 30 outline the range of weights and heights normally found at various ages in infancy.

During the second year of life, the previously high rate of growth diminishes, the caloric requirement is smaller, and the baby will instinctively eat less. This almost always disturbs the parents, who may try to force the child to eat, which in turn may be the start of a feeding problem.

Feeding Problems

Feeding problems arise easily in early life. Many can be prevented by parental understanding. Many parents do not realize how quickly their own likes and dislikes are communicated to their offspring. A mother's involuntary grimaces when she feeds her infant cod-liver oil or a strained vegetable she does not like are well noticed by the baby, and it soon rejects the particular food.

Many parents have a preconceived idea of how much the infant should eat. They should be warned not to expect the baby to drain each bottle to the last drop since its appetite will vary from feeding to feeding. They must also be patient when newly introduced solid foods are rejected at first. When the baby grows older and its rate of weight gain decreases together with its appetite, and its attention begins to wander in contrast to its previous ravenous interest in food, that is the time when parental self-restraint, instead of forced feeding, will go a long way toward the prevention of future feeding problems.

Infant Feeding Practices and Future Development

Tables 29 and 30 illustrate the ranges of height and weight of "well-born" boys and girls from birth to the end of the second year of life. Normal, well-born, healthy, and well-cared-for infants will generally grow at the same rate whether breast-fed or formula-fed. In fact, even a 15 percent variation in protein intake does not appear to change their growth pattern significantly. Subject to the usual individual genetic variations, a certain consistency and predictability of linear growth exists within the framework of adequate nutrition within the percentile groups depicted in these tables. Thus, intentional overfeeding of an infant will lead only to a predictable increase in weight which is not necessarily desirable.

In recent years it has been demonstrated that overfeeding of *very* young infants may lay the foundation for predisposition to obesity in later life.

Table 29 Weight and Length of Boys from Birth to 2 Years

Age	Measurement		Percentile						
			3	10	25	50	75	90	97
Birth	Weight	pounds	5.8	6.3	6.9	7.5	8.3	9.1	10.1
		kilograms	2.63	2.86	3.13	3.4	3.76	4.13	4.58
	Length	inches	18.2	18.9	19.4	19.9	20.5	21.0	21.5
		centimeters	46.3	48.1	49.3	50.6	52.0	53.3	54.6
3 months	Weight	pounds	10.6	11.1	11.8	12.6	13.6	14.5	16.4
		kilograms	4.81	5.03	5.35	5.72	6.17	6.58	7.44
	Length	inches	22.4	22.8	23.3	23.8	24.3	24.7	25.1
		centimeters	56.8	57.8	59.3	60.4	61.8	62.8	63.7
6 months	Weight	pounds	14.0	14.8	15.6	16.7	18.0	19.2	20.8
		kilograms	6.35	6.71	7.08	7.58	8.16	8.71	9.43
	Length	inches	24.8	25.2	25.7	26.1	26.7	27.3	27.7
		centimeters	63.0	63.9	65.2	66.4	67.8	69.3	70.4
9 months	Weight	pounds	16.6	17.8	18.7	20.0	21.5	22.9	24.4
		kilograms	7.53	8.07	8.48	9.07	9.75	10.39	11.07
	Length	inches	26.6	27.0	27.5	28.0	28.7	29.2	29.9
		centimeters	67.7	68.6	69.8	71.2	72.9	74.2	75.9
12 months	Weight	pounds	18.5	19.6	20.9	22.2	23.8	25.4	27.3
		kilograms	8.39	8.89	9.48	10.07	10.8	11.52	12.38
	Length	inches	28.1	28.5	29.0	29.6	30.3	30.7	31.6
		centimeters	71.3	72.4	73.7	75.2	76.9	78.1	80.3
15 months	Weight	pounds	19.8	21.0	22.4	23.7	25.4	27.2	29.4
		kilograms	8.98	9.53	10.16	10.75	11.52	12.34	13.33
	Length	inches	29.3	29.8	30.3	30.9	31.6	32.1	33.1
		centimeters	74.4	75.6	77.0	78.5	80.3	81.5	84.2
18 months	Weight	pounds	21.1	22.3	23.8	25.2	26.9	29.0	31.5
		kilograms	9.57	10.12	10.8	11.43	12.2	13.15	14.29
	Length	inches	30.5	31.0	31.6	32.2	32.9	33.5	34.7
		centimeters	77.5	78.8	80.3	81.8	83.7	85.0	88.2
2 years	Weight	pounds	23.3	24.7	26.3	27.7	29.7	31.9	34.9
		kilograms	10.57	11.2	11.93	12.56	13.47	14.47	15.83
	Length	inches	32.6	33.1	33.8	34.4	35.2	35.9	37.2
		centimeters	82.7	84.2	85.8	87.5	89.4	91.1	94.6

Source: H. C. Stuart, in Nelson, "Textbook of Pediatrics," 8th ed., W. B. Saunders Company, Philadelphia, 1964.

Normally nourished infants develop a fixed number of fat cells in their adipose tissues which does not change with increasing age. Later in life in the presence of a positive calorie balance, excess calories are stored in the form of fat in the

Table 30   Weight and Length of Girls from Birth to 2 Years

Age	Measurement		Percentile						
			3	10	25	50	75	90	97
Birth	Weight	pounds	5.8	6.2	6.9	7.4	8.1	8.6	9.4
		kilograms	2.63	2.81	3.13	3.36	3.67	3.9	4.26
	Length	inches	18.5	18.8	19.3	19.8	20.1	20.4	21.1
		centimeters	47.1	47.8	49.0	50.2	51.0	51.9	53.6
3 months	Weight	pounds	9.8	10.7	11.4	12.4	13.2	14.0	14.9
		kilograms	4.45	4.85	5.17	5.62	5.99	6.35	6.76
	Length	inches	22.0	22.4	22.8	23.4	23.9	24.3	24.8
		centimeters	55.8	56.9	57.9	59.5	60.7	61.7	63.1
6 months	Weight	pounds	12.7	14.1	15.0	16.0	17.5	18.6	20.0
		kilograms	5.76	6.4	6.8	7.26	7.94	8.44	9.07
	Length	inches	24.0	24.6	25.1	25.7	26.2	26.7	27.1
		centimeters	61.1	62.5	63.7	65.2	66.6	67.8	68.8
9 months	Weight	pounds	15.1	16.6	17.8	19.2	20.8	22.4	24.2
		kilograms	6.85	7.53	8.03	8.71	9.43	10.16	10.98
	Length	inches	25.7	26.4	26.9	27.6	28.2	28.7	29.2
		centimeters	65.4	67.0	68.4	70.1	71.7	72.9	74.1
12 months	Weight	pounds	16.8	18.4	19.8	21.5	23.0	24.8	27.1
		kilograms	7.62	8.35	8.98	9.75	10.43	11.25	12.29
	Length	inches	27.1	27.8	28.5	29.2	29.9	30.3	31.0
		centimeters	68.9	70.6	72.3	74.2	75.9	77.1	78.8
15 months	Weight	pounds	18.1	19.8	21.3	23.0	24.6	26.6	29.0
		kilograms	8.21	8.98	9.66	10.43	11.16	12.07	13.15
	Length	inches	28.3	29.0	29.8	30.5	31.3	31.8	32.6
		centimeters	71.9	73.7	75.6	77.6	79.4	80.8	82.8
18 months	Weight	pounds	19.4	21.2	22.7	24.5	26.2	28.3	30.9
		kilograms	8.8	9.62	10.3	11.11	11.88	12.84	14.02
	Length	inches	29.5	30.2	31.1	31.8	32.6	33.3	34.1
		centimeters	74.9	76.8	79.0	80.9	82.9	84.5	86.7
2 years	Weight	pounds	21.6	23.5	25.3	27.1	29.2	31.7	34.4
		kilograms	9.8	10.66	11.48	12.29	13.25	14.38	15.6
	Length	inches	31.5	32.3	33.3	34.1	35.0	35.8	36.7
		centimeters	80.1	82.0	84.7	86.6	88.9	91.0	93.3

Source: H. C. Stuart, in Nelson, "Textbook of Pediatrics," 8th ed., W. B. Saunders Company, Philadelphia, 1964.

existing fat cells, each one of which increases in size as it stores more fat. During a period of negative calorie balance (as when the individual purposefully limits his food intake), the adipose tissues will shrink again as each fat cell decreases in size as it releases stored depot fat for provision of needed energy. Overfeeding of a young infant stimulates the development of a significantly greater than normal number of fat cells in such an individual, which in turn facilitates the future ready elaboration of larger masses of adipose tissue during later life with a tendency to greater difficulty in regaining of normal weight— especially if this is coupled with a *continued* habit of overfeeding and overeating during childhood and adolescence.

Chapter 18

Nutrition in Childhood and Adolescence

The nutritional needs of children and adolescents are unique and demand special attention. These requirements are conditioned primarily by the building and maintenance of new body tissue, by the demands of a high order of physical activity, and to some extent by interrelated intrinsic and environmental factors, such as emotional changes as the growing child reacts to his maturation and his surroundings. In general, the growing child and adolescent require a high caloric intake because of their great activity and an abundance of good-quality protein and minerals because of their rapid growth. The need for vitamins is enhanced beyond that of a sedentary adult because of the characteristic high metabolic activity of this period in the life cycle.

One means of judging the adequacy of the diet in childhood is the plotting of height and corresponding weight with progressing age. Such a record is also helpful in the clinical evaluation of general health. Tables 31 to 34 outline the range of height and weight data normally encountered at different ages in childhood and adolescence.

Physiologic Considerations

Between the ages of 2 and 12, growth is a more or less gradual process which poses its enhanced nutritive requirements in a relatively conservative fashion.

The pace is accelerated during adolescence when the growing individual advances from childhood to manhood or womanhood. Adolescence is a period of highly accelerated physical growth, development of secondary sex characteristics and eventual sexual maturation, and a change in mental attitudes, interests, and emotional responses. In terms of nutrition, this period introduces not only greatly enhanced needs for nutrients to meet the demands of physical growth, but also a shift in the food habits of the child to the concepts of the adult of what constitutes an adult choice of foods.

Adolescent growth exhibits a maximum acceleration just before sexual maturation, with deceleration almost immediately thereafter. The concurrent basal metabolism increases when growth is more intense and drops soon after sexual maturation. In extreme instances the premenarcheal rise in basal metabolism in girls may approach the limits of a hyperthyroid state while the subsequent fall may approach the levels of a hypothyroid state. The prepubescent growth acceleration and maturation occur earlier in girls than in boys and thus make for a different nutritional timetable for each sex from the twelfth year on.

Growth rates differ from individual to individual, and the onset of physiologic maturation may come at any time between the eleventh and sixteenth years. Hence judicious caution is indicated in using an "average" figure in the evaluation of individual growth and dietary adequacy.

Caloric Requirements

The dietary allowances recommended by the Food and Nutrition Board for childhood and adolescence are summarized in Table 22. Average caloric requirements increase from 1300 cal for boys and girls 1 to 3 years of age to 2400 cal at the age of 7 to 10. The average requirement for boys 11 to 14 years old is 2800 cal; it increases to 3000 cal between the fifteenth and eighteenth years, in contrast to 2700 between the ages of 23 and 50, and 2400 in those over 51. In girls, the picture is similar, though here maturation, and thus maximal caloric need, occurs at an earlier age. On the average, girls 11 to 14 years old require 2400 cal—more than at any other time during their life cycle, except for periods of pregnancy and lactation. The difference between the energy requirements of adolescent boys and girls exists primarily because boys ordinarily grow to a larger stature and are physically more more active.

Protein and Mineral Requirements

The protein and mineral requirements in childhood and adolescence exhibit a trend similar to caloric needs. While linear skeletal growth is most obvious, the skeleton mineralizes progressively throughout childhood and early adult life and continues to become heavier long after linear growth has ceased. Calcium and phosphorus, the main constituents of mature bone, must be adequately provided by food for normal skeletal development. The recommended calcium allowance for boys and girls rises from 0.8 g per day at the age of 1 to 1.2 g between the ages of 11 and 18. This value contrasts considerably with the recommended allowances of 0.8 g for adult men or nonpregnant, nonlactating adult women.

In the growing body frame, muscle growth should keep pace with skeletal growth. This calls for active elaboration of muscle tissue, an increase in blood volume and blood constituents, and a continuous positive nitrogen balance. Optimal growth and nitrogen assimilation can take place only if the child's food provides an abundance of all the essential amino acids and other nutrients required for growth and sufficient calories from nonprotein food sources to spare the protein so that it is not utilized for the creation of energy but for tissue synthesis. While growing children may continue to gain in height and weight on suboptimal food intakes, this is likely to result in mineral-poor bone, nitrogen-poor soft tissues, borderline or frank anemia, a depressed metabolism, a decrease in physical activity, and an increased susceptibility to infection. Loss of resistance to disease at the time of puberty is seen particularly in girls, whose growth spurt is less prolonged and more rapid. The hormonal changes which occur at this time are also partially responsible for much of this loss of resistance; nevertheless an increased intake of protective foods, with particular emphasis on protein, is essential with the first signs of puberty.

The recommended daily allowance for protein rises gradually through the ages of 1 to 10 from 23 g to 36 g. The allowance for boys 11 to 14 years old is 44 g and rises to 54 g between the ages of 15 and 22 (in contrast to 56 g for adult and elderly men). The corresponding recommended allowances for girls are 44 g for ages 11 to 14, 48 g for ages 15 to 18, and 46 g thereafter.

The daily iron allowance rises from early infancy (10 mg) to 15 mg from the middle of the first to the fourth year. It drops to 10 mg per day between the fourth and the tenth years. Thereafter, in males it rises to 18 mg during adolescence and stabilizes at 10 mg in males of subsequent ages—reflecting the increased requirement of adolescence and its rapid growth. The recommended allowance for girls and women, 11 to 51 years old, is 18 mg of iron daily, and subsides to 10 mg thereafter—reflecting the increased iron demands of menstruation and childbearing.

Other Nutrients

Vitamin D is essential for optimal calcium and phosphorus assimilation. Though many children receive sufficient sunshine in the summer for endogenous vitamin D synthesis, few receive enough in the winter. Giving some sort of vitamin D preparation in early infancy has become routine in most households; however, too few parents realize the importance of continuation of vitamin D supplementation through the balance of childhood. To ensure a daily supply of 400 IU of vitamin D, it is appropriate to consider the routine consumption of vitamin D milk, a quart of which will not only supply this amount but also satisfy the daily calcium requirement.

The allowances for thiamin, riboflavin, niacin, and ascorbic acid follow the trend exhibited by the caloric need; these daily requirements increase gradually during early childhood, to spurt to a lifetime high during adolescence (Table 22). The vitamin A requirement is primarily proportional to body weight. It thus increases gradually through early childhood and reaches its high level in adolescence; it remains at this level throughout the remainder of adult life.

Food Patterns during School Age

The diets of children have improved in many ways over those of the past. In the United States, today's children and adolescents are taller and heavier than they were a generation or two ago. The reason for this is not wholly nutritional since freedom from disease and other unfavorable environmental factors has played an important part in this development. Nevertheless, within the limits imposed by the genetic potential of the individual, the improvement in the quality of diets has permitted growth to reach approximately maximal levels.

While general overall averages of per capita food consumption appear satisfactory, there is abundant evidence of unequal distribution of food and dietary essentials. Ascorbic acid, calcium, thiamin, riboflavin, and iron are the nutrients most commonly deficient in juvenile diets. The increased caloric need of the growing youngster is ordinarily reflected in his appetite. Unless additional food is provided during scheduled mealtimes, the individual resorts to between-meal snacks. Much of this extra food consists of candy and soft drinks which abound in calories but may make little contribution of other nutrients to the diet.

Practices commonly found among youngsters of school age which set the stage for dietary inadequacy are (1) small, poorly chosen, or omitted breakfasts, (2) inadequate lunches eaten away from home, (3) choice of food left to the child, without adult guidance, (4) failure to eat enough meats, eggs, vegetables, and fruits, (5) expenditure of school lunch money on candy and soft drinks, which constitues a substitution of "empty" calories for what might have been a well-balanced diet. To this list may be added occasional self-imposed dieting on the part of girls who attempt to achieve artificial standards of slimness and on the part of boys who follow ill-advised diets in an effort to improve unsightly acne. Obesity may also present a problem in the adolescent. Many adolescent girls have often been chubby throughout their early childhood, but vanity—coming with pubescence—makes them conscious of their appearance and they attempt to adjust their food intake. In some girls, however, there may develop an attitude of defeatism with gradual withdrawal from sports and social activities and compensatory overindulgence in food. A similar cycle may be found in the male, though perhaps to a smaller extent.

Optimal nutrition for female teen-agers is of particular importance since in recent years the age of the first pregnancy has been decreasing progressively. Consequently a growing percentage of girls in the late teens not only have a suboptimal dietary intake for themselves, but are not equipped with sufficient

Table 31   Weight and Height of Boys from 2 to 5 Years

Age	Measurement		Percentile						
			3	10	25	50	75	90	97
2 years	Weight	pounds	23.3	24.7	26.3	27.7	29.7	31.9	34.9
		kilograms	10.57	11.2	11.93	12.56	13.47	14.47	15.83
	Height	inches	32.6	33.1	33.8	34.4	35.2	35.9	37.2
		centimeters	82.7	84.2	85.8	87.5	89.4	91.1	94.6
2½ years	Weight	pounds	25.2	26.6	28.4	30.0	32.2	34.5	37.0
		kilograms	11.43	12.07	12.88	13.61	14.61	15.65	16.78
	Height	inches	34.2	34.8	35.5	36.3	37.0	37.9	39.2
		centimeters	86.9	88.5	90.2	92.1	94.1	96.2	99.5
3 years	Weight	pounds	27.0	28.7	30.3	32.2	34.5	36.8	39.2
		kilograms	12.25	13.02	13.74	14.61	15.65	16.69	17.78
	Height	inches	35.7	36.3	37.0	37.9	38.8	39.6	40.5
		centimeters	90.6	92.3	93.9	96.2	98.5	100.5	102.8
3½ years	Weight	pounds	28.5	30.4	32.3	34.3	36.7	39.1	41.5
		kilograms	12.93	13.79	14.65	15.56	16.65	17.74	18.82
	Height	inches	37.1	37.8	38.4	39.3	40.3	41.1	41.9
		centimeters	94.3	96.0	97.5	99.8	102.5	104.5	106.5
4 years	Weight	pounds	30.1	32.1	34.0	36.4	39.0	41.4	44.3
		kilograms	13.65	14.56	15.42	16.51	17.69	18.78	20.09
	Height	inches	38.4	39.1	39.7	40.7	41.9	42.7	43.5
		centimeters	97.5	99.3	100.8	103.4	106.5	108.5	110.4
4½ years	Weight	pounds	31.6	33.8	35.7	38.4	41.4	43.9	47.4
		kilograms	14.33	15.33	16.19	17.42	18.78	19.91	21.5
	Height	inches	39.6	40.3	40.9	42.0	43.3	44.2	45.0
		centimeters	100.6	102.4	104.0	106.7	109.9	112.3	114.3
5 years	Weight	pounds	33.6	35.5	37.5	40.5	44.1	46.7	50.4
		kilograms	15.24	16.1	17.01	18.37	20.0	21.18	22.86
	Height	inches	40.2	40.8	41.7	42.8	44.2	45.2	46.1
		centimeters	102.0	103.7	105.9	108.7	112.3	114.7	117.1

Source: H. C. Stuart, in Nelson, "Textbook of Pediatrics," 8th ed., W. B. Saunders Company, Philadelphia, 1964.

nutritional reserve for their future infants. Since many times they are also at the peak of the emotional instability of adolescence, there is little likelihood that a sudden improvement of their diet will take place once a pregnancy has been established.

Evidence from dietary surveys indicates that many adolescents are ill-nourished and that their food intake is more variable and less adequate than that of any other age group. While family commensality exerts the most

Table 32 Weight and Height of Girls from 2 to 5 Years

Age	Measurement		Percentile						
			3	10	25	50	75	90	97
2 years	Weight	pounds	21.6	23.5	25.3	27.1	29.2	31.7	34.4
		kilograms	9.8	10.66	11.48	12.29	13.25	14.38	15.6
	Height	inches	31.5	32.3	33.3	34.1	35.0	35.8	36.7
		centimeters	80.1	82.0	84.7	86.6	88.9	91.0	93.3
2½ years	Weight	pounds	23.6	25.5	27.4	29.6	31.9	34.6	38.2
		kilograms	10.7	11.57	12.43	13.43	14.47	15.69	17.33
	Height	inches	33.3	34.0	35.2	36.0	36.9	37.9	38.9
		centimeters	84.5	86.3	89.3	91.4	93.8	96.4	98.7
3 years	Weight	pounds	25.6	27.6	29.6	31.8	34.6	37.4	41.8
		kilograms	11.61	12.52	13.43	14.42	15.69	16.96	18.96
	Height	inches	34.8	35.6	36.8	37.7	38.6	39.8	40.7
		centimeters	88.4	90.5	93.4	95.7	98.1	101.1	103.5
3½ years	Weight	pounds	27.5	29.5	31.5	33.9	37.0	40.4	45.3
		kilograms	12.47	13.38	14.29	15.38	16.78	18.33	20.55
	Height	inches	36.2	37.1	38.1	39.2	40.2	41.5	42.5
		centimeters	92.0	94.2	96.9	99.5	102.0	105.4	108.0
4 years	Weight	pounds	29.2	31.2	33.5	36.2	39.6	43.5	48.2
		kilograms	13.25	14.15	15.2	16.42	17.96	19.73	21.86
	Height	inches	37.5	38.4	39.5	40.6	41.6	43.1	44.2
		centimeters	95.2	97.6	100.3	103.2	105.8	109.6	112.3
4½ years	Weight	pounds	30.7	32.9	35.3	38.5	42.1	46.7	50.9
		kilograms	13.93	14.92	16.01	17.46	19.1	21.18	23.09
	Height	inches	38.6	39.7	40.8	42.0	43.0	44.7	45.7
		centimeters	98.1	100.9	103.6	106.8	109.3	113.5	116.2
5 years	Weight	pounds	32.1	34.8	37.4	40.5	44.8	49.2	52.8
		kilograms	14.56	15.79	16.96	18.37	20.32	22.32	23.95
	Height	inches	39.4	40.5	41.6	42.9	44.0	45.4	46.8
		centimeters	100.0	103.0	105.7	109.1	111.7	115.4	118.8

Source: H. C. Stuart, in Nelson, "Textbook of Pediatrics," 8th ed., W. B. Saunders Company, Philadelphia, 1964.

important influence on the dietary habits of the child, as the adolescent moves toward independence, the influence of the family meal pattern wanes. More meals are eaten away from home, the adolescent's attitudes and routines are changed with peer acceptance a paramount goal, and too often this leads to the development of limited dietary habits and the restriction of food choices to a relatively small number of favorite "in" items. The influence of sometimes misleading commercial advertising and food faddism and misinformation

Table 33 Weight and Height of Boys from 5 to 18 Years

Age	Measurement		Percentile						
			3	10	25	50	75	90	97
5 years*	Weight	pounds	34.5	36.6	39.6	42.8	46.5	49.7	53.2
		kilograms	15.65	16.6	17.96	19.41	21.09	22.54	24.13
	Height	inches	40.2	41.5	42.6	43.8	45.0	45.9	47.0
		centimeters	102.1	105.3	108.3	111.3	114.2	116.7	119.5
6 years	Weight	pounds	38.5	40.9	44.4	48.3	52.1	56.4	61.1
		kilograms	17.46	18.55	20.14	21.91	23.63	25.58	27.71
	Height	inches	42.7	43.8	44.9	46.3	47.6	48.6	49.7
		centimeters	108.5	111.2	114.1	117.5	120.8	123.5	126.2
7 years	Weight	pounds	43.0	45.8	49.7	54.1	58.7	64.4	69.9
		kilograms	19.5	20.77	22.54	24.54	26.63	29.21	31.71
	Height	inches	44.9	46.0	47.4	48.9	50.2	51.4	52.5
		centimeters	114.0	116.9	120.3	124.1	127.6	130.5	133.4
8 years	Weight	pounds	48.0	51.2	55.5	60.1	65.5	73.0	79.4
		kilograms	21.77	23.22	25.17	27.76	29.71	33.11	36.02
	Height	inches	47.1	48.5	49.8	51.2	52.8	54.0	55.2
		centimeters	119.6	123.1	126.6	130.0	134.2	137.3	140.2
9 years	Weight	pounds	52.5	56.3	61.1	66.0	72.3	81.0	89.8
		kilograms	23.81	25.54	27.71	29.94	32.8	36.74	40.73
	Height	inches	48.9	50.5	51.8	53.3	55.0	56.1	57.2
		centimeters	124.2	128.3	131.6	135.5	139.8	142.6	145.3
10 years	Weight	pounds	56.8	61.1	66.3	71.9	79.6	89.9	100.0
		kilograms	25.76	27.71	30.07	32.61	36.11	40.78	45.36
	Height	inches	50.7	52.3	53.7	55.2	56.8	58.1	59.2
		centimeters	128.7	132.8	136.3	140.3	144.4	147.5	150.3
11 years	Weight	pounds	61.8	66.3	71.6	77.6	87.2	99.3	111.7
		kilograms	28.03	30.07	32.48	35.2	39.55	45.04	50.67
	Height	inches	52.5	54.0	55.3	56.8	58.7	59.8	60.8
		centimeters	133.4	137.3	140.5	144.2	149.2	151.8	154.4
12 years	Weight	pounds	67.2	72.0	77.5	84.4	96.0	109.6	124.2
		kilograms	30.48	32.66	35.15	38.28	43.55	49.71	56.34
	Height	inches	54.4	56.1	57.2	58.9	60.4	62.2	63.7
		centimeters	138.1	142.4	145.2	149.6	153.5	157.9	161.9
13 years	Weight	pounds	72.0	77.1	83.7	93.0	107.9	123.2	138.0
		kilograms	32.66	34.97	37.97	42.18	48.94	55.88	62.6
	Height	inches	56.0	57.7	58.9	61.0	63.3	65.1	66.7
		centimeters	142.2	146.6	149.7	155.0	160.8	165.3	169.5

Table 33—Cont'd. Weight and Height of Boys from 5 to 18 Years

Age	Measurement		Percentile						
			3	10	25	50	75	90	97
14 years	Weight	pounds	79.8	87.2	95.5	107.6	123.1	136.9	150.6
		kilograms	36.2	39.55	43.32	48.81	55.84	62.1	68.31
	Height	inches	57.6	59.9	61.6	64.0	66.3	67.9	69.7
		centimeters	146.4	152.1	156.5	162.7	168.4	172.4	177.1
15 years	Weight	pounds	91.3	99.4	108.2	120.1	135.0	147.8	161.6
		kilograms	41.41	45.09	49.08	54.48	61.23	67.04	73.3
	Height	inches	59.7	62.1	63.9	66.1	68.1	69.6	71.6
		centimeters	151.7	157.8	162.3	167.8	173.0	176.7	181.8
16 years	Weight	pounds	103.4	111.0	118.7	129.7	144.4	157.3	170.5
		kilograms	46.9	50.35	53.84	58.83	65.5	71.35	77.34
	Height	inches	61.6	64.1	65.8	67.8	69.5	70.7	73.1
		centimeters	156.5	162.8	167.1	171.6	176.6	179.7	185.6
17 years	Weight	pounds	110.5	117.5	124.5	136.2	151.4	164.6	175.6
		kilograms	50.12	53.3	56.47	61.78	68.67	74.66	79.65
	Height	inches	62.6	65.2	66.8	68.4	70.1	71.5	73.5
		centimeters	159.0	165.5	169.7	173.7	178.1	181.6	186.6
18 years	Weight.	pounds	113.0	120.0	127.1	139.0	155.7	169.0	179.0
		kilograms	51.26	54.43	57.65	63.05	70.62	76.66	81.19
	Height	inches	62.8	65.5	67.0	68.7	70.4	71.8	73.9
		centimeters	159.6	166.3	170.5	174.5	178.9	182.4	187.6

*Several measurements at 5 years differ slightly from their counterparts in Table 31 because they were obtained from a different population of children.

Source: The data in this table are from studies by and are reproduced by courtesy of Howard V. Meredith, Ph.D., Iowa Child Welfare Research Station, State University of Iowa.

among teen-agers has become a significant factor, and concern for ecology and distrust of scientific progress (often equated with the "establishment" in many adolescent minds) has led to an increased use of "natural" or "organic" foods. Today's teen-agers are largely intelligent, more sophisticated, inquisitive, and critical; they are also less well-nourished and need and deserve objective, straightforward nutrition information in a nonpedantic fashion which will help them understand their nutritional needs and problems.

Dietary Recommendations

The essential nutrients as well as calories must be amply provided if the growing child is to achieve his maximum growth potential and well-being and the physical equipment to meet adolescent and adult life. This is best achieved

Table 34 Weight and Height of Girls from 5 to 18 Years

Age	Measurement		Percentile						
			3	10	25	50	75	90	97
5 years*	Weight	pounds	33.7	36.1	38.6	41.4	44.2	48.2	51.8
		kilograms	15.29	16.37	17.51	18.78	20.05	21.86	23.5
	Height	inches	40.4	41.3	42.2	43.2	44.4	45.4	46.5
		centimeters	102.6	105.0	107.2	109.7	112.9	115.4	118.0
6 years	Weight	pounds	37.2	39.6	42.9	46.5	50.2	54.2	58.7
		kilograms	16.87	17.96	19.46	21.09	22.77	24.58	26.63
	Height	inches	42.5	43.5	44.6	45.6	47.0	48.1	49.4
		centimeters	108.0	110.6	113.2	115.9	119.3	122.3	125.4
7 years	Weight.	pounds	41.3	44.5	48.1	52.2	56.3	61.2	67.3
		kilograms	18.73	20.19	21.82	23.68	25.54	27.76	30.53
	Height	inches	44.9	46.0	46.9	48.1	49.6	50.7	51.9
		centimeters	114.0	116.8	119.2	122.3	125.9	128.9	131.7
8 years	Weight	pounds	45.3	48.6	53.1	58.1	63.3	69.9	78.9
		kilograms	20.55	22.04	24.09	26.35	28.71	31.71	35.79
	Height	inches	46.9	48.1	49.1	50.4	51.8	53.0	54.1
		centimeters	119.1	122.1	124.8	128.0	131.6	134.6	137.4
9 years	Weight	pounds	49.1	52.6	57.9	63.8	70.5	79.1	89.9
		kilograms	22.27	23.86	26.26	28.94	31.98	35.88	40.78
	Height	inches	48.7	50.0	51.1	52.3	54.0	55.3	56.5
		centimeters	123.6	127.0	129.7	132.9	137.1	140.4	143.4
10 years	Weight	pounds	53.2	57.1	62.8	70.3	79.1	89.7	101.9
		kilograms	24.13	25.9	28.49	31.89	35.88	40.69	46.22
	Height	inches	50.3	51.8	53.0	54.6	56.1	57.5	58.8
		centimeters	127.7	131.7	134.6	138.6	142.6	146.0	149.3
11 years	Weight	pounds	57.9	62.6	69.9	78.8	89.1	100.4	112.9
		kilograms	26.26	28.4	31.71	35.74	40.42	45.54	51.21
	Height	inches	52.1	53.9	55.2	57.0	58.7	60.4	62.0
		centimeters	132.3	137.0	140.3	144.7	149.2	153.4	157.4
12 years	Weight	pounds	63.6	69.5	78.0	87.6	98.8	111.5	127.7
		kilograms	28.85	31.52	35.38	39.74	44.82	50.58	57.92
	Height	inches	54.3	56.1	57.4	59.8	61.6	63.2	64.8
		centimeters	137.8	142.6	145.9	151.9	156.6	160.6	164.6
13 years	Weight	pounds	72.2	79.9	89.4	99.1	111.0	124.5	142.3
		kilograms	32.75	36.24	40.55	44.95	50.35	56.47	64.55
		inches	56.6	58.7	60.1	61.8	63.6	64.9	66.3
	Height	centimeters	143.7	149.1	152.6	157.1	161.5	164.8	168.4

Table 34—Cont'd. Weight and Height of Girls from 5 to 18 Years

Age	Measurement		Percentile						
			3	10	25	50	75	90	97
14 years	Weight	pounds	83.1	91.0	99.8	108.4	119.7	133.3	150.8
		kilograms	37.69	41.28	45.27	49.17	54.29	60.46	68.4
	Height	inches	58.3	60.2	61.5	62.8	64.4	65.7	67.2
		centimeters	148.2	153.0	156.1	159.6	163.7	167.0	170.7
15 years	Weight	pounds	89.0	97.4	105.1	113.5	123.9	138.1	155.2
		kilograms	40.37	44.18	47.67	51.48	56.2	62.64	70.4
	Height	inches	59.1	61.1	62.1	63.4	64.9	66.2	67.6
		centimeters	150.2	155.2	157.7	161.1	164.9	168.1	171.6
16 years	Weight	pounds	91.8	100.9	108.4	117.0	127.2	141.1	157.7
		kilograms	41.64	45.77	49.17	53.07	57.7	64.0	71.53
	Height	inches	59.4	61.5	62.4	63.9	65.2	66.5	67.7
		centimeters	150.8	156.1	158.6	162.2	165.7	169.0	172.0
17 years	Weight	pounds	93.9	102.8	110.4	119.1	129.6	143.3	159.5
		kilograms	42.59	46.63	50.08	54.02	58.79	65.0	72.35
	Height	inches	59.4	61.5	62.6	64.0	65.4	66.7	67.8
		centimeters	151.0	156.3	159.0	162.5	166.1	169.4	172.2
18 years	Weight	pounds	94.5	103.5	111.2	119.9	130.8	144.5	160.7
		kilograms	42.87	46.95	50.44	54.39	59.33	65.54	72.89
	Height	inches	59.4	61.5	62.6	64.0	65.4	66.7	67.8
		centimeters	151.0	156.3	159.0	162.5	166.1	169.4	172.2

*Several measurements at 5 years differ slightly from their counterparts in Table 32 because they were obtained from a different population of children.

Source: The data in this table are from studies by and are reproduced by courtesy of Howard V. Meredith, Ph.D., Iowa Child Welfare Research Station, State University of Iowa.

with the aid of three satisfying meals per day, to provide the protective foods at adequate levels, and afternoon and bedtime snacks which include milk or a flavored milk drink. The meal plan should follow the outline given in Chap. 15.

Emphasis should be placed on an adequate breakfast, since this meal follows a prolonged period of fasting, and a skimpy breakfast or its outright omission may lead to a decrease in attention span and efficiency in school or at work during the late morning hours. A breakfast which contributes substantial amounts of protein, fat, and carbohydrate facilitates the maintenance of blood sugar levels above the fasting level in the late morning hours and tends to sustain mental alertness and physical activity until lunchtime. Comparison experiments have indicated that among schoolchildren the habitual omission of breakfast results in decreased efficiency in the late morning; it runs parallel with a poorer attitude toward schoolwork and appears to detract from scholastic attainments. In this connection, the precise food-item content of breakfast does not seem to be a determining factor in its efficiency as long as it is basically adequate and balanced from the standpoint of nutritional content. In this respect, a breakfast may be considered optimal if it provides one-third of the daily caloric requirement and one-third, or more, of the daily protein allowance.

In view of the high protein requirement in adolescence, the meat, fish, or poultry servings should be large and at least one egg should be eaten each day, especially by teen-age girls to help supply them with much needed dietary iron to compensate for blood-iron losses during menstruation and to prevent progressive anemia, particularly if they become mothers at an early age.

If at all possible, a milk quota of 2 pints should be observed because milk serves as the main source of calcium and a major source of protein and riboflavin. It may be consumed as whole milk or in the form of cocoa or chocolate milk; it may be made into custards and puddings, or it may be taken in the form of cheese; but it should never be ignored. When fresh milk is not readily available, the dried or canned evaporated article is quite suitable. Simple desserts are acceptable if taken in moderation and at the right time. They should be eaten only at the end of the meal since otherwise they will satiate the youngster before the more essential food items are consumed. If the outline in Chap. 15 is followed at mealtime, snack items and social eating may be considered chiefly a supplementary source of calories. Sweets and between-meal snacks should be permitted only if there is no indication that they interfere with appetite for the scheduled main meals of good nutritive rating.

Variety should be maintained in the diet, and the child must be taught to eat portions of everything reasonable and wholesome which is served at the table. Permitting a child to develop peculiarities of taste is a mistake of convenience which may turn into a definite handicap in adult life. Whereas the toddler and very young children tend to dawdle over their food, many preadolescents prefer to rush through their meals in order to leave the table and return to their own pursuits. Regularity of meals and lack of haste are important, and the child or adolescent should never be permitted to "wolf" a meal. An atmosphere of courtesy, pleasantry, and interest at mealtime is important in creating behavior and meal patterns which become increasingly important with the years.

Good food, exercise, recreation, and rest are all important factors in a program of healthful living. When the growing youngster does not respond to such a regimen with overt evidence of good nourishment, the problem may be a metabolic disorder, an infection, or an emotional disturbance and may require medical attention beyond the realm of dietetic adjustment.

Chapter 19

Geriatric Nutrition

Sound nutrition in the elderly is not fundamentally different from normal nutrition in the mature adult. The basic requirements for satisfactory metabolism are essentially similar throughout life. However, certain characteristics inherent in the process of aging and peculiar to the elderly add unique facets to geriatric nutrition. The major factors which affect the nutritional status of the aged are discussed below.

Inadequate Dentition

Most individuals do not reach old age with a full complement of teeth. Inadequate dentition and ill-fitting uncomfortable dentures are important contributors to undernutrition in old age. In the absence of normal mastication, food is inadequately prepared for digestion. Poor dentition results in avoidance of foods which require thorough mastication and tends to limit the diet to softer foods. As time goes by important food items are automatically excluded from the diet, especially meats and the normal sources of bulk, fruits and vegetables.

Social and Economic Status

Economic factors are of paramount significance in the food pattern of most elderly people. There is a tendency to eat the cheaper carbohydrate foods and to bypass the nutritionally more important, but also more expensive, protein foods. Packaged bakery goods are cheap and require no further preparation and thus enjoy a popularity among the elderly which is not justifiable from the standpoint of nutritional well-being. Many elderly people live alone and lack the facilities to properly prepare meals and keep foods. Moreover, under such lonely circumstances there is little incentive to have organized meals at all. Some elderly persons have family conflicts and nurse justified or imaginary grievances which are reflected in their refusal to eat properly, while others are physically unable to take care of themselves and to get around with enough ease to obtain proper food.

Habits

Eating habits are one of the greatest obstacles to the establishment of optimal diets among the majority of persons. Habits, good, bad, or indifferent, are acquired and fixed by repetition. The longer food habits have been indulged in, the more rigid and ingrained they become. The dietary pattern of many elderly persons is thus a formidable structure, difficult to modify, and in too many cases it is based on gustatory preference, self-indulgence, prejudice, indifference, lack of appetite, poor fluid intake, apathy, and fear—fear of the "wrong" foods, fear of constipation, or fear of "indigestion." Moreover, the present-day ready availability of milk, fruits, and vegetables did not exist when most 70-year-olds were young and were forming their personal food habits.

Physiologic Factors

With advancing age there is a diminishing sensitivity to taste and smell which interferes with the normal pleasure associated with eating. Secretion of hydrochloric acid in the stomach and digestive enzymes in general also diminishes, and the total volume of secretions of the gastrointestinal tract decreases. Thus digestion and absorption may not be optimal in many elderly persons. Biliary impairment is not infrequent; it interferes with normal digestion and utilization of fats and may result in gaseousness and discomfort after the ingestion of fatty foods. Low stores of the fat-soluble vitamins are not uncommon, either because of voluntary abstention from fats (and the associated fat-soluble vitamins) or because of poor intestinal absorption resulting from biliary insufficiency.

Constipation is frequent among the elderly. It is partially due to the atonic intestinal musculature, but decreased physical activity and unwise dietary habits, such as an inadequate intake of fluids and the avoidance of fruits and vegetables—the normal source of bulk—underlie much of it.

The nitrogen balance tends to become negative in old age as the dietary protein intake diminishes and nitrogen assimilation becomes less efficient, while tissue protein catabolism remains unabated. The ill effects of hypoproteinemia—retarded bone and wound repair, predisposition to anemia, and decreased resistance to infection—are thus more conspicuous in advanced age.

Caloric Imbalance

The basal metabolic rate decreases in old age, and fewer calories are needed to satisfy the body's energy requirements for the upkeep of its vital functions. Hand in hand with the drop in metabolic rate, physical activity decreases in the later years as well, thus diminishing considerably the total caloric requirement. Nevertheless, in too many aging individuals the previous eating habits persist, though the energy expenditure is markedly reduced, and obesity becomes a frequent problem in late middle age. The obese are more susceptible to the degenerative disorders. Obesity increases surgical risk, predisposes to cardiovascular disease and the emergence of latent diabetes, and has a deleterious effect in osteoarthritis of the weight-bearing joints; the prognosis for the diabetic or cardiac patient is also poorer in the presence of obesity.

Actually, because of the increased incidence of degenerative disease among the obese and the detrimental effect of obesity on longevity, overweight is not a frequent problem among the truly aged; the obese do not tend to survive to a very advanced age. Among septuagenarians and octogenarians, caloric deprivation and emaciation are more prevalent than obesity. Extreme underweight and undernutrition are equally undesirable since they lessen the oldster's vigor and sense of well-being. Adjustment of the caloric intake and body weight of the elderly person is thus one of the basic principles of a sound geriatric nutritional regimen.

Vitamin and Mineral Requirements

The metabolic vitamin requirement is not markedly changed in old age, but apparently greater attention must be paid to an adequate dietary supply, since a diminished total food intake, poor qualitative selection of food items, and, possibly, less efficient absorption set the stage for inadequate vitamin stores.

The mineral requirements do not decrease because of age. Among the elderly, calcium and iron intakes are most apt to be deficient. The risk of chronic iron-deficiency anemia is increased by the diminished gastric hydrochloric acid secretion, which makes for the decreased absorption of dietary iron.

In the United States, in dietary surveys of the aged, deficiencies in calcium, iron, vitamin A, ascorbic acid, and the B complex vitamins have been found most frequently. In other Western countries the most common deficiencies seem to relate to calcium, iron, vitamin A, riboflavin, and ascorbic acid.

Many retired persons and old-age pensioners tend to have excessive calorie intakes with emphasis on higher-than-needed fat intakes.

Osteoporosis (or postmenopausal demineralization of bones) is a disorder of middle and old age which results in a gradual decrease in the amount and strength of bone tissue in the body. By virtue of the demineralized, weak, porous bones which it produces, osteoporosis sets the stage for many of the fractures and spine deformities which victimize elderly persons, since it predisposes bone to ready breakage even under relatively minor mechanical stress. The disorder is widespread among the aging, especially among women, and constitutes a major, basic cause of physical disability in old age. A variety of factors are believed to set the stage for osteoporosis. In the past, emphasis was primarily on the hormonal changes of advancing age; decreased secretion of the partially anabolic sex hormones results in decreased elaboration and maintenance of the proteinaceous bone matrix which is the precursor of the subsequent, mineralized bone structure. Progressive skeletal disuse—the greater inactivity and immobilization of old age—also contributes to the demineralization of bone in the elderly. In recent years, chronic calcium undernutrition has also been recognized as a major factor, as evidence has accumulated that the skeletal demineralization of osteoporosis may be the end result of prolonged negative calcium balance occurring in persons with a higher than normal calcium requirement, with decreased absorption, or with an inability to adapt to an inadequate calcium intake.

The most rational preventive measure is a reasonably high calcium intake throughout life, with special attention to a *continued high dietary calcium supply from age 40 on.* When osteoporosis is manifest in old age, restoration of the waning hormone levels is in the realm of the physician, but the negative calcium balance may and should be prevented by the generous inclusion of calcium-rich items in the diet, especially milk, against which there exists a strong prejudice among many older people.

Dietary Recommendations

The desired diet in later years is moderate to high in proteins, moderate in carbohydrates, relatively low in fats, and rich in vitamins and minerals. The total caloric intake should suffice to maintain a level of body weight consistent with, or slightly below, the values given in Table 35 in Chap. 21. Any existing overweight or underweight should be corrected gradually.

The intake of fats should be less than the present national average, which amounts to 40 to 45 percent of the total caloric intake. In advanced age about 25 percent of the caloric intake should come from fat. The diet should be rich in all vitamins and minerals, since in old age these may be absorbed less efficiently and the total amount of food eaten may be smaller. Sufficient iron and calcium should be provided to correct existing deficiencies and to maintain normal balance.

The fluid intake should be generous. Enough liquids should be consumed to permit excretion of at least 1½ liters of urine per day. Except in warm weather and under conditions of excessive perspiration this requires a daily intake of about 2 liters of fluid. A liberal intake of water, juices, milk, coffee, and tea, spaced throughout the day, helps to maintain a normal flow of urine and counteracts tendencies to constipation. The mild stimulating effects of caffeine from coffee and tea are not harmful, except in specific illnesses or idiosyncrasies, and have a salutary effect on older persons. When insomnia is a problem, caffeine late in the day is to be discouraged. Judicious and moderate use of alcoholic beverages is often regarded as helpful in the nutritional care of the aged. A glass of wine before dinner increases a lagging appetite and has a laudatory, protective, vasodilating effect; its relaxing properties are also valuable at bedtime.

A large proportion of patients who have been placed on salt-restricted diets for the management of cardiovascular disorders belong to the older age group. In these persons salt depletion is dangerous and must be watched for, particularly during hot weather and sickness with fever, when sodium and chloride loss by perspiration tends to become critical.

The elderly do not take willingly to abrupt changes. To avoid emotional disturbance and outright rejection of the advice by the elderly subject, any alterations in the dietary should be gradual and fitted to the individual as much as possible. For instance, since fluid milk is rejected by many aged persons, dried skim milk may be introduced into well-accepted foods to avoid mealtime problems.

When chewing is difficult, ground or chopped meat or tender fish is preferable and soft fruits or juices are best substituted for hard fruits. The emphasis should turn to egg or cheese dishes, finely chopped vegetables, and puddings and soups (which may be enriched with milk or dry milk solids). Strained and junior infant foods present a large selection of nutritious items, and they require no preparation.

Meal Plan in Old Age

To ensure a well-balanced diet, the following should be had every day:

LEAN MEAT, FISH, OR POULTRY
1 or more servings (4 oz or more). Occasionally beans, peas, lentils, or peanut butter may be substituted in order to meet a tight budget. In such a case, some milk, cheese, or an egg should be taken during the same meal.

MILK
1 pt. This may be taken as whole or skim milk or in the form of cheese, puddings, custards, creamed soups, and other foods which contain fluid or dried milk. 1½ oz cured cheese is roughly the nutritional equivalent of ½ pt milk.

EGGS
3 to 5 eggs per week.

FRUITS
2 helpings, a helping of citrus fruit (or 4 oz of the juice) or of fresh tomatoes,
    berries, or cantaloupe and a helping of other fruits.

VEGETABLES
1 helping of deep yellow or dark green leafy vegetables and 1 other serving,
    which may include other vegetables or a potato.

WHOLE-GRAIN OR ENRICHED CEREALS OR BREAD
2 servings. This may be alternated with noodles or rice.

BUTTER OR MARGARINE
2 tbsp.

Sample Menus

Inexpensive and light

BREAKFAST
Breakfast cereal with glass of milk
Orange (or orange juice)
Coffee or tea optional

LUNCH
Chicken soup and crackers
Egg or cheese sandwich
Sliced tomatoes
Beverage

DINNER
Hamburger steak
Mashed potatoes
Salad or vegetable
Bread and butter
Pudding
Beverage

BEDTIME SNACK
Chocolate milk or cheese; occasionally soft fruit

More elaborate and hearty

BREAKFAST
Egg

Buttered toast
Milk
Orange (or orange juice)

LUNCH
Hot beef or ham sandwich
Tomato and cottage cheese salad
Jello
Beverage

DINNER
Fruit cocktail
Tender Swiss steak
Baked potato
Spinach loaf or chopped spinach
Roll and butter
Ice cream (small serving)
Beverage

BEDTIME SNACK
Chocolate milk or cheese; occasionally soft fruit

Chapter 20

Nutrition and Dental Health

By reason of the anatomic structure and function of the oral cavity, its tissues are subject to a much wider variety of environmental stresses than other, more protected tissues in the body. In contrast to most other tissues which are normally sterile, the mouth is an ideal location for the growth and multiplication of a wide range of microorganisms. The teeth and gums are subject to recurrent physical and chemical trauma by a variety of foods which differ considerably in temperature, consistency, texture, and acidity. The soft tissues of the mouth—gums, tongue, and the oral and labial mucosa—are very susceptible to metabolic abnormalities of nutritional origin. (The classic signs of nutritional deficiencies in these tissues are discussed in Chaps. 10 and 11, Vitamins, and Chap. 22, Malnutrition and Deficiency Diseases.) In the past few decades, as frank nutritional deficiencies like scurvy, pellagra, beriberi, and rickets are seen less in dental practice, attention has shifted in particular to the relationship between nutrition and the teeth proper. Since then, a correlation between specific nutritional abnormalities which occur during tooth development and the incidence of tooth decay has been recognized, and the daily dietary influences on dental caries have come under study as well.

The Present-Day Concept of Tooth Decay

Everytooth has an individual degree of susceptibility to decay which depends on its histologic and chemical makeup, which in turn is controlled by genetic and nutritional factors active during its development. This caries susceptibility or caries resistance of the tooth tends to remain basically unchanged during its lifetime.

The activity of microorganisms is necessary to bring about destruction of tooth substance. This is presumably due to the action on the tooth of the acid end products of microbial fermentation. The oral cavity must contain an easily metabolized substrate which supports the metabolism and reproduction of the etiologic organisms; of all dietary components, carbohydrates are most implicated in enhancing tooth decay. The carbohydrates must be present in a form which prevents a speedy clearance from the mouth. Large amounts of sugar solution do not increase the incidence of decay significantly, but the same quantity of sucrose in the form of sticky candy or jam, closely applied to the tooth surfaces, will.

To produce damage to the tooth structure, cariogenic organisms must colonize and grow in close association with the tooth surface. This they do in "dental plaque," a viscous, bacteria-laden film in which bacteria grow, multiply, metabolize food debris, and convert carbohydrates, particularly sucrose, to organic acids (especially lactic acid) which dissolve tooth minerals. Another reason for the high caries-producing potential of sucrose is its ease of conversion by bacteria to viscous polysaccharides (dextrans and levans) which are the structural basis of the dental plaque and also serve as a reserve energy source for plaque bacteria which can utilize them and continue to form acid even when traces of food from former meals have disappeared from the mouth.

The physical consistency and quantity of saliva also mediate the caries rate; it is yet undetermined whether this is due to the direct mechanical flushing action which removes the fermentation-supporting carbohydrates, through some other suppressive action on the responsible microorganism, or to inorganic ions contributed by the saliva and incorporated into the outer tooth structure.

Nature and Development of Dental Tissues

Any discussion of the influence of nutrition on tooth decay must be preceded by a consideration of the characteristics of dental structure and development. The teeth are composed of three hard, calcified tissues: the bony mass, or dentin; the hard, glossy, visible outer coating of the dentin, the enamel; and a thin, hard coating of the dentin below the gum level, the cementum. The dental pulp (commonly referred to as the "nerve" of the tooth) is located in the center of the dentin; it is made up of highly vascularized and innervated connective tissue which extends into the interior of each tooth from the trabecular part of the jaw. Though capillary and lymph vessels thus lead into the center of the tooth, there appears to be no connection between them and the dentin and enamel. In reality, very minute tubules penetrate the bony part of the dentin and very fine organic fibrils are located within the enamel, and these noncalcified structures may serve the dental tissues as channels of transport. Neither dentin nor enamel has the ability to repair mechanical injury, to replace decayed portions, or to re-form structures which have developed improperly.

The life history of a tooth has three main subdivisions: the period during which the crown of the tooth is being formed and calcified in the jaw; a period of maturation during which the tooth is gradually erupting into the oral cavity and the roots are formed; and the long period during which the mature tooth functions in the mouth. In the case of the first molar, the life cycle may be illustrated as follows: (1) The first histologic forerunners of the crown are present at the time of birth. (2) During the next $2^{1}/_{2}$ to 3 years the organic precursors of the crown develop and are being calcified. (3) During the sixth or seventh year the crown erupts into the oral cavity, while the roots continue to develop until the ninth or tenth year. (4) The long, postdevelopmental period of maintenance of the tooth in the mouth follows.

The Role of Nutritional Factors during Dental Development

During the developmental period, the genetic makeup of the individual largely determines the peculiarities of the tooth structure and its composition; concurrently, the general health of the individual and the availability of specific nutrients influence and modify the process of development.

Characteristic malformations of tooth structures may occur as a result of vitamin A deficiency. In such cases, the enamel is hypoplastic and may be malformed; the dentin is poorly calcified, and at times the pulp is invaded by small calcified concretions. In severe vitamin C deficiency, dentin is laid down irregularly or not at all, and rarefaction and weakness develop in the supporting alveolar jawbone, with resulting looseness of the teeth. In human teeth, neither vitamin A nor vitamin C deficiency during the developmental phase has been clearly shown to result in subsequent increased caries susceptibility of the teeth. However, observations in experimental animals would indicate that such a result might follow. Deficiency in vitamin D leads to disturbed calcification of the dentin and hypoplasia in the enamel of the permanent teeth. Most important, there appears to be a definite correlation between vitamin D deficiency during tooth development and incidence of later tooth decay.

Fluorine is one of the most important dietary factors which influences the chemical composition of the developing tooth and its eventual susceptibility to decay. Ingestion of optimal amounts of fluoride ion during tooth development results in increased amount of fluoride in the enamel and dentin. Surface enamel routinely contains approximately 10 times as much fluoride as the internal layers of enamel. The fluoride content of the outer surface continues to increase during the first decade after the tooth erupts, provided that the diet or drinking water supplies adequate amounts. Once the developing tooth has erupted into the oral cavity, it is possible to incorporate significant amounts of fluoride into the surface layer of the enamel by topical applications of fluoride-containing solutions or gels to children's teeth, at intervals, by the dentist.

How fluorine confers protection against caries is still debated. It has been suggested that the production of the less soluble calcium fluoroapatite is the main factor. Whatever the mode of action, the ingestion of fluoride ion during tooth development provides a high degree of protection against the caries process whether the fluoride ion occurs in the food or water naturally or has been added to the public water supply.

Extensive epidemiologic surveys have shown decisively that within the limits of 0 to 1 part per million (ppm) there is an inverse relationship between the amount of fluoride ion ingested during the developmental phase and the incidence of tooth decay during subsequent childhood and adult life (Chap. 12). Wherever the water supply contains about 1 ppm of fluorine, the nonerupted and erupted teeth also contain a higher level of fluorine than in regions with fluorine-poor water. The safety of the controlled addition of fluoride to public water supplies to the extent of 1 to 1.2 ppm has been repeatedly demonstrated, as well as the distinctly lower rate of dental caries (50 to 60 percent less tooth decay) which accompanies this procedure. At the present time approximately 80 million people in the United States receive optimal levels of fluoride in their drinking water. While water fluoridation is by far the preferable method in urban areas, fluoride ingestion from pharmaceutic preparations or foods is a useful substitute.

An excessive intake of fluorine may lead to mottling of the enamel of the teeth. In extreme cases the enamel may become pitted and the teeth appear stained and corroded. Such dental fluorosis may be seen in a number of communities (particularly in the Texas panhandle and Colorado) where the natural water supply contains 2 to 6 ppm of fluorine.

The Role of Dietary Factors during the Postdevelopmental Period

The degree to which tooth decay will occur during the long functional period, after development and maturation are complete, depends to a large extent on the inherent qualities of the tooth; however, the oral environment and systemic dietary conditions serve as powerful influences, and the ultimate fate of the tooth is determined by both sets of factors. A diet rich in sticky carbohydrates with a poor clearance encourages cariogenesis by creating conditions on the surface of the tooth and in its crevices which are favorable to microbial activity. Supplements of sugar when given *with* meals are less harmful than those administered *between* meals. Thus the form of the ingested carbohydrate and the length of its retention on the tooth are more important than the total amount of carbohydrate eaten. The following list of carbohydrate foods is presented in decreasing order of oral retention to illustrate the type of food item most likely to support cariogenesis if consumed at the conclusion of meals or in the form of in-between-meal snacks: fig cookies, chocolate, ice cream, sweet pastry, caramel, crackers, white bread, potato, apple, orange soda, orange juice, boiled carrot.

One of the most interesting, yet not fully explored aspects of dental caries is the influence of overall systemic nutrition on teeth after their maturation. Recent experimental work, primarily with laboratory animals, indicates that dietary postdevelopmental influences cannot be ascribed solely to the accumulation of readily fermentable foodstuffs on the tooth surface. Apparently the quality of the diet has a profound influence on the well-being of fully matured teeth through systemic pathways, whether this is mediated by way of the general circulation and the pulp of the tooth or through the composition of the saliva.

Less is known about the relation of nutrition to periodontal disease (gingivitis) than to dental caries. Periodontal disease affects a large percentage of individuals in middle and advanced age. Once started, it progresses more rapidly in patients whose nutrition is poor; chronic deficiency of vitamin C may be a contributing factor. However, the picture is not clear because oral hygiene (removal of plaque and calculus) is another important factor influencing the degree and prevalence of periodontal disease.

Dietary Recommendations

Present knowledge may be summarized in the following recommendations. During the developmental period, the diet should be well balanced and should include foods from all basic categories. Special attention should be given to an ample supply of vitamin D, calcium, and phosphorus. The available drinking water should contain about 1 ppm of fluorine, whether natural or attained through controlled fluoridation. (If the fluorine content of the natural water supply exceeds 2 ppm, as it does in certain regions, it may be desirable to look for alternate sources of water or for methods to decrease the fluorine concentration.) Once the teeth have formed, sticky high-carbohydrate foods with a slow clearance from the mouth should be avoided, and ingestion of such snacks between meals is best interdicted. At the same time, foods that furnish a detergent or cleansing effect on dental plaque (such as raw carrots or apples) should be encouraged. Physical removal of dental plaque between meals by brushing is, of course, another important aid in combating caries formation. An optimal, overall nutritional status is desirable from the standpoint of continued dental well-being, as it is for general health considerations.

Chapter 21

Obesity and Leanness

Obesity and Health

In recent years obesity has become a public health problem of considerable importance in the United States. About 20 percent of all adults (and 35 percent of adults over 40) are overweight to a degree that may interfere with optimal health and longevity, and obesity is becoming more important as more people live to an age when fat is easily acquired and hard to lose and chronic degenerative diseases are common. Aside from the general problem of physical fitness, diet and obesity are now recognized as important factors in the causation, prevention, and treatment of many diseases. Obesity aggravates cardiovascular disease and osteoarthritis and increases the liability to hypertension, atherosclerosis, hernia, and gallbladder disease. Overweight also facilitates the emergence of latent diabetes in predisposed individuals as they approach an advanced age and adds to the hazards of surgery; it makes for postural derangement, and in extreme cases it is the cause of obesity dyspnea with pulmonary insufficiency. It is also of interest that the mortality from cirrhosis of the liver in obese males is 249 percent of the expected.

Medicoactuarial statistics make it quite clear that the obese do not live as long as the lean, lending support to the old proverb, "He who eats to satisfy his palate digs his grave with his teeth" (or "there is death in the pot," II Kings 4:40). The chief causes of death among overweight individuals are cardiovascular-renal diseases, diabetes, and disorders of the liver and biliary tract.

The burden of obesity is not borne equally among all segments of society. In the United States, it is more likely to be found in the lower socioeconomic strata. This association is particularly marked in women; surveys have shown the prevalence of obesity in adult urban women in the lower, middle, and upper socioeconomic levels to be 30 percent, 16 percent, and 5 percent, respectively. The most recent federal survey among poor rural and urban population strata has found an obesity rate of about 50 percent among black women.

In this chapter the term *overweight* applies to persons whose weight is 10 percent or more above the desirable body weight (based on height and build), and the term *obesity* refers to an excess of 20 percent or more over the desirable body weight.

Causes of Obesity

Obesity is frequently blamed on anything rather than ingestion of food: endocrine factors, body build, or heredity. Actually, obesity caused by endocrine dysfunction is exceptionally rare, and "familial" obesity, when scrutinized closely, is essentially of environmental rather than hereditary origin. What appears to be a genetically induced condition is more often merely a passing on of food habits from one generation to the next. Children tend to imitate their overeating parents, and once their food intake pattern has been established, the familial tendency to overweight is perpetuated.

The essential, basic cause of obesity is an intake of calories in excess of metabolic requirements. Obesity may be caused by an increased caloric intake in the presence of a constant energy output, or by a decreased energy expenditure in the presence of a constant caloric intake, or by any relative variation of the two factors which makes for a caloric excess. A person need not be a "heavy eater" to have a positive caloric balance; individual caloric requirements vary enormously, and it is possible for a person of low metabolic rate, small size, and sedentary habits to be in positive caloric balance on what appears to be a very moderate food intake. The important fact is that small increments of caloric excess over a prolonged period of time can result in pronounced obesity.

The youth of 18 in rigorous athletic training needs approximately 4200 cal because he is still growing, his basal metabolic rate is relatively high, and his physical energy expenditure is very great. The man of 22 who has stopped growing but does similar work needs about 3600 cal; his counterpart working in an office may need only 2400 cal, and while bedridden, approximately 2000 cal would more than suffice. As he becomes older and more sedentary and his metabolic rate decreases, 2000 to 2400 cal per day may well result in considerable overweight in this person, whose food habits have long since become ingrained and have remained unchanged despite his decreased caloric requirement.

Present-day environmental conditions encourage overeating and a drop in physical activity. Mechanization has decreased hard physical labor in industry, farming, and the home. The workday is shorter, and the 5-day workweek has become the norm. The automobile and modern communications have done their share to decrease caloric expenditure, and recreation has become increasingly less active, descending the caloric ladder from participating sports to spectator sports to the viewing of spectator sports on television, preferably while recumbent and incorporating refreshments.

The rising standard of living has also encouraged an increased food intake. Since income has risen, more money is spent on food and more emphasis is being placed on the tastier, calorie-rich foods. At the same time, modern food processing and packaging and the convenience of food shopping and eating out have not served to curtail individual food intakes.

Obesity-facilitating Mechanisms

Lack of physical activity encourages the development of obesity through two mechanisms—one direct and obvious, the other indirect and less well known. The first mechanism is based on the fact that in the absence of sufficient exercise, only a relatively small proportion of generously ingested food calories is used up to provide energy for physical activity; thus any unused calories are converted into fat storage depots in the body. With respect to the second mechanism, there is now evidence that the normal internal mechanisms which regulate appetite and satiety (Chap. 6) will not operate properly at the low levels of energy expenditure which characterize large numbers of individuals in today's civilization. Thus given the many exogenous inducements for eating which impinge on the individual from his environment, and an impaired internal cutoff mechanism, the tide is in favor of excessive food intake.

Recent research on obesity has emphasized increasingly the importance of "internal" and "external" signals which serve as determining cues for the individual's eating behavior. The internal cues are physiologic and encompass gastric contraction and distention, blood glucose (and probably amino acid) concentration, dryness of the mouth, weakness, changes in body temperature, irritability, and the like. External cues are nonphysiologic and primarily psychosensory and environmental; they include factors such as the sight, appearance, aroma, proximity, and taste of food, and food-related factors such as the time of day (relation to customary eating time) and setting ("while watching a television food advertisement"; "we were near the cafeteria") and others. It has been proposed that eating behavior in lean persons (and those ordinarily engaged in some measure of physical exercise, see above) is controlled principally by internal signals which constantly and effectively supply physiologic cues as to their state of hunger and satiety. In lean persons presumably the influence of internal cues outweighs most of the time that of external signals, and thus they are able to regulate their energy balance and to maintain a fairly constant body weight with the passage of time.

In contrast, most obese individuals appear to be relatively insensitive to internal signals related to satiety and hunger, and are overly responsive to food-related external cues. When the food is dull and the eating situation uninteresting, the obese subject actually limits his food intake; ordinarily, however, he will follow his own established eating pattern and will respond to positive food-related cues such as flavor of the meal, and he appears to be unable to perceive internal signals that announce that the point of physical and metabolic satiety is reached. This, perhaps, is one key to understanding the notorious long-run ineffectiveness of most attempts to treat obesity.

Motives for Overeating

On the average, most eating patterns are determined by the social environment, primarily the immediate family and secondarily the regional or ethnic group. Though the cultural pattern and family training are important factors, individual preference is nevertheless the most important consideration, and the pleasures of the table being gratifying indeed, there is little reason why most individuals would instinctively or consciously restrain their food intake. It is to be expected that many will indulge in this form of physical pleasure, which demands few prerequisites on the part of the participant and may be had at a moment's notice and without the collaboration of others. Indeed, as the individual ages, food is one of the few pleasures easily attainable, and it is readily understood why the middle-aged person instinctively preserves his customary mealtime habits and finds food of more importance than ever.

The motives which induce people to overeat beyond actual needs are not always as simple as implied above. The importance of emotional and psychologic motivation has become increasingly accepted in considering obesity. The psychology of food intake is discussed in detail in Chap. 6; suffice it to mention here that the gratification of conscious or unconscious emotional needs is behind many more cases of overeating than would be suspected on cursory observation.

Psychologic obesity may be broadly divided into two forms; developmental and reactive. Developmental obesity, the common childhood variety, involves the entire growing personality. Such an individual shuns ordinary activities and tends to have few social contacts. Eating and the consequent obesity are a compensating refuge from insecurity, anxiety, impotence, defeat, and a feeling of loneliness and social isolation. The resultant ungainly appearance frequently serves as the excuse for failures.

Reactive obesity generally does not begin in childhood. It has its roots in some upsetting experience, such as homesickness, breaking up of a love affair, illness, or death of a dear person. Here too, overeating may constitute the compensating, balancing factor in adjustment to life and may prevent more serious disturbances.

Adipose Tissue—the Organ of Obesity

During the last few years considerable new knowledge has been obtained concerning the "organ" of obesity—the adipose tissue of the overweight individual. Apparently human obesity may be characterized according to the cellular pattern of the adipose tissue of the obese subject.

Given a normal balance between caloric intake and expenditure since infancy, an individual will have a fairly fixed number of fat cells which does not change markedly throughout the life cycle. During the adult years, when an excess of food calories is consumed and not used up through a parallel energy expenditure, fat accumulates in the individual fat cells and these grow *in size*; however, there is *no* increase in the total *number* of fat cells in the body. When such an individual readjusts his caloric intake downward (as when he follows a weight-reducing diet) or when his physical energy output increases considerably, and he now must draw on his fat depots to obtain the required fuel for his daily energy expenditure, the *size* of his adipose cells *decreases* as he draws on his fat reserves. There is, however, *no* reduction in *number* of existing fat cells.

In brief, it appears that normally, in the adult, there is a fairly fixed number of fat cells (the magnitude of this number varies with the individual) which, like tiny balloons which are capable of being inflated and deflated according to need, will increase in size as they store excess fat and decrease in size as existing fat stores are being used up.

This total number of fat cells in the body of an individual is fixed by mid to late adolescence. During infancy and early adolescence, however, overfeeding with rapid weight gain can induce a substantial (two to five times normal) *increase* in fat cell *number* in the still-developing adipose tissues. Once such adipose hyperplasia has been established, the *number* of fat cells in such an individual will not decrease in later life; it is irreversible even under conditions of active weight reduction.

It has been proposed that there are two types of obesity, one characterized by a normal number of (reversibly) hypertrophied fat cells, and the other by hyperplastic (hypercellular) adipose tissues. The former may be looked upon as adult-onset obesity, the latter as growth-onset or developmental. A genetic predisposition to adipose hypercellularity may also play a role in the latter category. Individuals with very considerable obesity usually also have an abnormally increased number of fat cells; this type of obesity is a more severe form which is less amenable to weight reduction. This is also consistent with the fact that the majority of obese children become hard-core, obese adults.

Obesity and Diabetes

The cellular character of adipose tissue is of more than just morphologic interest. It determines important metabolic aspects of the internal environment. It is known that large fat cells are more refractory to the action of insulin than small ones. Thus more insulin is required to facilitate normal glucose metabolism in a body composed in part of insulin-resistant large fat cells (in an obese person) than in one containing insulin-responsive smaller fat cells (in a lean person). This will explain why obese subjects usually have elevated plasma insulin levels and respond to a challenge with glucose with increased insulin secretion in comparison with normal subjects. In fact, the degree of hyperinsulinemia in obesity increases in proportion to the quantity of total body fat and decreases (and glucose tolerance improves) after weight reduction.

Since most maturity-onset diabetics are obese just before or at the time their disease emerges—i.e., they have many abnormally large (insulin-resistant) fat cells—this may explain why weight reduction (decrease in adipose cell size and increased responsiveness to insulin) in such patients suffices, in many cases, to control their diabetic symptoms. This will explain why, in adult individuals genetically predisposed to diabetes who walk a tightrope with respect to their overall insulin economy, obesity as an added stress factor will stimulate the frank emergence of the previously latent disease.

The Obese Child

In our culture it appears difficult for the obese person to translate into effective action his resolve to eat less and exercise more. It is also a fact that an increasing proportion of school children (10 to 40 percent) are overweight, and that 50 to 85 percent of obese children remain obese as adults. This lends added gravity to the need to understand, and if possible, prevent, the development of obesity in childhood. The most effective measures for prevention should be taken during the early years. The fat infant is not a paragon of future health, and too rapid weight gain in infancy should be avoided. Physical activity must be encouraged early to permit it to become an integral part of the child's daily life. This is particularly important where there is a family history of obesity. Among many adolescents, obesity is not necessarily based on an extreme degree of overeating, but rather on a striking pattern of physical inactivity involving an almost ingenious avoidance of unessential physical exertion.

Psychologic factors play a larger part in juvenile obesity than in the adult counterpart. Poor adjustment to home and school and other emotional problems can lead to an excessive, compensatory interest in food. Early recognition by the parents of a slow, almost imperceptible tendency toward weight gain is an important factor in successful prevention of what may become an irreversible situation. For the adolescent who appears to be motivated and ready to lose weight, a reducing program should be outlined, involving guidance by an understanding and knowledgeable physician, cooperation of schoolteachers (particularly the physical education instructor) and the school nurse, and tactful devotion and interest on the part of both parents.

Treatment

The treatment of obesity should be considered a long-range project; no one method is applicable to all persons, and setbacks, either temporary or permanent, must be expected. The immediate object of treatment is to reverse the state of caloric excess and to obtain a negative caloric balance. Such a caloric deficiency forces the body to metabolize endogenous materials in order to obtain the energy required for its vital activities. At first the readily available glycogen reserves are used up. This is followed by the simultaneous utilization of small amounts of protein from the body's metabolic pool and of fat from its fat depots. Eventually, while increasingly smaller quantities of protein are catabolized, the caloric deficit is made up primarily by energy obtained from the breakdown of fat reserves. A general, gradual shrinkage of adipose tissues takes place, and the body weight continues to decrease as long as the negative caloric balance is maintained. Once the undesirable excess weight has been lost, the caloric intake and expenditure may then be adjusted to maintain the desirable body weight.

Exercise

The desired caloric deficit may be brought about through a decrease in caloric intake or an increase in physical activity. In theory, an increase in physical activity, without a major compensatory adjustment of the food intake, is bound to accelerate the correction of obesity. In practice, a sudden increase in physical exercise alone is sometimes a disappointing measure. Walking a mile uses up only about 92 cal, representing the caloric value of 1.1 ounces of bread or 1.5 ounces of ice cream.

It has been said that sporadic attempts at unaccustomed physical exercise may serve to stimulate the appetite of the individual and thus may ultimately defeat the desired purpose.

Actually, the performance of exercise is not automatically followed by an increase in food intake. This increase in food intake appears to take place only if the individual was fairly active to start with. If he was sedentary, his physical activity may be stepped up in many cases with little or no increase in appetite. (Conversely, if activity is decreased below a certain point, which depends on the individual, appetite does not decrease correspondingly; the result, of course, is accumulation of fat.)

The energy cost of moving or supporting the body is proportional to body weight; hence the caloric expenditure of a given physical activity is greater for the obese person. Exercise tends to improve muscle tone and circulation and is thus desirable as a general health measure. Physically active persons tend to have a more stable weight than inactive individuals. In brief, regular, sustained, mild-to-moderate exercise plays a desirable role in the correction of over-weight, provided a control is simultaneously exercised over caloric intake.

Low-Calorie Diets

Decreasing the intake of food calories is generally the major factor in obtaining a negative caloric balance. There are two prerequisites to any beneficial reducing diet: (1) It must supply the nutritional requirements of the individual; i.e., it must contain all essential nutrients in preferably optimal, and at least minimal, quantities. (2) It must supply fewer calories than the individual expends each day. Unless both requirements are met, the particular regimen is not a bona fide reducing diet and may be either ineffective or harmful when used over a prolonged period. (Exceptions to this are extremely low-calorie diets accompanied by physician-prescribed, specific nutritional supplementa-tion. It is sometimes difficult or impractical to supply optimal amounts of all essential micronutrients in an 800- to 1000-cal diet; in such cases the physician will often prescribe a specific preparation to prevent any possible mineral or vitamin deprivation.) Many widely publicized fad diets are based on bizarre intake patterns or emphasize the exclusive use of a small number of food items ("steak diet," "egg diet"). Such diets belong in the domain of the nutrition faddist of the birdseed-and-molasses school.

Reducing diets which are used for limited periods of time may be quite useless at times; in many cases, the individual—his limited objective achieved—will revert to his habitual pattern of food intake and the temporary gain will soon be wiped out. To achieve permanent results, the goal must be a permanent lifelong change in food habits.

A workable reducing diet can be based on the recommendations for the adult diet in Chap. 15. These recommendations make provisions for adequate supplies of proteins, vitamins, and minerals. Adherence to these recommenda-tions ensures adequate nutrition without providing an excess of calories. The caloric intake may be decreased further by the judicious reduction in the quantity of food items which are primarily of fat or carboh.drate nature (butter, cream, gravy, salad oils, cake, noodles, rice) and by the elimination of food items not mentioned in Chap. 15 but which may make up a considerable percentage of the food intake of the average person: candy, carbonated beverages, pastries, alcoholic beverages (beer in particular), potato chips, and the like.

It is imperative that the diet selected be reasonably compatible with the food pattern to which the obese individual is accustomed. The changeover to a lowered caloric intake represents a physiologic and psychologic strain which should not be aggravated by the additional introduction of a major gustatory conflict into the picture. A reducing diet which conforms to the reducer's food preferences is one to which he becomes accustomed more easily and which is more likely to be adopted by him eventually, with inevitable personal adaptations, as a permanent food pattern. The qualitative makeup of the reducing diet must never tax the patience of its consumer, since the long-range success of the regimen depends on the fat person's permanent adoption of a more reasonable food pattern based, to a large extent, on his low-calorie diet.

The omission of entire meals is of no advantage in a weight reduction regimen. It serves only to accentuate the individual's discomfort and results in a ravenous appetite which induces overeating at the occasion of the next meal. The habitual omission of breakfast—the meal easiest to skip—not only accentuates noontime hunger, but may also lead to a significant loss of efficiency in the late morning hours. Extreme self-denial during the first half of the day rarely leads to a decreased overall daily caloric intake; individuals who skimp breakfast and lunch will almost invariably compensate for their earlier rigorous self-discipline at dinner and during the snack-rife period between dinner and bedtime.

In planning the weight reduction of an obese person the question of how much to reduce the caloric intake always arises. Some individuals have been habitual heavy eaters and have always had numerous snacks between meals. In their case, restriction to the three regular meals and black coffee might be sufficient. Many fat people, however, have already reduced their diet without success, and a drastic caloric limitation is necessary. The caloric content of the reducing diet will vary with the individual and his metabolic needs. In one case an 1800-cal diet, containing about 90 g protein, 60 g fat, and 225 g carbohydrate, might be indicated, while another more sedentary subject may require a 1200-cal diet, containing roughly 60 g protein, 40 g fat, and 150 g carbohydrate. Some workers consider it unnecessary to specify the respective amounts of protein, carbohydrate, fat, and calories, but give the subject printed diet lists. This is a very expedient method when a trained dietitian is available to formulate such diets. In hard-core cases and when a dietitian is not available, it may work out better to acquaint the subject thoroughly with the recommendations contained in Chap. 15 and to teach him the nutritive value of the major food groups (Chap. 14) as well as of individual food items—the latter with the aid of tables of food composition.

It is important to obtain some results as soon as possible; otherwise the subject becomes discouraged quickly and loses confidence in his reducing diet. On the other hand, too rapid a weight loss is undesirable since the individual will feel nervous, weak, and irritable and his skin will not be able to regain elasticity in step with the rapid reduction in the subcutaneous adipose tissues. If the total daily caloric intake of a person is reduced by 500 cal, he should normally lose about 1 pound weekly. (About 3500 cal is the equivalent of 1 pound of body weight.) Ideally the subject should lose weight at a slow but steady rate, 1 to 2 pounds per week, until a reasonable weight for his height and age is reached. At this point the caloric value of the diet may be gradually increased to stabilize the body weight at the desired level. A careful watch must be kept on the subject's weight and food intake for some time to come to prevent his backsliding into his previous pattern. It is important that the subject be seen regularly by a physician during any drastic attempt at reducing, so that any adverse symptoms which arise may be treated and the diet modified, and so that encouragement may be given.

In recent years, so-called complete formula diet products have been introduced to the public by pharmaceutical and food manufacturers. These preparations may be in solid or liquid form. They usually consist of protein from milk or soy flour, with added fats and carbohydrates. Vitamins and minerals are added at a level which equals or exceeds the known daily requirements, and the overall composition of the mixture is usually adjusted to yield approximately 900 cal per recommended daily dose. These formula diets appear to be effective and relatively safe means of weight reduction, if adhered to. (They are low-residue diets and should be supplemented with low-calorie foods high in residue, such as lettuce and celery, in order to maintain normal bulk in the lower intestine.) On the other hand, individuals who are excessively overweight and who may have additional ailments such as cardiovascular-renal disorders or diabetes mellitus should not undertake weight reduction without medical guidance. One of the important goals in any long-term weight control program is to educate the individual to adhere to better dietary habits. Since a ready-made therapeutic diet formula in no way resembles ordinary foods, the obese individual hardly learns improved eating habits through dependence on it for weight reduction. Furthermore, monotony of the formula "diet" may soon result in its abandonment—at which time the patient resumes his normal food intake pattern which originally led to his overweight. Though formula diets may have some adjunctive value in a weight control program, they should not be relied on as the mainstay of the reducing regimen. The dietary program which results in a lifetime maintenance of a desirable weight through permanent readjustment of the food intake pattern is the only one of genuine benefit to the obese individual.

Starvation

In recent years it has been recommended that weight loss be brought about in grossly obese, refractory patients by repeated periods of 10- to 14-day total fasts or even by longer-term starvation regimens. Proponents of total fasting have emphasized that prolonged starvation is easily tolerated since the subject usually loses appetite after 3 or 4 days, that little discomfort is experienced subsequently, and that no serious side effects are observed. Even though hunger is usually no problem after the first few days, *total* starvation is not an advisable procedure; if nevertheless it is decided upon, it is an obligatory in-hospital procedure since such a regimen may cause cardiac arrhythmias, orthostatic hypotension, and urate retention followed by acute gout. There are two weight-reduction starvation deaths on record (one due to development of idiopathic lactic acidosis in an obese diabetic patient). Prolonged starvation thus should be undertaken *only* under close medical supervision and is not advisable for obese patients with a history of cardiovascular disease, liver disease, or gout.

The procedure also results in the loss of considerable amounts of body protein and potassium, when the original intention is loss of fat—not lean tissue mass. Thus, weight reduction during the initial 2-week period is largely due to loss of protein and water, and relatively little fat is lost. Vitamin deficiencies and anemia may also set in without preventive supplementation. The encouraging rapid initial weight loss is soon nullified when the starved subject is permitted to eat again; even on a low-calorie diet (900 cal/day) there is a rapid weight gain initially which represents largely tissue rehydration. More important, the average cumulative fat loss during total starvation of 1 to 2 months is not significantly different from that experienced during a similar period on a diet of 900 cal per day. In most cases total fasting, when compared with a low-carbohydrate 900-cal diet, does not seem to result in any lasting benefit in terms of weight reduction.

Special Composition Diets

A variety of special diets emphasizing diverse proportions and/or preponderances of protein, fat, and carbohydrate have been advocated, but there is no evidence that any special combination of the three food sources of calories can nullify or reverse the basic law of conservation of energy. Special benefits have been claimed for diets which severely restrict carbohydrates while permitting a relatively high fat intake. Such diets may, at first, be more encouraging to the dieting patient since they tend to lead to a loss of sodium and water—and thus to an apparent rapid "weight loss." It has also been proposed that high-fat, low-carbohydrate diets lead to a mild ketosis which in turn is associated with an initial diuretic effect and thus with a consequent fairly rapid weight reduction due to loss of body water. The resulting ketosis also is said to inhibit appetite, which makes dieting easier. Nevertheless, in the *long* run such diets will result in a true weight reduction due to loss of fat no greater than that obtained with other low-calorie reducing diets since in all such regimens the long-range determining factor is a reduced intake of *calories*.

Surgery

When obesity is truly massive (body weight is twice the ideal weight), intractable, and of long standing, when a correctable endocrine abnormality has been ruled out, and for life-threatening obesity, as in the Pickwickian syndrome, drastic approaches may be necessary. For such patients the surgical creation of an intestinal bypass may be considered. The basis for this treatment is the deliberate induction of a malabsorption syndrome by surgical bypass of most of the small intestine through an anastomosis of the jejunum to the terminal ileum.

Such surgery will produce a dramatic weight loss in all patients which continues over a period of many years. The possible side effects include incapacitating diarrhea, electrolyte imbalance, vitamin deficiencies, urinary tract oxalate stones, and fatty degeneration of the liver. The latter complication may be serious, and a continuous medical follow-up of such patients is essential. Several post-bypass deaths due to hepatic cirrhosis with irreversible hepatic failure have been reported. The hepatic fatty degeneration is reversible by restoration of bowel continuity, and a renewed intestinal hookup may be necessary after several years (with consequent partial return of the obese state).

Psychiatric Support

For many persons, being overweight is a mechanism which permits adjustment to life. In cases where emotional motivations underlie the obesity, correction may be extremely difficult and even dangerous, since overeating may prevent a more serious disturbance. Psychotherapy may well be necessary before the obesity can be corrected.

It is thus important to determine, to the degree that this is possible, the cause of the obesity and to examine critically the subject's motive for wanting to lose weight. Sometimes it is helpful to trace a weight curve through the individual's life and to attempt to relate high and low points to corresponding life circumstances and occurrences. Clarification of the reasons for failure to reduce before—or for possible relapses after previous attempts at weight reduction—should also be obtained.

Other Measures

The average obese individual will welcome any preparation which will curb his appetite or assist in other ways his attempts to lose weight. A variety of such pharmaceutical aids exists, based on different principles of approach. (Most physicians do not regard these as desirable measures; they are mentioned here for the sake of completeness.) The most innocuous, though not necessarily desirable, are bulk-producing substances which act by filling the stomach and presumably curb hunger pangs without adding many calories to the body economy. These are usually nonmetabolized vegetable gums like methylcellulose; they are taken before regular mealtimes, followed by relatively large quantities of water. The wetted gum swells into a plastic mass which fills the stomach and may decrease the subsequent food intake at mealtime by producing a false feeling of satiety. In practice, these bulk-producing substances help less than half of those who try them, and they have only temporary value. They should not be used unless prescribed by a physician, since they are not always harmless. Their overzealous use may be accompanied by the production of nutritional deficiencies, and they are thus not desirable, especially in the wrong hands.

Other bona fide pharmaceutical preparations include appetite depressants of the amphetamine type. These produce a certain amount of euphoria, decrease the urge for excessive eating, and thus make dietary restrictions more tolerable. Their effect is only temporary, and the individual using them may become habituated to them. Being central nervous system stimulants, they have undesirable excitatory side effects ranging from insomia (when taken at dinnertime) to nervousness, increased pulse rate, palpitations, and a temporary rise in blood pressure. Such preparations should be used only on specific medical advice, especially since they constitute a certain risk to individuals who are nervous, hypertensive, or suffer from heart disease.

Amphetamine drugs for control of obesity are also available in combination with barbiturates, meprobamate, and similar tranquilizing or sedating drugs. Although the latter may counteract some of the stimulating effects of the amphetamines, they do not contribute otherwise to weight reduction. The belief seems firmly established that the use of appetite-depressing drugs makes it easier for the physician to educate the patient in the correction of his food intake pattern. However, by this emphasis on reliance on drugs rather than on diet alone, such use may be more harmful than helpful. In any event, the use of amphetamine and related drugs usually does not help weight control for more than a brief period, and at best these preparations may serve for some patients as a temporary adjunct to dieting, exercise, and psychotherapy. There is little if any evidence that the known appetite-depressing drugs contribute in any important measure to the long-term correction of obesity.

Substances which raise the basal metabolic rate and thus increase caloric expenditure (for instance, thyroid extract) have also been used in selected cases in an effort to reduce an obese individual who appears refractory to attempts at weight reduction by diet alone. Although such preparations may accelerate weight loss temporarily, because of the danger of undesirable side effects connected with their long-term administration, their use for reducing purposes is not justified.

Prevention

Prevention of obesity is much more desirable than treatment of the condition once it is established. Prevention is accomplished more easily, and it avoids the damage to the obese person's health as well as the unpleasantness and anguish associated with obesity and its subsequent treatment by dietary restriction. To be effective, prevention must start in early childhood. Parents who believe that large, fat children are invariably strong and healthy are mistaken; if overfeeding of the young child is followed by encouragement of overeating on the part of the growing youngster, the habit may persist and be carried into adulthood. It is especially important that overweight parents recognize their responsibility to their children in this respect. Parents should be informed of proper eating habits, and children and adolescents should be trained early. The key figure in the striving for future longevity and well-being is perhaps the teen-age girl. It is she who will probably soon bear children (and who will determine by her own dietetic practices to a large degree the start which they get in life), and it is she who will most probably be the cook and food purchaser and, thus, directly and indirectly, determine the food pattern of her entire family.

Outlook

Obesity is a widespread and complex disorder. Crash programs, special diets, and appetite-reducing drugs seldom lead to more than temporary results. The joke about the fat patient who has lost 500 pounds since he started dieting is tired but apropos. Practically nothing short of a lifetime commitment to dietary self-control can permanently control obesity. Thus a strong motivation is the keystone to long-term success.

The patient should be given valid nutritional information and sympathetic guidance in following a lifelong diet restricted in total calories, adequate in nutrients, and acceptable to his taste and life-style. Sometimes community self-help groups—not unlike Alcoholics Anonymous, in which the obese persons obtain additional motivation through a joint effort with others beset with the same problem—contribute the extra help which leads to long-term success. It can be anticipated that most successes will be short-term ones, and in cases with a repeated history of failure to maintain the hard-won gain, especially where psychiatric insight hints that the obesity may be a protective mechanism, the physician or dietitian may be well advised to help the patient accept his obesity.

Nibbling versus Gorging

Many obese people consume most of their food within a relatively short period each day. These people eat little or no breakfast or lunch, but eat voraciously during the evening. A large proportion of such individuals find it extremely difficult to shed their excess fat through limitation of food intake as long as they persist in their particular intake pattern. In recent years, investigations involving laboratory animals, and preliminary experiments involving man, have been undertaken to shed light on the question whether the *manner* or *periodicity* of eating, specifically the spacing and rate of ingestion, may produce changes in food metabolism and eventual body composition. Results of such experiments have shown that certain changes in intermediate metabolism and body composition may take place in animal species which ordinarily consume their food by ad lib nibbling throughout the waking hours, when these animals are adapted to eating their food during a few infrequent, widely spaced, "gorging" sessions. In general, in the species studied it was observed that a "stuff-and-starve" pattern of food intake (in contrast to "nibbling") is associated with increased fat production from ingested carbohydrates and permanently increased fat deposits in the body—subsequent to a shift in intermediate carbohydrate metabolism from the conventional pathway of glycolysis (see Chap. 8, Fig. 4) followed by the citric acid cycle (Fig. 5), to the hexose monophosphate shunt scheme of carbohydrate degradation (Fig. 6). Other observations included decreased body protein, a somewhat depressed thyroid activity, reduced glucose tolerance (blood glucose levels gravitated toward a diabetic pattern), increased blood cholesterol levels, and a somewhat increased overall food intake. Long-term consequences of this type of feeding program showed that animals fed in this fashion do get fat and that the feeding pattern tends to be self-perpetuating once established.

These observations may have a number of interesting implications in considering man's eating pattern in general ("meal eating" versus "nibbling"), and particularly the eating pattern observed in many obese persons. However, to date insufficient well-controlled studies involving human volunteers have been carried out to draw meaningful conclusions.

Underweight

Broadly speaking, any excess of food supplied to the body beyond its metabolic needs will be stored in the form of fat. However, some persons find it difficult to achieve a normal gain in weight, probably owing to overactivity, chronic lack of appetite, illness, malnutrition, or some deficiency in assimilative power.

As a rule, in order to assure the laying on of body fat, one has to supply an excess of food beyond the caloric expenditure of the individual. One important means of bringing about such a positive caloric balance is to diminish the expenditure of energy. For this reason, physical rest is an important aid for those who should gain weight. The diet should be built around the items mentioned in Chap. 15 and should supply quantities above and beyond what the lean person is used to consume. Respect should be paid to the gustatory preferences of the individual, since it would be useless to prescribe extra food which he refuses to eat.

Fat itself is the most concentrated of calorie-yielding foods. It may be given in the form of butter, gravies, cream, ice cream, pork, well-marbled meat, and fat poultry or fish. Carbohydrates are very useful since extra amounts may be added to the diet easily without becoming too repugnant to the subject and because they have a rapid gastrointestinal clearance, in contrast to fat, which slows gastric motility and imbues the person with a feeling of fullness and satiety for many hours. Protein yields fewer calories than fat, but during attempts to increase weight extra quantities are needed to establish a positive nitrogen equilibrium. Actually, protein will be assimilated in the form of muscle tissue primarily under conditions of increased muscular exercise or when the body musculature has previously wasted in the course of illness or undernutrition. Nevertheless, as new fat depots are laid down, new supporting tissues and a greater blood volume are needed as well, and a positive nitrogen balance is a prerequisite for the formation of such tissues and blood constituents.

Setting an arbitrary level for a high-calorie diet is obviously impossible, but the consumption of 500 cal in excess of the habitual intake should cause a gain of about 1 pound per week as long as the individual perseveres in such a regimen. One of the easiest ways of increasing the calorie intake without inducing a complete overhaul of the established eating habits is the introduction of additional margarine or butter to be used generously on vegetables, eggs, in hot cereals, on rice, noodles, and spaghetti, and in cooking and baking in general. Between-meal feedings may frequently leave the patient with little desire for food at mealtimes; however, highly flavored additional snacks (such as nuts, potato chips, dips, hors d'oeuvres, and extra desserts) may be added successfully to regular meals to increase the calorie intake of a person with a jaded appetitie.

The dietary change and its attendant calorie increments should be introduced gradually. A stepwise increase is much more realistic and practical in achieving the calorie optimum than a sudden, major increase in the customary intake. The appetite of the subject should be encouraged by any effective means. At times a glass of dry wine serves as an efficacious appetizer; if the subject is a heavy smoker, reduction of smoking or outright cessation will often initiate a gain in weight. The high-calorie regimen should be kept up until the desired weight for the subject's height is reached. At this point the caloric intake is gradually reduced to a level which permits maintenance of the new body weight.

Desirable Body Weights and Caloric Intakes

Table 35 details average normal weight for men and women over 25, graded according to body frame. The table allows about 8 pounds for men's clothing and 4 pounds for women's. Age is not specified; the values are for persons 25 to 30 years of age, and the premise is that no further weight change with age is desirable. The normal weight of girls 18 to 25 may be arrived at by subtracting about 1 pound for each year under 25. The table recognizes the fact that, within the same height class, body weights must differ in accordance with relative skeletal breadth; unfortunately there is no accepted system for evaluating into which frame classification a particular individual belongs.

Table 36 gives calorie allowances for individuals of various ages and body weight, as recommended by the Food and Nutrition Board of the National

Table 35   Desirable Body Weights

(The following are desirable weights for men and women over 25, graded according to body frame. These tables, prepared by the Metropolitan Life Insurance Company, are based on weights associated with the lowest mortality. The charts allow about 8 pounds for men's clothing and 4 pounds for women's. To arrive at the normal weight of girls 18 to 25, subtract 1 pound for each year under 25.)

Men

Height (with shoes on)		Weight in pounds, as ordinarily dressed, including shoes and suit		
Feet	Inches	Small frame	Medium frame	Large frame
5	2	112–120	118–129	126–141
5	3	115–123	121–133	129–144
5	4	118–126	124–136	132–148
5	5	121–129	127–139	135–152
5	6	124–133	130–143	138–156
5	7	128–137	134–147	142–161
5	8	132–141	138–152	147–166
5	9	136–145	142–156	151–170
5	10	140–150	146–160	155–174
5	11	144–154	150–165	159–179
6	0	148–158	154–170	164–184
6	1	152–162	158–175	168–189
6	2	156–167	162–180	173–194
6	3	160–171	167–185	178–199
6	4	164–175	172–190	182–204

Women

Height (with shoes on; 2-in heels)		Weight in pounds, as ordinarily dressed, including shoes and dress		
Feet	Inches	Small frame	Medium frame	Large frame
4	10	92–98	96–107	104–119
4	11	94–101	98–110	106–122
5	0	96–104	101–113	109–125
5	1	99–107	104–116	112–128
5	2	102–110	107–119	115–131
5	3	105–113	110–122	118–134
5	4	108–116	113–126	121–138
5	5	111–119	116–130	125–142
5	6	114–123	120–135	129–146
5	7	118–127	124–139	133–150
5	8	122–131	128–143	137–154
5	9	126–135	132–147	141–158
5	10	130–140	136–151	145–163
5	11	134–144	140–155	149–168
6	0	138–148	144–159	153–173

Table 36   Calorie Allowances According to Body Weight and Age
(At Mean Environmental Temperature of 20°C and Assuming Light Physical Activity)

Body weight			Calorie allowance per age		
kg	lb		22	45	65
Men:					
50	110		2200	2000	1850
55	121		2350	2150	1950
60	132		2500	2300	2100
65	143		2650	2400	2200
70	154		2800	2600	2400
75	165		2950	2700	2500
80	176		3050	2800	2600
85	187		3200	2950	2700
90	198		3350	3100	2800
95	209		3500	3200	2900
100	220		3700	3400	3100
Women:					
40	88		1550	1450	1300
45	99		1700	1550	1450
50	110		1800	1650	1500
55	121		1950	1800	1650
58	128		2000	1850	1700
60	132		2050	1900	1700
65	143		2200	2000	1850
70	154		2300	2100	1950

Source: Food and Nutrition Board, National Research Council.

Research Council. Both tables may be used as guides to the desired body weight and caloric intake of individuals.

While such tables have their value, it must be emphasized that they may have less validity for general application than may be apparent at first glance. A muscular athlete or laborer may exceed his ideal body weight by as much as 30 to 40 percent, the "overweight" representing lean muscle tissue built up and maintained because of extraordinary physical exercise. Such an individual will manifest none of the metabolic aberrations characteristic of obesity which depend on degree of body-fat accumulation. Thus, in actual practice it is better to determine whether the individual is fat or lean, rather than decide whether he is overweight or underweight according to the chart. The skin fold thickness and the presence or absence of fat pads over the buttocks and abdomen may give a truer picture than the body weight as such.

Skin Fold Thickness

Measurement of skin fold thickness has emerged in recent years as a practical clinical method of estimating body fat. Measurement is made of the doubled thickness of pinched-up folded skin and subcutaneous adipose tissue in a specified locus of the body. This "fold" is held with the thumb and forefinger of the left hand and pulled away from the underlying muscle; simultaneously special calipers which exert a constant pressure between their two contact points are applied to the isolated "skin fold," and the distance between the caliper points is read on the caliper dial.

The sites usually measured are the triceps and subscapular skin folds. The former is located at the back of the right upper arm midway between the olecranon and acromion processes; the latter is located immediately below the angle of the right shoulder blade. In the clinic, for large field surveys and broad screening purposes, the triceps skin fold thickness is used often as an index of obesity since it is the easiest to measure, gives highly reproducible results, and has a high correlation with body density values—an index of total body fatness. It also involves a minimum of inconvenience and embarrassment to the subject since it does not require disrobing. Standard tables of skin fold thickness and their relation to obesity are now available. A triceps skin fold thickness in males of 25 mm and over, for instance, is characterized as an indication of obesity. Skin fold measurement can also be used as a rough index of body fat on a do-it-yourself basis; thus, nonobese, healthy young adults have a subcutaneous fat fold, squeezed firmly between finger and thumb, halfway between the umbilicus and pubis and about 1 inch from the midline, which corresponds to the thickness of the thumb in the female and the little finger in the male. Occult edema must be ruled out in what may otherwise be an undernourished person.

In general, with respect to desirable body weights and caloric intakes, once the nutritional state has been determined, clinical judgment may still overrule the dictates of the weight chart, as it may well be more desirable to keep the diabetic individual lean and the tuberculous patient fat or to preserve the emotional balance of the obese person with psychiatric problems. On the whole, though, these are the individual exceptions, not the rule.

Part Four

Nutrition in Disease

Chapter 22

Malnutrition and Deficiency Diseases

Malnutrition

Malnutrition is a state of impaired functional ability or deficient structural integrity or development brought about by a discrepancy between the supply to the body tissues of essential nutrients and the specific biologic demand for them. The causes of malnutrition are as manifold as its clinical and subclinical manifestations. Primary malnutrition is the result of insufficient intake of essential nutrients because of lack of food (crop failure, war, poverty), regional lack of availability, improper selection of foods, economic depression, edentia, prolonged imprisonment, and a host of other factors, many of which are concerned with the external environment. Many cases of malnutrition in individuals are not necessarily the result of a deficient dietary intake but are caused by physiologic failure beyond the ingestion stage; for example, a nutritional deficiency may develop as the result of failure to absorb normally an essential nutrient which is supplied by the diet in adequate quantities. Similarly, nutritional deficiencies may be brought about by impaired digestion, abnormal intermediate metabolism, excessive excretion, and increased biologic requirements. Such secondary or conditioned deficiencies may occur, in the face of what may otherwise be an adequate dietary intake, in the case of gastrointestinal diseases with rapid emptying time, vomiting, and diarrhea, in pancreatic or biliary diseases which interfere with normal digestion and absorption, in liver diseases with impaired hepatic function, or when rapid growth, closely spaced pregnancies, lactation, surgery, injuries, extensive burns, or febrile or metabolic diseases increase the body's requirements for one or more nutrients.

Not only are the conditions numerous which predispose to nutritional deficiency, but they are usually multiple and simultaneous in operation. Thus in underdeveloped areas of the world widespread malnutrition is not just the result of one factor—poverty—but ignorance, religious or cultural taboos, and intercurrent chronic parasitic infections play an important compounding role. Just as there is usually more than one predisposing condition at work, ordinarily more than one nutritional factor is in deficient supply. Thus the individual who suffers from a well-defined deficiency of a single essential nutrient is the exception; as a rule a number of deficiencies involving more than one dietary factor are at work concurrently and simultaneously or sequentially bring about an impaired nutritional status and multifaceted disease picture. For instance, the skid-row alcoholic who has neglected his diet for years usually bears multiple stigmata of malnutrition, from the polyneuritis of athiaminosis, through the pellagrous "wine sores" on his skin, to the hepatic damage which is secondary to a deficient intake of high-quality proteins. The occurrence of simultaneous multiple deficiencies complicates the nutritional rehabilitation of the malnourished individual considerably, and the treatment of single deficiencies in a generally and chronically malnourished patient is as effective in bringing about an improvement as the granting of a loan to settle a single debt of a business burdened by a long-standing accumulation of financial obligations.

Pathogenesis of Deficiency Diseases

Though it would be difficult to separate and pinpoint the individual stages, the pathogenesis of a deficiency disease may be looked upon as a continuous, progressive development which, if not interrupted at some point by remedial action, may advance to the final full-blown clinical picture which characterizes the specific disease.

This development starts with nutritional inadequacy because of primary or secondary factors (see above); eventually the body reserves of the nutrient (or nutrients) in inadequate supply become depleted. When tissue depletion has reached a critical point, it interferes with the normal biochemical reactions in selected tissues or in the body at large. This will initially result in functional changes such as increased fatigability or abnormal gastrointestinal or neurologic function. As the nutritional deficiency continues, minor, or eventually major, anatomic lesions develop and gross clinical signs and symptoms become manifest.

Manifestations of Malnutrition

The manifestations of nutritional deficiency are legion. The individual signs and symptoms have been described in the preceding chapters dealing with the food elements; they run the gamut from obscure changes in the composition of the body fluids to major skeletal deformities, from functional disabilities (like the night blindness of avitaminosis A) to the fatal protean disease picture of kwashiorkor. It is important to remember that at present the less dramatic, more generalized (and generally less appreciated) constitutional manifestations of nutritional neglect—retardation of growth, weakness, loss of weight, increased susceptibility to infection, retarded convalescence in disease, slight anemia, mental depression, decreased ability to handle biologic stress situations—are considerably more widespread and in toto probably more significant than the more impressive, but commonly less frequently seen, textbook pathologies of the classic nutritional deficiencies.

The major deficiency diseases, their clinical manifestations, and their treatment are individually described in the sections which follow. A detailed discussion of the biochemical and physiologic basis which underlies the clinical manifestations is found in Part 2 of this book.

AVITAMINOSIS A

Etiology

Primary vitamin A deficiency is due to inadequate intake of vitamin A or its precursors, the carotinoids. Secondary vitamin A deficiency is the result of impaired absorption of the fat-soluble vitamin, as is the case in the diseases associated with steatorrhea—sprue, celiac disease, cystic fibrosis (Chap. 26); secondary deficiency also occurs in the absence of sufficient bile in the intestine, after surgical removal of major portions of the bowel or as a result of the excessive use of mineral oil. Other causes for secondary or conditioned avitaminosis A are failure to convert dietary carotene into the biologically active vitamin A, as in severe liver diseases, diabetes, and hypothyroidism, and depletion of reserves, as in pregnancy and lactation. Vitamin A stores in previously well-nourished adults usually suffice to prevent clinical manifestations of avitaminosis A even after many months of complete deprivation. In contrast, vitamin A deficiency may be produced more readily in infants since they are born with relatively small reserves of the vitamin.

Signs and Symptoms

The basic pathology of avitaminosis A is hyperkeratinization of the skin at large and a keratinizing metaplasia in the linings of the respiratory, gastrointestinal, and genitourinary tracts and endocrine, salivary, sebaceous, and lacrimal glands. Avitaminosis A also results in night blindness since the vitamin is a component of the visual purple of the rods of the retina (Chap. 10).

In children, retarded growth may be a result of the deficiency, though night blindness and progressive xerophthalmia (dryness of the cornea and conjuncti-va) are more common. Xerophthalmia is the result of metaplasia of the paraocular glands with loss of their secretions and of metaplastic changes in the conjuctiva. The full-blown syndrome of xerophthalmia is characterized by a wrinkled and lusterless conjuctiva and haziness and dryness of the cornea with small erosions or punctate superficial infiltrations. Subsequently, perforation occurs and there may be prolapse of the iris, or the lens may be expelled. Inflammation resembling conjunctivitis may develop. This may progress to keratomalacia characterized by softening and destruction of the eyeball, and blindness. This is not seen in the United States, but is not uncommon elsewhere. Generalized dryness of the skin may be observed in infants, but follicular hyperkeratosis is rare in childhood.

Xerophthalmia occurs in many developing countries in Asia, the Middle East, the Caribbean, and Latin America principally in infants and young children and is often associated with protein-calorie malnutrition. It is a major cause of preventable blindness and occurs against a background of poverty, ignorance, and poor dietary practices. The transition from early symptoms of xerophthalmia—dryness of the conjunctiva and night blindness—to advanced xerophthalmia with bacterial infection, to soft and opaque cornea, to eventual total blindness occurs particularly rapidly in the child with clinical protein-calorie malnutrition and is often overlooked until it is too late. Seasonal prophylaxis by introducing green and yellow vegetables into the diet when they are available, and by the annual or semiannual recourse to an oral or intramuscular administration of a large quantity of water-dispersible vitamin A is highly advisable in known populations at risk.

It is particularly important to institute vitamin A supplementation in all children suspected of having a marginal vitamin A status who suffer from protein-calorie malnutrition and who are being given dietary protein supple-ments. It is known that the metabolic and general recuperation which follows protein supplementation will increase the improving child's previously de-pressed vitamin A requirement; it may have little or no vitamin A liver stores, or it may mobilize its last liver reserves and subsequently be plunged into rapid vitamin A deficiency. This is one of the reasons why skim milk powder used for improvement of the nutritional status of children in developing countries should always be fortified with vitamin A to assure that the improvement in protein nutrition is not accompanied by the appearance of the ocular lesions of suddenly activated vitamin A deficiency.

Xerophthalmia is rare in the adult, but decreased dark adaptation and eventual night blindness are common. Xeroderma (dryness and roughening of the skin, with some measure of itching) is followed by follicular hyperkeratosis on the lateral aspect of the arm and extensor surface of the thigh; associated thickening of the keratin layers of the skin on the palms and soles and accentuation of skin markings are not uncommon. However, not all cases of follicular hyperkeratosis in malnourished individuals are specifically due to vitamin A deficiency; nor is cutaneous hyperkeratinization an invariable result of vitamin A deprivation.

Treatment

Treatment consists of administration of therapeutic amounts of vitamin A, correction of the pattern of dietary intake, and in the case of secondary or conditioned deficiency, therapy of the underlying disease or correction of the responsible condition. In young children the daily oral administration of 10,000 IU of vitamin A for 1 to 2 weeks usually suffices; in adults, 25,000 IU is required. Where the possibility exists that dietary fat, including the fat-soluble vitamin A, is not properly absorbed, the newer water-miscible vitamin A preparations are indicated and a wetting agent (polysorbate 80) should be taken with each meal in capsule form. In the event that the deficiency does not respond to oral therapy, intramuscular supplementation is necessary at the rate of 40,000 to 80,000 IU daily for 1 week followed by 40,000 IU every 3 to 6 days.

Once treatment has been successful, a recurrence should be prevented by a prophylactic diet. It is not sufficient merely to prescribe a "well-balanced diet." Detailed dietary instruction is necessary which emphasizes the routine inclusion of foods high in vitamin A (Chap. 10) in the daily diet.

VITAMIN D DEFICIENCY (RICKETS, OSTEOMALACIA)

Etiology

Deficiency in vitamin D leads to inadequate intestinal absorption of calcium and phosphorus and an increased loss of both minerals via the urine and feces. There is usually an attendant moderate decrease in serum calcium and a pronounced fall in serum phosphorus levels; in an effort to maintain normal blood calcium levels, calcium is mobilized from bone. In adults the resultant generalized skeletal demineralization is referred to as osteomalacia.

In infants and children the disease entity caused by vitamin D deficiency, rickets, differs considerably from osteomalacia since here the skeleton is still in the process of active growth and development. Here the organic cartilaginous matrix which precedes hard bone formation is formed, but calcium and phosphorus salts are not deposited in it. Epiphyseal cartilage cells do not degenerate, as they do during normal bone formation, and there is no continued expansion of capillaries and subsequent mineralization along longitudinal growth lines. New cartilage continues to form, resulting in an irregularly widened epiphysis. In severe vitamin D deficiency of long standing, resorption of the cancellous bone of the diaphysis and of cortical bone may be observed. The combination of retarded or insufficient mineralization and the normal gravitational and mechanical stress eventually results in skeletal malformations.

Fundamentally, vitamin D deficiency results from inadequate exposure to ultraviolet light (Chap. 10). In the absence of sufficient endogenous production in the irradiated skin, the individual depends on dietary intake of the preformed exogenous vitamin, and primary vitamin D deficiency is thus the combined result of inadequate exposure to sunlight and deficient dietary intake. Because of interference of the skin pigment with optimal endogenous vitamin D synthesis, the need for dietary vitamin D in the dark-skinned races (particularly in temperate climates and northern locations) is especially great.

Secondary vitamin D deficiencies are the result of failure to absorb the vitamin adequately from the intestine and are usually caused by the same conditions enumerated in the section dealing with secondary avitaminosis A (see above).

Signs and Symptoms

In early rickets there may be few physical findings except irritability and restlessness during sleep. Closure of the cranial fontanelles is delayed, and the affected infant crawls or walks late. A soft, yielding skull (craniotabes) is one of the earliest physical signs; this is followed by beading of the ribs at the costochondral junction (*rachitic rosary*) and enlargement of the epiphyseal ends of the long bones. Eventually, weight bearing and mechanical stress cause bowing of the legs, knock-knee, lateral thoracic depressions at the sites of attachment of the diaphragm (*Harrison's grooves*), and the characteristic pigeon-chest deformity of the rib cage.

Roentgenologic examination may be diagnostic even before clinical signs appear. The most characteristic changes are diminished calcification of existing bone, cupping at the lower ends of the radius and ulna, and a frayed appearance of the diaphyseal ends of the long bones near the growing epiphysis. Cupping occurs because in rickets the cartilage-shaft junction is weak and yields under mechanical strain; as a result, the growing cartilage cells fan out to the periphery.

In osteomalacia of adults, demineralization is pronounced in the spine, pelvis, and legs. Gravitational stress on the softer bones causes compression of the affected vertebrae, bowing of the long bones, and a compression deformity of the pelvis.

In infants and adults alike, the hypocalcemia of rickets or osteomalacia predisposes to rachitic tetany. In most cases this is manifested by neuromuscular hyperirritability, but it may progress to carpopedal spasms, generalized spasticity, and even convulsive seizures as the serum calcium level drops below 7 mg per 100 ml.

Treatment

As long as the dietary calcium and phosphorus intake is adequate, uncomplicated rickets may be treated solely by administration of vitamin D. The recommended daily dosage varies from 2,000 IU on up, depending on the individual's response. The initial dosage of 2,000 IU may have to be increased to 20,000 IU in infants and 40,000 IU in children if the condition remains refractory and provided renal hyperparathyroidism (which does not respond to vitamin D) has been ruled out. The first sign of improvement is a rise in serum phosphorus, which is commonly observed by the second week; this is usually followed by bone mineralization within 2 to 4 weeks of initiation of treatment. Ossification may be demonstrated by x-ray examination. Once an initial response has been obtained, the therapeutic dosage of vitamin D may be gradually scaled down to the prophylactic level of 400 IU.

In the case of malabsorption, water-miscible vitamin D should be given, and if this fails, parenteral administration should be resorted to. When large therapeutic doses of vitamin D are given, the physician must be on the lookout for signs of hypervitaminosis D. If the serum calcium level reaches 12 mg per 100 ml or if calcium casts appear in the urine, vitamin D administration must be stopped immediately and the urine should be acidified to prevent calculus formation (Chap. 30).

If hypocalcemic tetany complicates infantile rickets, intravenous calcium should be given (10 ml of 10 percent calcium gluconate administered slowly, intravenously).

Prophylaxis

Vitamin D deficiency may be prevented by adequate exposure of the infant to sunlight or by feeding vitamin D. The latter is less subject to the vagaries of climate and season and thus more dependable. A minimum of 400 IU of vitamin D should be administered daily to the full-term infant. Premature infants' require the same amount; they should receive 400 IU of the water-miscible form of the vitamin, which will be absorbed even in the face of impaired fat absorption.

Vitamin D may be given in a variety of forms, as cod-liver oil, other fish-liver oils, or part of a pediatric multivitamin preparation. Vitamin D milk is whole milk which has been fortified to contain 400 IU of the vitamin per quart. Practically all commercial brands of nonsweetened evaporated milk are enriched with vitamin D to yield 400 IU per quart after proper dilution. Excessive administration of the pure vitamin may lead to hypervitaminosis D (Chap. 10) and must be cautioned against.

Adult osteomalacia due to vitamin D deficiency is not common. Osteomalacia due to deficiency in vitamin D and calcium may be found after prolonged starvation or in pregnancy complicating malnutrition of long standing. It is felt that adults whose diet is not deficient in calcium and who possess a well-mineralized skeleton do not require supplementary amounts of vitamin D above and beyond their tissue stores of this vitamin and the quantities supplied by endogenous synthesis and by an average diet. In all cases of suspected osteomalacia, postmenopausal osteoporosis must be ruled out.

THIAMIN DEFICIENCY (BERIBERI)

Etiology

Primary thiamin deficiency is the result of inadequate dietary supply. In Southeast Asia, where the dietary of the poor strata of the population consists primarily of polished rice and little else, beriberi is still common. Not only is the thiamin content of polished rice negligible, but the predominance of carbohydrate in the diet raises the metabolic thiamin requirement (Chap. 11) and helps to precipitate the disease. Beriberi is quite common when pregnancy and lactation raise the individual's thiamin requirement, and breast-fed infants may display symptomatology, since the milk of the malnourished mother may be deficient in thiamin. Most cases of thiamin deficiency in the United States and the Western world are found among chronic alcoholics who have a notoriously poor dietary intake owing to the replacement of potential thiamin-containing foods with alcohol, which may supply part of the caloric requirement of the individual.

In many instances, especially in the United States, where the diet is likely to contain more thiamin, conditioning factors are at work to precipitate the clinical manifestations of athiaminosis. These factors may be conditions which raise the thiamin requirement—pregnancy, lactation, pyrexia, hyperthyroidism—or diseases which interfere with proper absorption or utilization and hepatic disorders.

Signs and Symptoms

The earliest manifestation of thiamin deprivation is a syndrome of neurasthenia characterized by lack of initiative, anorexia, mental depression, irritability, poor memory, easy fatigability, inability to concentrate, and vague abdominal and cardiac complaints. With advancing deficiency, neurologic symptoms appear in the form of a bilateral, symmetrical peripheral neuropathy which involves at first the longest nerve pathways, the most distal parts of the lower extremities. The neuritis is characterized by paresthesias ("pins and needles") of the toes followed by burning sensations in the feet which are particularly pronounced at night. The symptomatology progresses with advancing degeneration of the peripheral neuronal pathways, to include decreased perception of light touch, calf muscle tenderness, loss of vibratory sense, loss of normal reflexes, and eventually motor weakness and secondary muscular atrophy, involving at first the distal leg and progressing proximally. Once the neuropathy in the lower extremities is advanced, the hands and arms may also become involved. (This usually happens after the sensory abnormalities have extended to the middle of the thigh.) In very advanced cases of athiaminosis Wernicke's syndrome may develop (Chap. 34).

Thiamin deficiency may also cause defects in the myocardium, and in beriberi the heart may show dilatation and enlargement, especially on the right side. Histologically the heart muscle shows focal or diffuse necrosis of muscle fibers with edema fluid in the interstitial spaces. In *wet beriberi* (in contrast to *dry beriberi*, which is characterized chiefly by peripheral polyneuritis, paralysis, and muscle atrophy) the clinical picture is to a large degree one of congestive heart failure with cardiac dilatation secondary to damage of the cardiac musculature and with serous effusions and dependent edema. Dyspnea, irregularities of heartbeat, and a large pulse pressure are commonly found. Serous effusions into the pericardium and pleural and peritoneal cavities with generalized edema may also be seen in beriberi when the heart is competent. The underlying mechanism of wet beriberi without etiologic cardiac involvement is not clearly understood and has been ascribed by some clinicians to concurrent hypoproteinemia.

Beriberi may be predominantly of the dry or wet type or may display a mixed symptomatology. In either case, anorexia, constipation, nausea, and vomiting are common. In infants an acute form of the disease may occur which runs a fulminating course and terminates in cardiac failure.

In the United States thiamin deficiency syndromes occur almost exclusively in alcoholics and are usually attributed to a poor dietary intake. It has recently been demonstrated that, in addition to the expected poor diet, in severe alcoholism there is also a specific impairment of intestinal absorption of thiamin which may play a determining role in alcoholic thiamin deficiency. In conjunction with this it should be mentioned that a new form of the vitamin— thiamin propyl disulfide—has intestinal absorption qualities greatly superior to the conventional thiamin hydrochloride, which is absorbed by a rate-limiting process and is often not absorbed well in malnourished subjects and alcoholics. (In such individuals oral administration of thiamin propyl disulfide yields superior therapeutic results.)

Treatment

The treatment of athiaminosis in any of its forms consists of prompt oral or parenteral administration of thiamin. The dosage depends on the clinical manifestations and varies from 10 to 15 mg of oral thiamin daily in divided doses in cases of neurasthenia or mild polyneuritis to twice this dosage in advanced neuropathy. Thiamin may also be administered parenterally; 10 to 20 mg once a day suffices in cases of peripheral neuritis. Patients with beriberi heart disease or Wernicke's syndrome should receive 10 to 20 mg parenterally, twice daily, until improvement is noted. Infantile beriberi, which is usually acute, is best treated by parenteral administration of 5 to 10 mg of thiamin daily.

Clinical nutritional deficiencies involving a single nutrient are rarely encountered; as a rule the patient is malnourished with regard to more than one essential nutrient and the clinical manifestations of the most acute deficiency are more prominent and are responsible for the major diagnostic label.

Consequently, in all cases of athiaminosis a prompt correction of the general dietary defect is mandatory and multiple therapy with other vitamins (particularly those of the B complex) is indicated. The extent of supportive multivitamin therapy will depend on the clinical judgment of the attending physician.

In addition to supplementation with other vitamins, a generous supply of high-quality proteins should be made available in the form of easily assimilable foods. The food cocktails mentioned in Chap. 23 in connection with the full liquid diet and tube feeding lend themselves particularly well to the feeding of weak, anorexic, malnourished patients.

Prophylaxis

Once the therapy of athiaminosis has been successful, a recurrence should be prevented by the establishment of an improved dietary pattern and, if possible, correction of the conditioning factors which led to the dietary neglect. It is not sufficient merely to prescribe a well-balanced diet, but detailed dietary instruction is essential which emphasizes the routine inclusion of foods high in thiamin (Chap. 11) in the daily diet.

NIACIN DEFICIENCY (PELLAGRA)

Etiology

The cause of pellagra is a severe deficiency of niacin and its precursor, the amino acid tryptophan. Primary niacin deficiency is usually associated with a diet based chiefly on corn and inadequate amounts of tryptophan-containing proteins. Milk and wheat protein contain sufficient tryptophan to compensate for a diet which is inadequate with respect to niacin. In contrast, corn protein is deficient in tryptophan and constitutes no protection against pellagra in the absence of adequate sources of niacin or tryptophan in the rest of the diet. Thus pellagra is not uncommon in areas where economic depression goes hand in hand with a traditional corn diet.

Pellagra is particularly likely to be found in the following predisposed groups:

1 The indigent and individuals with long-standing poor dietary habits. As a rule such individuals have subsisted for prolonged periods on a diet characterized by a low caloric intake; a high carbohydrate and fat content; a low protein, vitamin, and mineral content; and the glaring absence of fresh fruits and vegetables, lean meats, eggs, and milk.

2 Individuals afflicted with diseases which interfere with appetite or with the absorption and utilization of foods. Secondary niacin-tryptophan deficiencies may thus be found in chronic diarrheas, malabsorption diseases, hepatic cirrhosis, tuberculosis, and in disease states in which the metabolism is elevated.

3 Chronic alcoholics. The underlying etiology is the habitual, long-standing dietary neglect so often found in this group.

4 Occasionally patients treated with large doses of the drug isonicotinic acid hydrazide. This is a pyridoxine (vitamin B_6) antagonist and may create a deficiency in this vitamin, which is essential for the conversion of tryptophan to niacin.

Recently a mechanism other than simple niacin-tryptophan deficiency has been implicated in the causation of pellagra in population groups in India which consume large quantities of the millet cereal *jowar* as well as maize. Jowar has a very high leucine content (as maize does). Levo-leucine was found to interfere with tryptophan and niacin metabolism. Experimentally, leucine induced the canine equivalent of pellagra (blacktongue) in dogs and aggravated the symptoms of pellagra in pellagrous patients; the symptoms could be ameliorated by withholding the leucine supplements or by niacin supplementation.

Signs and Symptoms

Niacin deficiency may display the complete classic syndrome of pellagra with extensive dermatitis, glossitis, stomatitis, diarrhea, and mental disturbances, but in many cases it may manifest itself only with partial symptomatology, which features one deficiency sign alone or more in combination.

The cutaneous manifestations may be divided into four major types. The most acute lesion is characterized by erythema, which progresses through vesiculation and production of bullae to eventual crusting and healing. Sunlight appears to be one of the precipitating traumatic factors. Intertrigo with redness, maceration, and secondary infection is also found frequently. Another cutaneous manifestation is chronic hypertrophy with induration, fissuring, and pigmentation on pressure points. Chronic atrophic, ichthyotic changes with scaling and induration may be seen in pellagra cases of long standing.

The distribution of the skin lesions in pellagra is quite characteristic. They are usually found on parts of the body exposed to sunlight or mechanical trauma. Though unilateral lesions may be seen, a bilateral, symmetrical distribution is common. Thus lesions due to exposure to sunlight are found around the neck (*Casal's collar* or *necklace*), on the backs of hands, on the forearms, and on other uncovered parts of the body. Elbows and knees are common pressure points exposed to mechanical trauma and are frequently involved, as are the common intertriginous areas. In the Southern United States a definite seasonal influence on the severity of cutaneous manifestations has long been noted; this has been related to the increase in actinic trauma in the spring and summer.

The mucous membranes of the mouth are usually involved, displaying a scarlet glossitis and stomatitis with a swollen tongue and increased salivation.

The mouth may be very sore, with a burning sensation. In acute, long-term deficiency the buccal mucosa and underside of the tongue may be ulcerated. Pathologic changes in the gastrointestinal tract include atrophy of gastric mucosal cells, superficial ulcerations, and even petechial hemorrhages. Gastric and pancreatric secretions are diminished; this may be one of the underlying causes for the poor digestion and diarrhea characteristic of pellagra.

Gastrointestinal symptoms are at first limited to indeterminate burning sensations, postprandial epigastric discomfort, gaseous distention, eructation and flatulence, and occasional vomiting; these are followed by severe and extensive diarrhea, which may be bloody in cases of intestinal ulceration. The stools may be soft and watery (or even hard on occasion); their odor is invariably foul.

Central nervous system symptoms also occur and may consist of neurasthenia similar to the neurasthenic syndrome described above in connection with athiaminosis, or of a psychosis characterized by disorientation and confusion, anxiety, fear, hallucinations, occasional delirium, and paranoia, mania, or depression. A well-defined encephalopathic syndrome with lead-pipe rigidity of the extremities, sucking and grasping reflexes, and clouded consciousness is also recognized in severe niacin deficiency; it has been observed in severely malnourished patients following massive intravenous fluid therapy without adequate vitamin supplementation. The neurasthenia of niacin deficiency and the encephalopathic syndrome are discussed in greater detail in Chap. 34. The effects of niacin, thiamin, and other deficiencies are not always clearly distinguishable; thus in suspected pellagrins, concurrent thiamin deficiency may be responsible for some of the central nervous system symptomatology and is usually responsible for any evident peripheral neuropathy.

Treatment

The patient should be confined to bed until convalescence is well under way. Specific therapy consists of the oral administration of from 100 to 300 mg of niacinamide daily in divided doses. The amide is preferable since it does not precipitate the vasomotor disturbances resulting from administration of niacin (nicotinic acid) in large quantities. Niacinamide is given subcutaneously in multiple doses of 50 to 150 mg in cases where diarrhea or a noncooperating patient make oral administration ineffective or difficult. Since chances of concurrent multiple deficiencies are ever-present, multiple therapy with other vitamins (particularly those of the B complex) is indicated.

In conjunction with specific niacinamide therapy and supportive multivitamin supplementation, a well-balanced diet is given which contains 100 to 150 g of high-quality protein (preferably from meat, milk, and eggs) and provides about 3500 cal. In view of the gastrointestinal symptomatology, the diet should at first be a full liquid diet devoid of roughage. As the patient improves, a general diet high in good-quality proteins is given.

The treatment in cases of pellagrous central nervous system manifestations is discussed in detail in Chap. 34.

Prophylaxis

As in any other nutritional deficiency, effective prevention is more desirable than an eventual cure. Prophylaxis is especially important after successful treatment of pellagra since recurrences are common. An improved dietary pattern should be established, and if possible the conditioning factors which led to the dietary neglect should be corrected. It is important to remember that niacin will not become critical in an individual who consumes a diet which contains a variety of proteins including those from meat, eggs, and milk, since such food intake assures a supply of the precursor of niacin—tryptophan—in addition to the quantities of preformed niacin which are provided by such a diet.

RIBOFLAVIN DEFICIENCY

Etiology

Ariboflavinosis as a clinical syndrome may be found in individuals who consume a marginal diet devoid of dairy products, or other animal protein sources, and leafy vegetables. Secondary deficiencies may occur in chronic diarrheas, in malabsorption and liver diseases, and in states of increased metabolism. Riboflavin deficiency is not uncommonly found associated with pellagra.

Signs and Symptoms

The syndrome is characterized by cheilosis, angular stomatitis, glossitis, seborrheic dermatitis, and ocular manifestations—photophobia, itching, burning, and circumcorneal capillary engorgement with invasion of the superficial strata by blood vessels. The seborrheic dermatitis is usually found in the nasolabial region, near the inner and outer canthi of the eyes, behind the ears, and on the posterior surface of the scrotum. Any one of the symptoms when taken alone is not necessarily suggestive of ariboflavinosis; thus similar ocular lesions may have other etiologies, the seborrhea may be nonspecific, and angular stomatitis with fissuring may also be the result of edentia. However, the complete syndrome together with a suggestive history of a poor dietary intake is considered indicative of ariboflavinosis. A therapeutic trial will, in the end, confirm the diagnosis.

Treatment

The treatment of ariboflavinosis consists of administration of riboflavin coupled with improvement of the diet. From 10 to 20 mg of oral riboflavin is given daily in divided doses. Riboflavin supplementation should continue at the rate of 5 to 10 mg daily until complete recovery. A well-balanced diet rich in milk and milk products, organ meats, meat, and leafy vegetables should accompany the specific vitamin therapy. The remarks concerning multiple-vitamin therapy and prophylactic improvement of dietary habits which were made in previous sections dealing with other deficiencies are similarly valid with respect to ariboflavinosis.

VITAMIN C DEFICIENCY (SCURVY)

Etiology

Though subclinical vitamin C deficiency may be found in selected population groups, frank scurvy is relatively rare in the United States today. Classic scurvy was once widespread among sailors and explorers who depended on hardtack and salt-beef diets devoid of fresh fruits or vegetables. Today the greatest incidence of scurvy in the United States and Canada is found among infants who have been fed an exclusive cow's milk formula diet without supplementation with juices rich in vitamin C or other ascorbic acid supplements. As a rule, breast-fed infants have an extremely low incidence of vitamin C deficiency.

In later life, scurvy is limited to individuals who, for one reason or other, consume a diet devoid of fruits or vegetables which contribute vitamin C. Thus scurvy occurs at times in ulcer patients who consume diets which consist chiefly of milk, cream, eggs, and cereals. The disease is also found sporadically among elderly, impecunious bachelors, widows, and widowers who live alone and subsist on staple foods which can be stored and prepared easily and usually are extremely low in vitamin C content. The disease is still found in epidemic proportions among otherwise healthy individuals with a food intake restricted for prolonged periods to easily stored, nonperishable staple foods; thus the frequency of clinical signs of scurvy was considerable in soldiers of the South Korean Republic during and immediately after the Korean war, until a revision of the food pattern erased the condition almost completely.

Signs and Symptoms

The basic defect in vitamin C deficiency is an impairment of the normal formation of (primarily mesenchymal) intercellular ground matrix, be it collagen in the case of fibroblastic proliferation, chondroid or osteoid in the case of skeletal development, or the intercellular cement which is responsible for the cohesion of endothelial capillary cells. Thus defective collagen formation is responsible for impaired wound healing, the growing skeleton may exhibit an abnormal fragility due to the defect in osteoid formation and subsequent impaired calcification, and hemorrhages are possible in almost any tissue or organ owing to increased capillary fragility.

In infants scurvy usually develops between the fifth and fourteenth months. The patient fails to gain weight, is irritable and cries easily, has little appetite, and shows an aversion to moving the extremities because of pain connected with such motion. Hemorrhages due to increased capillary fragility may occur anywhere in the body. The costochondral junctions of the rib cage are usually beaded (*scorbutic rosary*), and x-ray examination shows a transverse enlargement and increased density at the ends of the long bones proximally to the epiphysis (the *scorbutic white line*) and a thin, nonmineralized, halolike distal epiphysis; a nonmineralized fibrous union between diaphysis and epiphysis is also discernible. A tendency to hemorrhage on minor trauma results in numerous ecchymoses, hemorrhages in the gums near erupting teeth (gums are very swollen, in such instances, and dark red in color), and subperiosteal hematomas or painful hemorrhages into the joints.

In adults, scurvy may not develop for many months after onset of vitamin C deprivation because the situation does not involve impaired growth and skeletal development and because of the presence of body reserves of ascorbic acid. Eventually weight loss, weakness, irritability, and nonspecific aches and pains in joints and muscles usher in frank clinical scurvy. This will happen when the overall ascorbic acid body pool size has dropped to less than 300 mg (at this point serum levels frequently approach 0.2 to 0.4 mg per 100 ml). Among the first and pathognomonic signs of frank scurvy are follicular hyperkeratoses (swelling and hardening of the depression from which skin hair grows), and perifollicular petechial hemorrhages. Petechial hemorrhages are found largely in the lower extremities. This is usually followed by gingival hemorrhages (loosening of the teeth is a later symptom in advanced cases) and hemorrhages in any tissue exposed to even minor mechanical trauma. Thus nonspecific petechiae, purpura, and ecchymoses are common. Bleeding into joints and muscles is not uncommon in advanced scurvy, and genitourinary, gastrointestinal, and cerebral hemorrhages occur occasionally in very severe cases. Except for hemorrhages into joints on trauma, there are no specific bone lesions in adults. Sometimes hemorrhages in the retina and bulbar conjunctiva are seen, and a drying up of the tear glands and salivary gland (Sjögren's syndrome) may be observed. In advanced cases emotional changes can be recognized, such as hypochondriasis, hysteria, depression, and decrements in psychomotor performance.

Treatment

Scorbutic patients respond dramatically and specifically to the administration of vitamin C. Infants should receive 150 to 300 mg of vitamin C daily by mouth, in divided doses, for 10 days, followed by 150 mg daily for a month. Thereafter it will suffice to ensure a daily intake of 30 to 60 mg of vitamin C in the form of fresh, unheated processed orange juice of standardized vitamin C content or in the form of noncitrus juices enriched with vitamin C. (Most canned strained juices for infants contain 40 mg of vitamin C per 100 ml.) In case of continued diarrhea or extensive vomiting, the recommended oral vitamin C dosages should be halved and administered intramuscularly or intravenously.

Adult patients should receive up to 800 mg of vitamin C daily, orally, in divided doses, for 1 week. This is followed by 400 mg daily until complete recovery. When parenteral therapy is indicated because of gastrointestinal disturbances, vitamin C is given intramuscularly or intravenously at the rate of half the recommended oral dosage.

Prophylaxis

In infants, the prevention of vitamin C deficiency lies in an early provision of dietary sources of ascorbic acid. Thus, beginning with the second week, infants should receive 1 to 2 teaspoons of strained orange juice daily; this amount should be gradually increased until the intake is 2 to 3 ounces by the end of the second month. The recommended daily dietary vitamin C allowance during the first year of life is 30 mg; since most strained orange juices for infants are standardized to contain 40 mg per 100 ml, a daily intake of 3 fluid ounces of these juices provides an adequate supply of the vitamin. Infants who are sensitive to orange juice may obtain their daily vitamin C quota in noncitrus infant juices which contain or are enriched with vitamin C or through supplementation with ascorbic acid or a multivitamin preparation containing ascorbic acid.

Prevention of vitamin C deficiency in adults lies in the establishment of good dietary habits or in correction of an existing defective food pattern. A well-balanced diet as outlined in Chap. 15 which contains the recommended quantities of citrus fruits (as well as tomatoes, green leafy vegetables, and potatoes) will supply adequate prophylactic amounts of vitamin C. The minimal amount of the vitamin necessary to prevent scurvy is 6.5 to 10 mg per day.

KWASHIORKOR (PROTEIN-CALORIE MALNUTRITION)

Etiology

Kwashiorkor, an African word coined by the Ga tribe in Ghana, is the name given to a clinical syndrome caused by severe protein deficiency in the postweaning stages of infancy and early childhood. Its literal meaning, "first-second," reveals a native insight into the epidemiology of this disorder since it refers to the fact that the condition is initiated in the first child when the second one is born. The disease is widely prevalent in the tropical and subtropical underdeveloped parts of the world and is a major health problem of young children among the poor strata of the population of Africa, India, Central and South America, the West Indies, Mexico, and Southeast Asia.

Kwashiorkor occurs most frequently in the young child soon after it has been weaned and is thereafter largely fed starchy paps; the underlying cause is failure to provide an adequate dietary source of protein to substitute for the protein of the breast milk which had been the child's only protein source before weaning—sometimes for the first 18 to 24 months of life.

There have been a few reports of kwashiorkor in adults. However, it occurs practically exclusively in young children, since the diet after weaning is especially likely to be deficient in protein and because the protein requirement in relation to caloric intake is much higher in early youth than at later periods in life.

Diarrhea or an intercurrent infection is often the precipitating factor which triggers the appearance of clinical symptomatology. Basically this is due to increased nitrogen excretion in disease, but in many cases the parent helps usher in the clinical syndrome by feeding the sick child nothing but thin, starchy gruels or by administering purgatives to rid the child of suspected intestinal parasites.

Signs and Symptoms

The symptoms of the disease are retarded growth, apathy, anorexia, hypoalbuminemia with edema, and characteristic hair and skin changes. The normal dark hair becomes fine, depigmented or reddish yellow, and may fall out in patches. The normally dark skin becomes flaky, peels, and leaves a reticulated, patchy surface ("crazy pavement dermatitis"). Hyperpigmentation and depigmentation of the skin are common. There is fatty infiltration and enlargement of the liver and, at times, fibrosis and cellular necrosis; the acini of the pancreas may show atrophic changes, and in many cases there is a manifest retardation in skeletal development and maturation, particularly around the knee, with subnormal mineralization, thinning of the cortices of the long bones, diminished trabecular pattern, and growth arrest. Severe diarrhea and steatorrhea, accompanied by electrolyte imbalance, potassium depletion, and anemia are part of the kwashiorkor syndrome.

The clinical picture is modified by the general state of nutrition; the classic ("sugar baby") type of kwashiorkor is based on severe protein deficiency in the face of an otherwise adequate caloric intake. A more marasmic picture with severe tissue wasting, loss of subcutaneous fat, and functional dehydration (despite the existing edema) is found where the basic protein deficiency is compounded by an acute or chronic deficiency in calories. In such infants the classic hair and skin changes are less apparent or absent, since the patient has been metabolizing his own tissues, which include endogenous proteins.

The mortality from kwashiorkor is high in the absence of proper treatment. On the other hand, recovery is common after protein repletion except where severe complications exist or where the condition is very advanced.

Other Defects

Severe protein malnutrition is capable of producing a clinically, biochemically, and histologically definable mild-to-moderate malabsorption syndrome. Gross and microscopic changes can be discerned in the small intestine, especially the jejunum. The gut mucosa becomes thin, the villi become flattened, broad, and fused, with atrophy of villi, increased cellularity of the lamina propria, and decreased height of epithelial cells. Concomitantly, the jejunum displays diminished enzyme activity; lactase, sucrase, and maltase activities tend to be low. The low disaccharidase activity is presumed to be an acquired deficit secondary to the mucosal damage. In severe protein-calorie malnutrition even glucose absorption may be abnormally low initially. The low disaccharidase activity makes for poor hydrolysis of disaccharides, especially lactose. In many children return of lactose absorption to normal may require one or more years after recovery.

Some patients also appear to have a defect of fat transport through the intestinal mucosa. Lipids seem to enter the mucosal cells normally, but further handling seems impaired with a resulting mild fat deposition in the cells. Generally, glucose absorption, lactose, and sucrose hydrolysis and fat transport all improve slowly and gradually after dietary treatment is initiated. Clinical recovery generally precedes the slow reveral of the intestinal mucosal defects.

In kwashiorkor, concomitant with a fatty liver, plasma triglyceride levels are low; a rise in blood triglyceride levels coincides, after dietary treatment is initiated, with a loss of liver lipids.

Children with severe kwashiorkor show a characteristic potassium depletion both in the body fluids and in muscle; magnesium deficiency—probably resulting from prolonged losses from diarrhea and vomiting, which also deplete potassium—is also found among the most severely affected children who tend to succumb to the disorder.

Children with protein-calorie malnutrition show an increased susceptibility to bacterial and viral infections. This is probably explained by a decreased bactericidal activity of leukocytes in kwashiorkor (which improves after treatment) and a demonstrated impaired antibody response to systemic viral diseases.

Diagnosis

In most cases, especially in areas where protein-calorie malnutrition is endemic, the presence of kwashiorkor is established by a combination of the medical history and the physical signs and symptoms. A low serum albumin level serves to confirm the diagnosis.

Also, the ratio of nonessential to essential amino acids in the serum is useful in confirming the presence of kwashiorkor and detecting borderline pre-kwashiorkor. In protein-calorie malnutrition there is a characteristic decrease of blood essential amino acid levels which precedes by many days the eventual diminished blood albumin levels which characterize the *advanced* disorder. The normal NEA/EA ratio varies from 1 to 2.1; in pre-kwashiorkor and kwashiorkor this ratio ranges from 2.5 to 4.

In kwashiorkor, depressed serum transferrin levels are related to the severity and course of the disease; a serum transferrin concentration of 0.33 mg/ml or less is related to a grave prognosis; children who recover usually have values above 0.6 mg/ml.

In recent years, examination of hair roots has been developed into a useful and inexpensive diagnostic tool in public health surveys for protein-calorie malnutrition, particularly in developing areas where sophisticated laboratory equipment is not available. Protein deprivation, even of relatively brief duration, results in atrophy of the external hair root sheath and marked atrophy with decrease in diameter and loss of pigment of the root bulb. In protein malnutrition, these changes precede the progressive downward changes in serum albumin and transferrin. Quantitative analytical methods have been developed and do not require highly specialized techniques. Aside from being useful in evaluation of populations known to be at risk in developing countries, these new techniques may also assist in the detection of borderline protein malnutrition in affluent societies where malnutrition is not commonly considered a major problem.

Treatment

Treatment is based on administration of proteins of high biologic value and on correction of any existing dehydration and electrolyte imbalance. A diet rich in milk protein has been the treatment of choice (primarily because of the ease of administration and ready digestibility of milk). Either skim milk powder, fresh skim milk, or whole milk may be used as a source of dietary protein.

During the first day of treatment, half-strength milk containing 5 percent sugar is given in 60- to 120-ml portions, 16 to 8 times per day. Tube feeding may be necessary in extremely anorexic children. Three-quarter-strength formula is fed during the second day, and full-strength formula by the third day. By this time there is less danger of gastric dilatation and vomiting or diarrhea, and the formula may be given in larger quantities at greater intervals. It is desirable to obtain a daily intake of 5 g of protein and 100 cal per kilogram of body weight. In the average 19- to 30-month-old patient this is accomplished by feeding 8 fluid ounces of full-strength milk, with 5 percent sugar, five times daily. Concurrently the child is given light solid foods (such as bananas), provided he can maintain the scheduled milk formula intake. Fruit juice, eggs, meat, vegetables, and cereals are gradually added to the diet throughout the period of recovery; an intake of 5 g or more of protein and 130 to 150 cal per kilogram body weight is the desired goal at this point.

A major problem in the early treatment of critically ill patients is the correction of the often severe dehydration and associated electrolyte imbalance, metabolic acidosis, and potassium depletion (the latter is not uncommonly the cause of sudden cardiac death). Slow intravenous administration of a solution made of one part of 1/6 *M* sodium lactate, two parts of Ringer's solution, and three parts of 5 percent glucose, at the rate of 40 to 50 ml/kg body weight, is helpful in correcting the potassium depletion and counteracts the acidosis, dehydration, and oliguria. In milder cases, potassium-containing fluids such as Darrow's solution should be given orally during the first day of treatment. Oral or intravenous magnesium supplements are beneficial in severe cases.

Specific therapy should also be given to treat or prevent any intercurrent infections. (Sulfonamides and penicillin are preferred to the broad-spectrum antibiotics because of the tendency of the latter to produce diarrhea.)

Special enzyme or lipotropic preparations are not indicated in the treatment of kwashiorkor, and the use of concentrated multivitamin preparations during the first weeks of therapy is not advantageous in most cases.

The rise of previously depressed serum albumin levels during therapeutic protein administration provides an index of progress and prognosis. Unless intercurrent infection or other complications occur, the main clinical signs and biochemical changes of kwashiorkor can be reversed in about 2 weeks, although repletion of normal nitrogen stores and recovery of weight for height usually require at least 3 months.

Prevention

Prevention of kwashiorkor lies in education toward general recognition of its dietary etiology and encouragement of a dietary pattern which supplies more proteins of high biologic quality. Though economic and regional agricultural factors are responsible to a large degree for kwashiorkor in the areas in which it is endemic, ignorance and custom play a significant role as well. Where adequate supplies of milk are not available, a properly selected mixture from available plant protein sources can be used to prevent and even treat the disease. One such mixture developed by the Institute of Nutrition of Central America and Panama (INCAP Vegetable Mixture 9B or Incaparina) contains 29 percent whole ground maize, 29 percent whole ground sorghum grain, 38 percent cottonseed flour, 3 percent torula yeast, 1 percent calcium carbonate, and 4,500 units of added vitamin A per 100 g. It has a protein content of 27.5 percent and is similar in protein quality to milk. It can be produced at a cost within economic reach of the population strata which display the highest incidence of kwashiorkor, and has proved highly acceptable in Central America in the form of a thin gruel (atole). This vegetable protein mixture has also been used successfully as the sole protein source in the therapy of established cases of kwashiorkor, where it produced a response similar to diets rich in animal protein. Other mixtures of slightly different composition have also been developed and used and have proved effective.

Similar inexpensive vegetable protein mixtures for human feeding which increase the quantity and improve the quality of dietary protein have been developed elsewhere, particularly at the Central Food Technological Research Institute in Mysore, India. Among these are Mysore Flour and Indian Multipurpose Food, based on peanut meal and Bengal gram (chick-pea).

The hope for prevention of kwashiorkor and widespread protein deficiency rests on the local development of similar inexpensive and available protein sources and a gradually diversified improved dietary pattern with greater availability of proteins of animal origin.

LONG-TERM CONSEQUENCES OF PROTEIN-CALORIE MALNUTRITION

Effect of Early Malnutrition on Somatic Growth

Despite a considerable body of research devoted to the etiology, pathologic and biochemical features, and diverse methods of treatment of protein-calorie malnutrition, relatively few well-controlled, long-term follow-up studies have been devoted to the effects of malnutrition in early life on subsequent growth and somatic development. There is more and more evidence to suggest that, in the long run, the *duration* of malnutrition has a more lasting effect on growth than the *severity* of malnutrition at any given time. Thus an incident of acute and even severe clinical kwashiorkor or marasmus may have little effect on growth and physical development in the long run provided the child's nutrition is normal and continues that way after the acute illness. In contrast, *continued* protein or calorie undernutrition *throughout* the childhood years can result in a definite stunting of height within the range of the individual's genetic endowment for potential physical growth. Most studies which followed former kwashiorkor patients for 10 or more years indicate that, given an equal nutritional chance and home environment, the slower-developing erstwhile kwashiorkor patients eventually catch up with well-matched controls (such as siblings); at the end of 10 or more years no significant physical differences were noticeable.

Effect of Early Malnutrition on Mental Development

A number of experiments with laboratory animals which were nutritionally severely restricted during fetal life, or very early during the development of their central nervous system, have shown that such deprivation can cause long-lasting or permanent retardation in the development of learning behavior. In recent years attempts have been made to establish whether a valid extrapolation can be made from animals to man.

Early studies have shown that children known to have been afflicted with severe malnutrition in early life did less well in intelligence tests and learning ability than children of similar age and sex who had no history of nutritional deprivation. It has also been shown that this effect is more prounounced in children in whom the episode of clinical malnutrition took place *very* early in life—before the sixth month after parturition. Children in whom malnutrition was manifested later in life showed a progressively diminished intellectual deficit, the later in life the nutritional deprivation took place. Malnutrition *beyond* the third year of life probably has no direct permanent effect on mental development, and starvation studies in adults and concentration camp experiences of World War II indicate that the mental depression and loss of ambition accompanying starvation are wholly reversed after refeeding.

By analogy with animal experiments, the earlier in development the malnutrition occurs, the greater the likelihood of some permanent damage due to interference with orderly organic development of the individual's brain. When brain growth is considered in cellular terms, it is indeed plausible that the brain is at great risk from severe malnutrition during *fetal* development and during the first 6 months of extrauterine life since it completes much of its physical development during this period. It also stands to reason that a severe nutritional deficit prior to completion of somatic brain growth may leave it with a permanent deficit in cell number, which can be the basis of a decreased mentation potential later in life. The as-yet-unanswered question is how malnourished a woman must be to jeopardize fetal nutrition and brain development.

To date studies have established that a high incidence of retardation in psychomotor development can be observed in malnourished children from the lower socioeconomic strata of different countries. The degree of retardation appears to be related to the amount of animal protein consumed and also to retardation in cranial growth. What is known to date does not permit the formulation of definite conclusions, but suggests that chronic undernutrition in the very young may act in a negative fashion upon mental and psychomotor maturation.

Very formidable arguments exist against a pat cause-and-effect relationship between early malnutrition and eventual mental achievement. In contrast to laboratory animals, in children it is difficult to separate the effects of malnutrition on subsequent intelligence from the effects of the social environment, and particularly from the genetic endowment of intelligence inherited from the parents. (None of the studies to date has determined the intelligence quotients of both parents of the children—malnourished and "normal"—whose intelligence was being tested and compared.) Rarely is a child at risk afflicted only with malnutrition. Extreme poverty and disease (and in more affluent countries, parental neglect) accompany and even cause it. Other factors determine the child's learning capacity; these include genetic disadvantages, lack of external stimulation to learn, lack of emotional stimulation and affection, a nonmotivating and nonintellectual environment, and low intelligence quotient and poor education of the parents. For underprivileged children in industrialized and affluent countries such factors are likely to override any effects of nutritional status.

Currently available evidence supports the conclusion that early severe malnutrition is *associated* with intellectual impairment. However, carefully controlled studies are needed to determine whether any effect is due solely to nutritional deprivation or to the constellation of environmental and genetic factors which simultaneously impinge on the malnourished child.

Chapter 23

Diets in Disease

Principles of Therapeutic Diets

Modifications of the normal pattern of food intake are advisable and even essential in the case of a number of diseases. The reasons for this are manifold. In some pathological conditions the quantitative nutritive requirements of the individual may be altered, as is the case in febrile diseases. Other conditions may require changes in the qualitative makeup of the diet; thus curtailment of sodium may be advisable in congestive cardiac failure. In other situations changes in the physical characteristics of the diet may be desirable, as is the case with liquid, soft, or bland diets advisable in certain gastrointestinal disorders.

In deciding on the dietary management of a disease certain general principles should govern the prescription and formulation of any special diet.

1 The diet should provide all essential nutrients as generously as its special characteristics permit.

2 The special therapeutic regimen should be patterned as much as possible after a normal diet.

3 The special diet should be flexible; it should consider the patient's gustatory habits and preferences, his economic status, and any religious rules which may govern his food intake.

4 A diet should be adapted to the patient's habits with regard to work and exercise.

5 The foods which are included in the special diet must agree with the patient.

6 The diet should emphasize natural, commonly used foods which are readily available and easily prepared at home.

7 A simple and clear explanation of the purpose of the diet and reason for it should be given to the patient and to the members of his family who are responsible for the preparation of his meals.

8 Except for cases where a maintenance diet must be adhered to for life, patients should be taken off special diets as soon as possible. Practically anybody required to follow a therapeutic diet feels conspicuous and set apart; this is especially important in the case of young children, who are more impressionable and for whom a prolonged special diet may be the making of an emotional problem.

9 The diet must be absolutely justified and defensible. Hospitals, patients, and patients's family alike will benefit if the number of special diets is reduced to those which are really necessary.

10 Feeding by mouth is always the method of choice; only when the patient is incapable or will not eat and drink enough should tube feeding or, if this is contraindicated, parenteral feeding be resorted to.

The Full Liquid Diet

Liquid diets are usually prescribed after surgery, in acute infections, and in cases where the patient has difficulty in swallowing or suffers from an acute inflammatory condition of the gastrointestinal tract. With subsequent recovery, the liquid diet is modified to a soft diet, which in turn gives way to a full, general diet. As the name implies, the liquid diet consists primarily of liquids or strained, semiliquid foods. Its purpose is to satisfy the normal requirements for all nutrients in a form which requires minimum physiologic effort for digestion and absorption. The full liquid diet consists of milk, milk drinks, carbonated beverages, coffee, tea, strained fruit juices, tomato juice, broth, strained cream soups, raw eggs, cream, melted butter and margarine, strained precooked infant cereals in milk, thin custards, gelatin desserts, ice cream, sherbet, strained vegetables (in soups), honey, syrups, and sugar and dry skim milk dissolved in liquids.

Fortified eggnogs and milk shakes are important nutritional mainstays of the liquid diet. The caloric value of milk is easily increased by the addition of sugar, syrups, honey, or cream; its protein content may be increased inexpensively by admixing dry skim milk powder (2 or more tablespoons per 8 ounces of milk). When blended into such a milk shake, enriched precooked infant cereals contribute significant amounts of iron, thiamin, and niacin, in addition to protein and calories. Raw eggs are easily homogenized with such milk drinks in a food blender and contribute protein, fat, iron, and vitamins.

Because liquid diets are ordinarily used for relatively brief periods, too little thought is given to their nutritional adequacy. Actually, the liquid diet may be used for prolonged periods, as is the case in conditions like esophageal stricture, terminal esophageal malignancy, or progressive bulbar paralysis. If a liquid diet is to be used for more than a few days, it should fully satisfy the nutritional requirements of the patient. Such a goal is readily met if the following items, or their equivalents, are incorporated into the daily diet:

1 qt whole milk
4 eggs
$3^1/2$ oz dried skim milk
$4/5$ oz (25 g) precooked enriched oatmeal for infants
7 oz 20% cream
1 tbsp dried brewer's yeast
1 cup sugar
1 cup orange juice

These food items contribute 2500 cal, 112 g protein, 3,160 mg calcium, 25 mg iron, 5,750 IU vitamin A, 4.7 mg thiamin, 5.4 mg riboflavin, 19.6 mg niacin, and 99 mg vitamin C; this more than meets the average daily dietary allowances for sedentary adults recommended by the Food and Nutrition Board. All ingredients, with or without the orange juice, can be made into a tasty food cocktail in a food blender with the addition of a flavoring agent (chocolate or vanilla) and, if desired, additional sugar. The mixture yields about 3 pints and should be served in six feedings of 1 cup each. At each of the mealtimes, coffee or tea, sherbet, orange or tomato juice, or broth or strained soup may be added for additional variety and flavor.

Sample Menu: Full Liquid Diet

(Contains approximately 115 g protein, 125 g fat, 320 g carbohydrate, and 2865 kcal)

BREAKFAST
Orange juice ($^1/2$ cup)
Food cocktail (1 cup)
Coffee

MIDMORNING
Food cocktail (1 cup)

LUNCH
Tomato juice ($^1/2$ cup)
Consommé
Food cocktail (1 cup)
Sherbert (3 oz)
Tea

MIDAFTERNOON
Food cocktail (1 cup)
Ginger ale

DINNER
Grapefruit juice ($^1/_2$ cup)
Consommé
Food cocktail (1 cup)
Gelatin dessert ($^1/_2$ cup)
Coffee

BEDTIME SNACK
Food cocktail (1 cup)
Grape juice

Elemental Diets

For the sake of completeness one should mention at this point a class of soluble liquid formula diets ("elemental diets") which are nutritionally complete and require little or no digestion; they are more fully described in Chap. 25 as a minimal-residue formula diet.

The Clear Liquid Diet

This standard hospital item should not be credited with the designation "diet." The clear liquid diet provides a minimal residue and consists primarily of dissolved sugar and flavored fluids. It contains no milk, and it supplies fluid (its main objective) in the form of ginger ale, sweetened tea or coffee, fat-free broth, plain gelatin desserts, and strained fruit juices. The caloric contribution of the clear liquid diet depends on the amount of dissolved sugar which it contains and is usually noticeably deficient when compared with the total body requirements.

Tube Feeding

A number of conditions preclude the taking of food by mouth and necessitate tube feeding or even parenteral feeding. Among these are coma or semiconsciousness, mental disease (especially when temporary restraint is required), terminal malignancy, overwhelming acute or chronic infection, severe burns, paralysis of swallowing muscles, oral pathology or surgery, and reintroduction of food after prolonged, extreme starvation.

Tube feedings may be needed for long periods, and it is therefore essential that they satisfy all nutritional requirements. Any food or food mixture which passes readily through a tube may be used. A number of special mixtures are commercially available; they usually combine ease of preparation with a rather high cost, and several among them fail to satisfy the full range of daily nutritional requirements.

The accompanying tube feeding formula is easily prepared from common food items and supplies considerably more than the average daily dietary allowances for sedentary adults recommended by the Food and Nutrition Board. This formula contributes 2700 cal, 129 g protein, 113 g fat, 300 g protein, 3,520 mg calcium, 18.5 mg iron, 6,700 IU vitamin A, 6.35 mg thiamin, 8.0 mg riboflavin, 21.1 mg niacin, and 102 mg ascorbic acid. If desired, a vitamin supplement may be substituted for part or all of the brewers' yeast and the orange juice. The salt may be omitted in the case of patients requiring a controlled sodium intake.

The formula is homogenized in a covered food blender and is stored in closed bottles in the refrigerator. Prior to feeding, the required portion is heated in a double boiler to about 100°F (temperatures which exceed 100°F may cause curdling). It is not advisable to give tube feedings in excess of 200 ml at any one time. Usually about 150 ml (5 fluid ounces) is given every 2 hours, ten times daily. The formula supplies about 1,500 ml of fluid daily, and the remainder of the patient's fluid requirement may be administered in divided doses in the form of water run through the tube immediately after each feeding. Important: If the ability of the stomach to empty is questionable, clear liquid feedings must be given initially and the remaining contents aspirated every 2 or 3 hours.

	Weight, g	Approximate household measure
Whole milk	1,000	4 cups
Egg yolks	100	5 yolks
Dried skim milk	150	5$^1/_3$ oz
Cream, 20%	200	1 cup
Sugar	125	4$^1/_3$ oz
Orange juice	200	7 fl oz
Dried brewers' yeast	50	3$^1/_2$ tbsp
Salt	5	1 tsp

Though rubber tubes of Levin type can be used, the smooth, thin polyvinyl or polyethylene tubes (No. 8, French, 38 inches long) are preferable; they lend themselves well to nasal and gastric passage, are well tolerated, and usually do not produce tissue irritation even if left in place for several weeks.

The Soft Diet

The soft diet is an easily digested intermediate between a full liquid diet and a light general diet. It usually follows the full liquid diet in the transition to a normal food pattern. As the name implies, only mechanically soft foods are included in the diet; fried foods, foods which contribute a significant indigestible residue (crude fiber), strongly flavored cooked vegetables, all raw vegetables, most raw fruits, whole-grain cereal products, and nuts are excluded.

Permissible foods	*Foods excluded*
Milk and milk drinks, coffee, tea, soft drinks, fruit juices	All other beverages
Precooked infant cereals, other refined cereals which do not contain bran	Whole-grain cereals
Fine, enriched white or rye bread, soda crackers	Whole-grain breads, rolls, or crackers; pancakes, waffles
Ground or tender meat, fish, or fowl, roasted, baked, or stewed; canned fish (without bones); cottage cheese, cream cheese, and very mild aged cheeses; soft-boiled and poached eggs	Fried, salted, smoked, or tough meat, fish, or fowl; sausages, luncheon meats; fried eggs; cured, aged cheese
Potatoes (except as noted on the right), macaroni, spaghetti, noodles, rice	Fried potatoes, potato chips; skins of baked potatoes should not be eaten
Butter, margarine, cream, oils	
Soft-cooked, strained, or chopped carrots, peas, beets, spinach, sweet potatoes, squash, asparagus tips, tomatoes; tomato juice	All raw vegetables; also cooked onions, cabbage, cauliflower, brussels sprouts, cucumbers, peppers, turnips, radishes, corn, dried beans, and peas
Soft-cooked or canned apples, peaches, apricots, pears (all without skins or seeds); other soft-cooked fruits if strained; raw bananas, avocados, fruit juices	All raw fruits except as noted on the left; also canned or cooked figs, pineapple, berries
Soups made from permissible foods	All other soups
Bland puddings, junkets, custards, gelatin desserts, ice cream, sherbet; soft, unspiced cakes and cookies	Pies, pastries, doughnuts, spiced baked goods, desserts containing fruits or nuts
Soft sweets, honey, jelly, spices, herbs, vinegar, gravies	Hard candy, candy containing nuts or fruit; marmalade, pickles, popcorn, nuts

Diet in Febrile Diseases and Infections

In contrast to the custom prevalent before the turn of the century, present-day clinical opinion holds that the fever patient should be generously fed to the limits of his digestive ability, except in the case of specific abdominal conditions. The free administration of food does not, as was once believed, raise the temperature of the febrile patient, and the digestion and absorption of a light diet goes on as well and undisturbed in the febrile as in the nonfebrile state. Moreover, during fever the basal metabolism increases significantly; in typhoid fever it has been found to increase 40 to 50 percent at a temperature of 104°F. It is a safe working assumption that the basal metabolic rate increases about 7 percent for each degree Fahrenheit in excess of the normal 98.6°F, and in the absence of a compensatory dietary caloric supply, tissue catabolism must furnish the required energy. As a result the underfed febrile patient is thrown into a negative nitrogen balance, which is far from desirable since it predisposes to hypoproteinemia and anemia, interferes with the body's anabolic defense mechanisms, and delays convalescence.

In the treatment of short-lived, acute febrile conditions, such as upper respiratory infections, it often suffices to supply a normal diet ad libitum and to maintain the patient's fluid intake to prevent dehydration. However, if the febrile illness is more serious and of several days' duration, the dietary management of the patient assumes a new significance.

Nitrogen losses precipitated by infectious illnesses may be quite extensive and tend to continue far beyond clinical recovery. In general, nitrogen losses are exhibited increasingly by the patient with infectious diseases as the conditions reach their clinical peaks. Maximum deficits, however, often occur after the period of highest fever. After serious systemic bacterial or viral infections, a negative nitrogen balance may persist up to several weeks after apparent return to "normal" health.

The dietary support of patients in prolonged, high-febrile states calls for a caloric intake of up to 80 cal/kg body weight (3500 to 5000 cal per average adult). A protein intake of 1.15 to 1.6 g/kg is required to maintain nitrogen equilibrium (80 to 110 g protein per average adult). Since they pose a smaller digestive and absorptive burden, carbohydrates should supply 55 to 60 percent of the total caloric intake. Because the febrile patient has often little appetite and lacks strength or desire to chew a normal diet, a liquid diet should be provided; this may be supplemented with soft-boiled eggs, custards, and cooked cereals. The caloric intake may be raised considerably by the use of supplementary sugar dissolved in fruit juices. With subsequent improvement a soft diet is introduced, and as convalescence progresses this gives way to a light, general diet.

Specific Therapeutic Diets

Specific methods of therapeutic dietary management, their principles, rationale, indications, and makeup are described in detail in the subsequent chapters. In all instances an attempt has been made to represent the convergent trend of current clinical thought.

Chapter 24

Nutrition in Diabetes Mellitus

Diabetes mellitus is a hereditary metabolic disorder characterized by deficient endogenous production or utilization of insulin, a hormone normally produced by the island cells of the pancreas. The presence of insulin in adequate amounts is essential for normal carbohydrate, or more specifically, glucose metabolism. Insulin deficiency results in impaired intracellular glucose breakdown, decreased conversion to fat, and defective glycogen formation. Consequently, glucose accumulates in the bloodstream (hyperglycemia) and spills over into the urine (glycosuria). Polyuria, polydypsia, polyphagia, and pruritis are secondary attendant symptoms. As the disease progresses, abnormal catabolism of protein and fat becomes part of the picture since carbohydrates are not utilized in a normal fashion for the production of energy. Eventually fat metabolism becomes deranged with abnormal accumulation of the end products of incomplete fat breakdown: acetoacetic acid, hydroxybutyric acid, and acetone. Unchecked accumulation of these ketone bodies leads to ketosis and acidosis, and eventually acidotic coma, the most serious acute complication of diabetes.

In its severe form (occurring more frequently in juvenile diabetes) the untreated disease rapidly progresses to a grave metabolic disorder, ketoacidosis, which may result in coma and death unless controlled by insulin administration and specific supportive therapy. Although the disease can be fatal unless properly treated, in most cases it can be well controlled. Today, with proper treatment, most diabetics can lead a near-normal life. Despite control of clinical symptoms, however, and the usual ability to hold in check the abnormal blood sugar level, in too many cases the long-term complications of diabetes, primarily those affecting blood vessels, peripheral nerves, kidneys, and the eyes, develop relentlessly. As a result, patients in whom the disease developed in early life usually have an abbreviated life-span and suffer progressive disability from the complications of the disease, usually beginning in early middle age.

In addition to changes in capillaries and small blood vessels characteristic of diabetes, the diabetic state also encourages accelerated changes in larger blood vessels akin to those found in atherosclerosis. The combination of these types of progressive blood vessel damage can result in ultimately fatal kidney failure, in narrowing and obstruction of the circulation in the extremities (which most commonly results in gangrene of the toes or foot and may require amputation), and in premature heart attacks. Particularly distressing is the progressive blood vessel damage in the retina of the eye, which in many cases will result in gradual blindness or in retinal detachment with sudden loss of sight. The characteristic progressive nerve damage of diabetes leads to a multitude of serious disabilities including impotence in the male.

In its less severe form, the so-called "maturity-onset diabetes," the disease gradually emerges in later life. This type of diabetes usually does not require treatment by daily insulin injection; in most cases, a diet which reduces the patient's body weight to the lean side of normal, and which avoids sugars, suffices to maintain the patient free of direct clinical symptoms. Nevertheless, even here patients will progressively suffer from complications such as accelerated degeneration of the blood vessels and thus may be subject to premature heart disease and a decreased life expectancy.

Therapy

The principal treatment of diabetes aims at amelioration of the key defect, inability to utilize carbohydrates normally, and at prevention of hyperglycemia and glycosuria by dietary regulation and drug therapy and avoidance of the symptoms of ketosis. Medical therapy is based on the parenteral supply of insulin which is lacking. Insulin may be given in the soluble, crystalline form which acts immediately but has no long-lasting effect or in forms which liberate the active hormone in a delayed, gradual fashion, such as protamine-zinc-insulin, globin-insulin, or isophane (NPH) insulin. Combinations of soluble, quick-acting insulin and the various prolonged-action preparations are also used, depending on the individual. A number of orally administered hypoglycemic drugs (tolbutamide, phenformin, etc.), used singly or in combination, are effective in controlling elevated blood sugar levels and glycosuria in mild maturity-onset diabetes. In recent years, however, there have been indications that the *long-term* use of the oral antidiabetic drugs leads to an increased mortality from cardiovascular disease, and it is now recommended that mild maturity-onset diabetes which does not require insulin injections be treated primarily by diet.

Diet in Diabetes

There is no one proper "diabetic diet." Dietary requirements of diabetics differ with the individual, the severity of the disease, the type and extent of insulin therapy received, and the amount of exercise performed. Also, the caloric content of a diabetic diet depends on the patient's weight and how it compares with his desirable weight. The obese diabetic requires a gradual reducing regimen, followed by a diet that will maintain him at a diabetic "ideal weight," which is about 10 percent lower than his statistical desirable weight (Table 35).

Special dietary regulation is essential for the diabetic, whether or not insulin or oral drug therapy is used. Insulin treatment unaccompanied by a coordinated dietary regimen is undesirable because of the constant possibility of insulin-induced hypoglycemic shock.

DIET FOR PATIENTS WITH MATURITY-ONSET DIABETES

A well-observed diabetic diet obviates the use of insulin (or oral antidiabetic drugs) in a majority of the diabetic population, which is composed to a large extent of individuals with maturity-onset diabetes. Moreover, a large number of asymptomatic individuals with the hereditary potential for diabetes will not develop the overt disease in later life (as is the common trend) if they manage to maintain a normal body weight, or preferably if they keep their weight below "normal." If an asymptomatic latent diabetic is permitted to gain weight as he grows older, he commonly develops frank symptomatology at an advanced age. Such persons respond quite well to diet therapy, and many—once stabilized with initial insulin or hypoglycemic drug support and reduced in weight—may be maintained for years without the need for continuous insulin or oral drug therapy.

Weight Reduction

The prime reason why the single most important objective in diet therapy of maturity-onset diabetes is the attainment of ideal body weight is that the responsiveness to insulin of fat cells depends largely on their size. In man, once the early days of infancy have passed, the total number of fat cells in the body is fixed and no longer increases in response to the needs of additional fat storage. In obese persons, to accommodate the need to store abnormal quantities of fat, the individual fat cells which make up adipose tissue depots enlarge considerably. The larger adipose cells are, the less responsive to insulin they are. Thus, adipose tissue of obese individuals, with enlarged fat cells, shows a diminished response to insulin and requires abnormally large quantities of insulin to sustain normal carbohydrate metabolism and tolerance. In a person with a genetic predisposition to diabetes (or one in whom an impairment of insulin activity is already manifest), the presence of an excessive proportion of largely insulin-insensitive adipose tissue spells the difference between a continued metabolic balance and an inability of the body further to metabolize carbohydrates normally.

On the other hand, in such individuals, weight loss and reduction in adipose cell size, concomitant with the return of normal tissue insulin sensitivity, will reduce overall insulin needs to normal and permit near-normal carbohydrate, fat, and protein metabolism even in the person with a compromised insulin potential—the latent or diagnosed maturity-onset diabetic.

In maturity-onset diabetes, weight reduction to a "lean" body state is the only therapy that many need to control symptoms. Whether *asymptomatic* hyperglycemia should be corrected is controversial. With weight reduction, carbohydrate tolerance is likely to improve and glycosuria to disappear. Continued glycosuria, when accompanied by excessive urination, or excessive thirst, indicates that the disease is too severe to be treated by diet alone.

Limitation of Sugars

The other general caveat which must be observed in diabetes and applies both to mild maturity-onset diabetes and to insulin-dependent diabetes (which usually has its onset in the early years of life) concerns limiting the intake of refined carbohydrates. In view of the limited ability of diabetics to metabolize carbohydrates, and since hyperglycemia, glycosuria, and faulty fat metabolism with ketosis result when this ability is overtaxed, concentrated sources of quickly absorbable carbohydrates, like sugar, candy, and fruit juices, are avoided or limited as much as possible. Other carbohydrates are not avoided, since most diabetic patients can handle a modest supply of carbohydrates which are being absorbed very gradually from the intestinal tract, especially when they are on supportive insulin or oral drug therapy. Thus, most diabetics, especially those with maturity-onset diabetes, can handle adequately the unrefined carbohydrates, primarily starches, found in flour, cereals, and vegetables (potatoes, beans, and others). *Pure* sugars, however, should be avoided. This includes, as a general rule, sugar per se, or mixed with other foods (on grapefruit or in coffee) or in the form of honey, or in candy, soft drinks, sweet pastry, ice cream, sherbet, canned or frozen fruits, or sugar-containing breakfast cereals. There exists a belief that fruits can be used ad libitum by diabetic patients. This is a fallacy; the predominant sugar in most fruits, fructose, is metabolized to glucose in the liver, and therefore fruits, despite their reputation as a "natural" and "healthy" food, should be eaten by the diabetic in *limited* quantities at any one time.

DIET IN INSULIN-DEPENDENT DIABETES

General Principles

The diet should be nutritionally adequate, with a calorie content which will maintain the patient at his ideal weight or slightly below. Patients on insulin therapy require a regular spacing of food intake to prevent intermittent periods of hypoglycemia. Periods of fast or feast must be avoided, or—in the presence of regularly administered, measured doses of insulin—temporary hypoglycemia or hyperglycemia will result. Ingestion of sugars should be avoided or minimized to avert the associated hyperglycemic peaks.

Carbohydrate Allowance

Contrary to the beliefs of half a century, there no longer appears to be any need to restrict disproportionately the intake of carbohydrates in the diet of most diabetic patients. It has been shown that increasing the carbohydrate content of the diet of insulin-dependent patients without increasing the total caloric content will not increase the insulin requirements. Today, diets containing 45 percent of their calories as carbohydrate are considered suitable for most diabetics. Inclusion of more carbohydrate in the diabetic diet than was deemed prudent in the past provides greater flexibility in menu design and increases patient acceptance of the diet. Moreover, it lowers the previously prevalent extremely high fat content of the diabetic diet, and thus—since much of this was consumed in the form of saturated fats and foods containing cholesterol— may reduce factors predisposing to the development of atherosclerosis and coronary heart disease, the most prevalent cause of premature death and debility in the diabetic.

It is essential to adapt the diabetic diet to the specific needs of the individual; thus, patients with abnormally high blood triglyceride levels, whose disorder is aggravated by the ingestion of even standard quantities of carbohydrate (type IV, or endogenous hypertriglyceridemia; see Chap. 29), must reduce the proportion of this foodstuff in their diet.

If the patient receives insulin therapy, the diet attempts to integrate the intake of carbohydrates with the time course of the insulin preparation used to avoid the risk of a hypoglycemic insulin reaction and to permit as complete and normal a utilization of the ingested carbohydrate through the action of both endogenous (if any) and administered insulin. Thus if long-acting insulin preparations are used, late bedtime feedings are needed to supply glucose during the night hours to reduce the risk of hypoglycemia induced by the gradually liberated insulin (which would otherwise be "unopposed"). In general, to avoid the risk of hypoglycemic reactions, the size and timing of snacks throughout the day or evening must be adjusted to the needs of the individual patient; they depend, among other things, on the amount of physical exercise and the type and dosage of insulin.

Protein and Fat Allowance

In most instances, the potential synthesis of carbohydrate from dietary protein and fat may be disregarded when one considers the relationship between carbohydrates contributed by each meal and the insulin therapy. Protein and fat provide a supply of potential glucose which is made available very gradually by metabolic processes; consequently, these nutrients may ordinarily be distributed as desired among the three meals. However, experience has shown that the gradual glucogenesis from protein eaten during dinner or at bedtime may be useful in preventing insulin-induced hypoglycemia at night or in the early morning hours whenever potent long-acting insulin preparations are used. It is therefore customary to allocate larger amounts of protein to the evening meal and to have another feeding at bedtime.

The protein allowance of the diabetic is the same as that for the normal individual or slightly higher. The protein intake should lie between 1.0 and 1.5 g/kg of desirable body weight. An increased protein intake is desirable after periods of poor control or marked weight loss. Children require more protein than adults, and an intake of 2 to 3 g of protein per kilogram of body weight is proper. Augmented protein allowances are also required during pregnancy and lactation (1.5 to 2 g/kg). If 20 percent of the total calories are provided in the form of protein, then carbohydrate and fat calories are set at 45 and 35 percent, respectively. In low-calorie diets this is easily achieved, but in high-calorie diets the expensive share of protein calories is best reduced to 15 percent, leaving the remaining calories approximately divided between fat and carbohydrate at a 38:47 ratio.

There is some evidence that the nature of fatty acids ingested influences the blood lipid levels of the individual and, by inference, the likelihood of atherogenesis (Chaps. 9 and 29). If the etiologic relationship between the excessive intake of saturated fatty acids and atherosclerosis is proved, then physicians in charge of diabetic patients will do well to consider the prescribed inclusion of fats rich in the polyunsaturated fatty acids in their patients' diets, since the average diabetic is particularly prone to development of atherosclerosis.

Calculating the Basic Requirements

The following will serve as an illustration of how to arrive at the basic dietary prescription. Except in cases of extreme obesity, the ideal weight of the patient is used as the basis of the calculation. (In the case of the diabetic, "ideal" means "normal" less 10 percent.) A moderately active patient who measures 5 feet 10 inches with his shoes on and has a small frame has a normally desirable weight of 145 pounds according to Table 35. His ideal weight as a diabetic is 10 percent less, or approximately 130 pounds. Turning to Table 36, we find that at the age of 65, this patient's daily caloric intake should be about 2100.

The protein allowance is arrived at on the basis of the patient's ideal weight—130 pounds (59kg); allowing 1.5 g protein per kilogram ideal body weight, his daily protein intake should be about 88.5 g. This allowance of 88.5 g protein provides 88.5 × 4, or 354 kcal—about 17 percent of the total requirement. The remaining requirement, 1746 kcal, may now be divided between fat and carbohydrate at an approximate ratio of 36 to 47 percent. This will yield 757 kcal to be supplied by fat and 988 kcal by carbohydrate. Thus 757 kcal may be supplied by 757/9, or about 84 g fat; the other 988 kcal is supplied by 988/4, or 247 g carbohydrate. Since the diet prescription is usually rounded off to the nearest figure 5, the daily dietary recommendation for this patient may be set at 90 g protein, 85 g fat, and 250 g carbohydrate. The physician's clinical judgment will now determine whether the patient is to have the full 250 g of carbohydrate or whether a smaller amount will be allocated and compensated for with an appropriate increase in the fat or protein intake.

Selection of Menu

In addition to meeting the physiologic requirements of the patient, the diet prescription should meet the economic, gastronomic, and social needs of the patient. To limit the patient to a stereotyped menu sheet with no consideration for these factors is to defeat the purpose of the diet, since in all likelihood it will not be adhered to. Thus the translation of the basic diet prescription into a suitable meal plan is an important aspect of planning a diabetic diet.

A simplified method of formulating diabetic diets has been published by a committee made up of representatives from the American Diabetes Association, the U.S. Public Health Service, and the American Dietetic Association. This method permits the planning of diabetic menus by the average layman on the basis of a protein/fat/carbohydrate prescription. The system is flexible enough to allow for a very large number of food combinations and is simple enough to permit restaurant eating without difficulty. All common foods are divided into six groups, or "exchange lists," on the basis of their composition. Milk in its various forms makes up the first list. The next three groups, the vegetable exchanges, fruit exchanges, and bread exchanges, contain foods of increasing carbohydrate content. The major protein-rich foods are found in the fifth group, and the fat exchanges in the sixth.

Each exchange list is characterized by a set protein/fat/carbohydrate composition which holds true, approximately, for all the foods included in the group. Thus members of the same exchange list are freely interchangeable in the menu without basically altering the amounts of protein, fat, and carbohydrate ultimately provided by the meal. The physician or dietitian needs only to supply the patient with the protein/fat/carbohydrate diet prescription, and armed with it and the list of foods included in the exchange lists, the patient can easily make up a variety of menus which add up to his basic prescription.[1] Naturally, the patient must be taught to select his foods wisely so that all the protective foods are represented in his daily diet (Chap 15). Thus the following should be included in the daily menu: at least one good source of vitamin C, 16 to 24 fluid ounces of milk, at least 5 ounces of meat or its equivalent, two servings each of fruits and vegetables, and adequate amounts of fats and enriched cereal products.

Other systems of diabetic dietary management exist and are of definite value. Emphasis has been placed on meal planning with the exchange list system because of the simplicity of the method; however, this should not reflect lack of merit on any of the other systems in use at present.

Juvenile Diabetes

The treatment of diabetes in the child is governed by the same general principles as treatment of adult diabetes, but special consideration must be given to certain peculiar facets of the disease in children: (1) as a rule, juvenile diabetes is of a more severe type; (2) insulin is an obligatory part of the treatment; (3) the blood sugar level is much more labile, and both hyperglycemia and hypoglycemic insulin shock are more easily produced; (4) the nutritional requirements of the growing child are greater and are subject to gradual change; (5) physical activity is more erratic in the child; (6) emotional factors, particularly during adolescence, are less predictable and are likely to influence the course of the disease; (7) intercurrent infections may throw the young diabetic into acidosis quickly and unexpectedly.

Whereas many of the older patients are obese, and a majority have a gradual onset of the disease, most children and young adult diabetics experience a relatively sudden onset of the disease and they tend to be undernourished when the condition is first diagnosed. During the initial period of treatment, provisions must be made for rebuilding the young diabetic's body tissues and nutritional stores. It is thus desirable to provide 3 or more grams of protein and 80 or more calories per kilogram of ideal body weight. Supplementation of the diet with up to five times the normal vitamin requirements is also highly desirable during the initial period. Once the patient has become stabilized, the Recommended Dietary Allowances of the Food and Nutrition Board (Table 22 in Chap. 13) are a good criterion for his nutritional requirements, and a meal plan based on the principles of the dietary diabetic management in adults may be adopted. However, several points must be emphasized at all times: (1) milk and milk products should be included in

---

[1]An illustrated brochure, "Meal Planning with Exchange Lists," together with meal plans of varying carbohydrate content, is available at nominal cost from the American Dietetic Association (620 North Michigan Avenue, Chicago 60611) or the American Diabetes Association, Inc. (1 West 48th Street, New York 10020).

generous quantities since otherwise calcium, the chief mineral requiring special attention in childhood, may not be supplied in adequate amounts: (2) continued supplementation with 400 IU of vitamin D daily is desirable: (3) the distribution of carbohydrates throughout the day should be relatively uniform, and this should include between-meal snacks and a late bedtime snack; (4) the use of concentrated sweets must be avoided since the margin between hyperglycemia and hypoglycemia is very narrow in the juvenile diabetic; (5) the food intake must be adjusted by experience according to the amount and type of insulin used and in conformance with the pattern of physical exercise of the young patient. In the last analysis it is this latter adjustment, based on a certain amount of hit-or-miss juggling, which will teach the parent and the young patient how to walk the narrow path between glycosuria and hypoglycemic reaction to insulin therapy.

Artificial Sweeteners and Diabetic Foods

Saccharin and the cyclamates have become standard aids to diabetics who have to avoid the use of sugar. Sodium cyclamate may contribute more sodium than is desirable to patients on a controlled sodium intake; the use of calcium cyclamate is preferable in such cases. The artificial sweeteners are either added to foods by the diabetic (i.e., to coffee) or are incorporated by the manufacturer into special "dietetic" foods or sugar-free, low-calorie beverages. Canned and frozen fruits have presented a problem to the diabetic in the past because of the sugar or syrup used in their preparation. Water-packed fruits are now quite readily available. In general, as the trend today is to permit the patient to eat ordinary foods as far as possible, aside from sugar-free artificially sweetened beverages and canned fruits, the use of special diabetic foods is decreasing.

Chapter 25

Nutrition and Diet in Diseases of the Gastrointestinal Tract

Diet Therapy in Gastrointestinal Disorders

Numerous diets are currently in use for the treatment of gastrointestinal disorders. Many were introduced early in the present century and have become part of medical tradition. There is a growing recognition that some of these diets may be based more on fancy than on fact; they have become part and parcel of medical lore and many may only exert a placebo effect. In some cases diets traditionally prescribed for specific gastrointestinal disorders are not based on scientific facts and objective measurements known or available today. Some, though no longer rationally defensible, may have satisfied the urge of some patients to be given and to follow a specific treatment (and of some physicians to do something for the patient). This chapter describes dietary regimens currently recognized as therapeutically useful; it mentions briefly a few diets primarily for historic reasons and labels them as such.

Gastric Indigestion (Dyspepsia)

Gastric "indigestion" refers to a syndrome which includes heartburn, nausea, upper abdominal discomfort, loss of appetite, distention, belching, and flatulence. The syndrome occurs either during or following the ingestion of food. Indigestion may be the result of organic disease of the gastrointestinal tract, or by reflex, of organic diseases originating elsewhere in the body. The majority of complaints occur in the absence of demonstrable organic pathology and are of "functional" character. Excessive or rapid eating, inadequate chewing, air swallowing, ingestion of poorly cooked or very fatty foods, ingestion of gas-forming vegetables (onions, radishes, cabbage, beans, brussels sprouts, cauliflower, turnips), and mental strain and emotional upsets are among common causes of the condition. Dyspepsia due to nervous and psychoneurotic causes is probably the most frequently encountered type.

Dietary Recommendations

If the dyspepsia is of organic origin, the underlying disease process must be treated to obtain relief. In the majority of cases the disorder is of nervous origin and a certain amount of dietary regulation is beneficial. Each case must be treated on its own merit, and no simple dietary rule can be set down. Dietary regulation, when accompanied by excessive restriction of food, may actually be harmful. Many dyspeptics would avidly embrace certain food taboos, if encouraged; and for psychologic reasons and to ensure adequate nutrition, the patient should be given a well-balanced diet without much emphasis on restriction. Exceptions to this are cases where a patient is truly allergic to certain foods or where a patient with an abnormally sensitive digestive tract cannot tolerate known specific foods or excessive amounts of roughage.

The patient is given a normal diet with a caloric intake adjusted according to his (desirable) body weight and physical activity. He should be told that his is a normal, well-balanced diet, and he should be instructed exactly how much to eat and when. If arrangements are left to him, the dietary regimen is likely to be unsuccessful.

Recommendations can be based on the food plan in Chap. 15, and initially a few daily menus may be given in detail. Emphasis should be on appetizing, well-cooked foods; excessive spicing and the delicatessen type of meal should be discouraged. Mealtimes should be set according to the patient's needs and should be kept at all times. At least an hour should be allowed for dinner. Meals should be taken in a pleasant and relaxed atmosphere. Foods must be thoroughly chewed, and haste should not be permitted. Excitement after a meal is definitely detrimental, and a period of rest and relaxation should be encouraged after each meal for peaceful digestion. Nicotine in the form of cigarettes is objectionable, especially before meals, and alcohol is contraindicated for patients complaining of dyspepsia. (In selected cases, moderate quantities of alcohol may be beneficial because of its relaxant effects.) Because of the nature of the disorder, the successful treatment of functional or nervous dyspepsia depends to a large degree on the physician's ability to act as psychologist and to individualize the dietary regimen of the patient.

Peptic Ulcer—Historic Treatment

Peptic ulcer is a localized erosion in the mucosa of the stomach or duodenum and at times in the lower end of the esophagus or on the jejunal portion of a surgical gastrojejunostomy. Excessive secretion of acid gastric juice is the immediate cause producing the lesion and in activating a previously healed ulcer. Because of the nature and location of the disorder, historically diet therapy has been an important part of the treatment.

For years the treatment of gastrointestinal disorders, including that of peptic ulcer, by special diets has been largely a matter of tradition and based on few scientific facts. A brief description of the traditional dietary treatment for peptic ulcer is given here primarily for historic reasons. The traditional peptic ulcer diet was described as one which (1) decreases secretion of gastric juice, (2) neutralizes stomach acidity, (3) decreases gastric motility, and (4) does not irritate the lesion mechanically. The ultimate in this respect was the Sippy diet. During the early days and even weeks of this regimen, the patient was given 3 ounces of a mixture of equal parts of milk and cream every hour. Between these feedings neutralizing alkaline powders were given every hour. Soft-boiled eggs and fine, cooked cereals were later added, and as the condition of the patient improved, cream soups and pureed vegetables were given. As the pain relief continued, the diet was permitted to become more diversified and gradually turned into the traditional "bland diet" (see below), and the patient returned to a schedule of three meals and a bedtime snack. At this point the patient usually continued on a bland diet permanently or until his physician pronounced him "cured."

Actually, the condition is such that permanent cures are rare and the personality of the ulcer patient makes for occasional recurrences and exacerbations. Anxiety, other emotional upsets, fatigue, infections, and alcohol are common factors precipitating a recurrence, which may occur whether the patient observes a bland diet or not. Rigid dietary ritualism is not desirable or necessary for satisfactory long-term management of peptic ulcer. The discipline of regularity and moderation in eating is, in itself, of value, and the psychologic circumstances under which the food is eaten approach in importance the actual choice of foods. In many cases a long-continued peptic ulcer diet only serves to make the patient an irritated or unhappy dietary cripple.

In recent years an increasing number of clinicians have expressed doubt about the need for a long-continued bland diet in peptic ulcer patients. Also, some physicians have become cognizant of the possible harmful effects of a long-term milk- or egg-rich bland diet in patients who have a proclivity to hypercalcemia and/or atherosclerosis. The tendency has been to liberalize the ulcer diet and to investigate, under well-controlled circumstances, the effectiveness of dietary restrictions in inducing healing of peptic ulcers or preventing recurrences. On the basis of numerous observations it now has been accepted that ulcer patients recover just as well on less-restricted or regular diets, and that recurrences of peptic ulcer are not prevented by a lifelong bland diet. On the contrary, the mental outlook (an important aspect in this disorder) and nutritional status of patients appear to improve more rapidly if patients are not forced to follow a restrictive dietary ritual.

Peptic Ulcer Diet Today

During the active stage of a recently diagnosed (or recurring) peptic ulcer, the physician may order a modified diet for a few days (see below, under Diet in Peptic Ulcer Hemorrhage) or may rely solely on frequently administered antacid preparations to relieve the patient's pain while permitting a near-normal food intake. (For prompt buffering of gastric acid and relief of pain, antacids are superior to milk, cream, or solid protein foods.) Experience has shown the clinical response and rate of healing of duodenal ulcers to be the same in either case. Pain is often minimized, however, by frequent small feedings instead of the usual three meals (for mechanical reasons and possibly because there is less stimulation for gastric acid secretion). This principle holds true during the acute stages as well as during borderline discomfort after subsidence or during recurrence of ulceration.

Once the acute condition has been stabilized, a regular diet is reinstituted (if it has been discontinued). Individual, specific foods to which the patient is intolerant should be avoided, but the physician will seldom be justified in routinely prohibiting certain classes of foods. Some patients feel discomfort following ingestion of specific food items—raw onions, sauerkraut, gas-producing beans, radishes, cabbage, citrus juices, or ice cream—and these are best avoided henceforth. With the exception of black pepper and chili peppers there is no good evidence that spices in moderation are harmful. There is also no reason to exclude roughage or coarse foods; there is no evidence that fruit with skins, lettuce, celery, or nuts, when they are well masticated and mixed with saliva, will bring about mechanical irritation or injury to the gastrointestinal mucosa.

Certain substances, however, act as specific secretagogues and *must* be avoided henceforth: caffeine-containing beverages (coffee, tea, and cola drinks) stimulate gastric acid secretion. Alcohol taken on an empty stomach likewise stimulates acid secretion. (For some patients, the relaxation induced by *limited* quantities of alcohol *well diluted* or *taken with meals,* however, may outweigh the possible harm of increased acid secretion.) Smoking, which also increases peptic secretory activity, aggravates the symptoms of gastric ulcer in particular (its effect on duodenal ulcers is less well studied) and is strongly contraindicated. The use of ulcerogenic drugs such as aspirin and the various salicylates, corticosteroids, phenylbutazone, oxyphenbutazone, indomethazine, and reserpine should be avoided.

In brief, the long-term diet of a peptic ulcer patient need not be restrictive except for the exclusion of specific foods of which he is intolerant and the specific items mentioned above which are *definitely* contraindicated. During periods of stress or beginning discomfort, frequent, small-volume feedings and use of antacids are helpful. Since there is a definite correlation between overt or covert mental-emotional stress and peptic ulcer, family and professional counseling and psychotherapy, or a change in stressful living or working habits, are more helpful to patients in minimizing the risk of recurrence than rigid diet therapy.

Diet in Peptic Ulcer Hemorrhage

Many clinicians today feel that ulcer hemorrhage cases are served better by feeding than by withholding food. If the patient is not vomiting, a feeding program is promptly instituted. Bland liquid feedings of milk and cream are given day and night every 2 hours. These are later supplemented by pureed bland foods. A full diet, completely pureed (Meulengracht diet) from the first day of the hemorrhage is also satisfactory. Vomiting or a state of shock which is not compatible with alimentation is a valid contraindication for food.

Diet during Pyloric Obstruction

The treatment of pyloric obstruction is that of the underlying disorder, and often it may be surgical. In the case of pylorospasm due to ulceration, a conservative approach may be tried. The nutritional status of the patient is usually poor because of the preceding nausea and limited food intake. Parenteral nourishment may be indicated at the onset of treatment to correct the dehydration, hypoproteinemia, and acid-base imbalance which is likely to be found in pyloric stenosis of several days' standing. The obstruction is overcome by continuous gastric suction or frequent lavage, night and morning. Between aspirations, the patient is first given small amounts of milk. Diminishing gastric residues between aspirations indicate clinical amelioration, returning gastric tone, and some passage of food through the pylorus.

Gradually, a pureed, bland diet is given in small amounts and gastric aspirations are spaced further apart as the need for them diminishes. The emphasis should be on a highly concentrated, protein-rich, low-fat diet for the first few days; fat tends to decrease gastric motility and tone, which is undesirable in this case, and the debilitated nutritional state of the patient should be corrected quickly.

The Bland Diet

The bland diet and its principles are described at this point primarily because it is still used in many medical centers routinely in the adjunctive treatment of a number of gastrointestinal disorders, such as gallbladder disease, diverticulosis and diverticulitis, idiopathic spastic constipation, ulcerative colitis, mucous colitis, and during postoperative care after abdominal surgery. An objective appraisal in the light of today's state of the art would probably reserve its use to trials of limited duration primarily in the case of patients with the last three conditions mentioned.

The bland diet is one which is mechanically, chemically, physiologically, and thermally nonirritating.

1   It has a smooth and bland consistency and texture. Coarse fibers may irritate sensitive mucous membranes: seeds, skins, and hard cell walls of plant foods constitute a major source of coarse fiber in the diet and are undesirable. Indigestible carbohydrates (cellulose, hemicellulose, lignin, protopectin) are reduced or modified by outright elimination, thorough cooking and hydrolysis, or mechanical pureeing. Hard-to-digest connective tissue in meats (cartilage, collagen, and elastin fibers) is reduced by trimming or modified by thorough cooking with moist heat. Cooking with moisture is used in order to avoid toughening or hardening of soluble proteins. Fried foods are avoided. Fish contains little connective tissue and need not be ground or chopped. Meat cuts other than tender roasts and steak are shaved, ground, or finely chopped. Strained baby foods are used in this diet since they save the labor of pureeing foods in the kitchen.

2   The diet has a bland taste and a chemically and physiologically nonirritating composition. An effort is made to reduce gastrointestinal stimulation and the resulting secretion and motility by eliminating strong spices and condiments. (Salt is permissible.) Meat extractives, found in consommés, meat broths, and gravies, stimulate gastric and enteric secretion and are avoided. Strongly flavored vegetables (onions, radishes, dried beans) and those belonging to the cabbage family (cabbage, brussels sprouts, cauliflower, etc.) are omitted because of their stimulating effect on the gastrointestinal tract and predisposition to gas formation.

Coffee and tea are contraindicated and their intake is limited in this diet because of the stimulating effects of caffeine. Alcohol is positively withheld, and smoking is interdicted.

3   The diet should be thermally nonirritating. Many physicians include the principle of moderate temperatures in their concept of a bland diet. Large quantities of very hot or very cold fluids (very hot drinks, iced tea, iced drinks) should be avoided. Smaller quantities of more slowly ingested hot or cold food items (e.g., ice cream, soup) are permissible.

Milk, having excellent acid-buffering qualities, is an important ingredient in any bland diet. On the other hand, prolonged dependence on milk may result in a deficient intake of nutrients not supplied by it, such as thiamin, vitamin C, and iron. Thus emphasis must be put on the inclusion of adequate amounts of eggs, meat, poultry, fish, and enriched fine cereals. It is important that foods high in vitamin C be included once or twice a day since all vegetables and practically all fruits must be cooked before they can be used in the bland diet. (Citrus juices may be taken on a full stomach without danger of irritating the gastric mucosa.)

Permissible foods	*Foods excluded*
Milk and milk products	Alcohol
	Carbonated beverages
Weak tea	Coffee or tea in any but minimal quantities
Bland cream soups	Consommé, meat stock
Enriched white or fine rye bread	Coarse, whole-grain bread
Bland crackers	Breads containing seeds
Precooked infant cereals	Whole-grain cereals
Fine, cooked cereals	Bran
Noodles, spaghetti, macaroni	
Cottage and cream cheese, very mild aged cheeses	Sharp cheddar and all other strongly flavored cheeses
Eggs, in any fashion except fried	
Butter, margarine, cream, vegetable oils	
Tender ground meats, poultry, or fish, roasted, broiled, baked, stewed	Fried, salted, smoked, or tough meats, frankfurters, luncheon meats
Potatoes in all forms except fried (skins of baked potatoes should not be eaten); soft-cooked, strained, or chopped carrots, peas, beets, spinach, sweet potato, squash, asparagus tips, tomatoes	All raw vegetables; also cooked onion, cabbage, cauliflower, brussels sprouts, cucumber, peppers, turnips, radishes, corn, dried beans and peas
Soft-cooked or canned apples, peaches, apricots, pears (without skins or seeds); other soft-cooked fruits, if strained; raw soft bananas, avocados, strained fruit juices	All raw fruits except soft bananas and avocados; also canned or cooked figs, pineapple, berries
Bland puddings, junkets, custards, gelatin desserts, ice cream, sherbet	Pies, pastries, doughnuts
Soft, unspiced cakes and cookies	Spiced baked goods
	Nuts, pickles, condiments

Sample Menu: Bland Diet

(Contains approximately 100 g protein, 90 g fat, 250 g carbohydrate, and 2210 kcal)

BREAKFAST
Milk (1 cup)
2 soft-boiled or poached eggs
1 slice white toast
Butter, apple jelly
Orange juice

LUNCH
Macaroni and (mild) cheese (1 cup)

Very soft, diced (or pureed) buttered carrots (¹/₂ cup)
Cream of tomato soup (1 cup)
Plain soda crackers, butter
Custard or butterscotch pudding

DINNER
Tender roast beef, trimmed, no gravy (5 oz)
Buttered noodles (¹/₂ cup)
White bread, butter, jelly
Tomato juice (¹/₂ cup)
Orange sherbet (3 oz)

BEDTIME SNACK
Whole or chocolate-flavored milk (1 cup)

The Irritable Colon Syndrome

This name describes a common functional disorder in which the dehydrating, mucus-secreting, and motor activities of the colon are deranged. Terms like *mucous colitis* and *spastic colitis* are used to describe particular aspects of the general condition. The cause of this drder may be related to any one or a combination of the following: psychogenic stimuli in anxious, hypertonic, tense, or harried individuals, chronic faulty habits with regard to food intake or elimination (rapid or irregular eating, repeated failure to respond to the urge to defecate, frequent ill-advised use of enemas and laxatives), and possibly allergy to specific foods. Usually the patient is constipated, but he may have periodic loose stools and even occasional severe diarrhea. In some cases pure mucus is produced on straining at stool.

Treatment must include the psychologic as well as physical aspects of the disorders. Mental and physical rest and the regaining of emotional stability are prime therapeutic prerequisites and usually more important than dietary regulation. The patient must be broken of any existing laxative or enema habits. He is instructed to observe regular meal hours in order to encourage regular bowel movements. No meal should be omitted. The food should be eaten slowly and, unless pureed, should be chewed well. Since the ingestion of food on an empty stomach serves as a stimulant for intestinal peristalsis, the patient is encouraged to move his bowels, without excessive straining, at the same propitious time every day, namely, 15 to 40 minutes after breakfast. The severely constipated patient may be helped initially with small quantities of mineral oil. On the other hand, diarrheal episodes may be treated with demulcent substances to thicken the excreta.

Obviously, no single dietary program is satisfactory for the divergent forms of the disorder. Many clinicians agree that in the face of recurring diarrhea, it is well to begin management with a low-residue diet (see below) which would allow the irritated colon the greatest possible rest. Once the episodes of diarrhea have subsided and as improvement warrants, additional lean meat, toast, cottage cheese, banana, and potato may be added in the order given. Vitamin supplementation is necessary since the nutritional state of patients who have suffered from recurrent diarrhea is likely to be subnormal. It is advisable to offer tap water in liberal quantities between meals; a pinch of salt per glass is a wise precaution because of a possible prolonged electrolyte loss. Alcohol is best interdicted until after total recovery.

The treatment of persons with the irritable colon syndrome who are constipated differs from the above outline. These patients are given a bland, soft diet which is relatively high in residue. Only foods are used which are easily digested and not likely to irritate the bowel (see bland anticonstipation diet, below). Patients are urged to drink 6 to 12 glasses of tap water during the day to counteract excessive dehydration of the contents of the lower bowel.

It is important that true food allergy be ruled out in all cases of the irritable colon syndrome since allergy to specific foods calls for a different dietary regimen (Chap 39).

The Low-Residue Diet

The low-residue diet is described at this point though it is by no means restricted to use in the irritable colon syndrome. This diet is also a useful adjunct in the treatment of diarrheas and gastrointestinal inflammation of varied origin such as tuberculous colitis, regional ileitis, ulcerative colitis, amoebic and bacillary dysentery, and before and after gastrointestinal surgery—especially of the lower bowel.

A low-residue diet is one which will leave a small or minimal residue in the lower intestinal tract after digestion and absorption have taken place proximally. Such a diet is desirable in any condition where the presence of bulky fecal masses in the lower bowel would constitute a strain on this organ, particularly after surgery involving the lower intestine. An extreme form of the low-residue diet, the nonresidue diet, is used in preparation of the patient for intestinal surgery (see Chap. 38 for a brief discussion of the nonresidue diet and sample menu). Low or nonresidue diets tend to rehabilitate the diseased organ by easing obstruction, distention, edema, inflammation of the bowel wall, and dehydration.

Lean meat, white poultry meat, lean fish, liver, hard-boiled eggs, rice, gelatin, strained fruit juices, sugar, and other refined carbohydrates leave minimal residues. Milk, whether boiled or raw, produces a residue of medium bulk, whereas cottage cheese does not. Fruits and vegetables, rich fatty foods, potatoes, soft-boiled eggs, butter, lard, Swiss cheese, and lactose produce large residues. Experience has shown that less material will be carried into the colon if the diet is kept fairly dry. Consequently, fluids are omitted or limited at mealtime and given in small quantities between meals. Better absorption is obtained if food is given in small amounts several times during the day.

In consideration of the conditions for which the low-residue diet is prescribed, it also incorporates the basic features of a bland diet (see section on bland diet, in this chapter). Thus indigestible carbohydrates and proteins as found in fruits and vegetables (especially when raw), uncooked cereals, bran, skins, seeds, nuts, and fried foods are omitted, as are strong spices and condiments, relishes, and onions.

Elemental Diets

The most effective minimal or nonresidue diet is represented by recently developed commercial diet formulas, mentioned here for the sake of completeness, which are chemically defined and supply all known nutritional requirements in predigested, soluble form. (Vivonex is the best example.) They are administered as a clear solution which requires no further digestive effort or only minimal effort before total absorption in the small intestine. Such a preparation results in very little fecal residue (one small bowel movement per week). Originally designed to feed astronauts and to produce very little feces, the elemental formula diet is a mixture of pure amino acids, simple sugars, essential fatty acids, and chemically pure vitamins and minerals.

Sample Menu: Low-Residue Diet

(Contains approximately 90 g protein, 45 g fat, 235 g carbohydrate, and 1705 kcal. Serve only the listed fluids with each meal. Additional fluids are permitted between meals.)

BREAKFAST
Precooked infant rice cereal with sugar and a minimum of cream (¹/₂ cup)
2 scrambled eggs (well done)
Decaffeinated coffee, sugar (1 cup or less)

10:00 A.M.
Strained orange juice (¹/₂ cup)

LUNCH
Broiled fillet of haddock, lemon (4 oz)
Rice, lightly buttered (¹/₂ cup)
Cottage cheese (3 oz)
Raspberry jello
Decaffeinated coffee, sugar (1 cup or less)

3:00 P.M.
Sweetened, clear grapefruit juice (¹/₂ cup)

DINNER
Chopped broiled calf's liver patty (4 oz) on toast
Noodles, lightly buttered (¹/₂ cup)

Lime (or orange) sherbet (3 oz)
Vanilla wafers
Decaffeinated coffee, sugar (1 cup or less)

BEDTIME SNACK
Sweet cider ($^1/_2$ cup)
Ladyfingers

Bland Anticonstipation Diet

This diet combines the basic characteristics of the bland diet with the principle underlying any diet for relief of constipation, namely, to supply enough material which is nonabsorbable in the small intestine and will thus enter the large intestine and contribute bulk to aid in its evacuation. It is important that the diet be well balanced with respect to all essential nutrients because some chronically constipated patients also tend to be chronically malnourished.

The qualitative dietary pattern of the bland anticonstipation diet is essentially that of the bland diet; i.e., food items that are mechanically, chemically, physiologically, and thermally irritating are excluded. The foods to be avoided are listed in the section on the bland diet. However, coffee is permitted because of its peristalsis-inducing action. A quantitative difference exists inasmuch as six servings daily of fruits and vegetables are included because of their bulk-contributing propensity.

The permissible raw vegetables are chopped lettuce and ripe tomatoes. Other permissible vegetables are soft-cooked or canned carrots, asparagus, beets, mushrooms, pumpkin, spinach, peas, squash, tomatoes, and pureed lima beans or corn. Three servings of vegetables are given each day. The permissible raw fruits are bananas and avocados. Other permissible fruits are soft-cooked or canned apples, apricots, pears, peaches, cherries, and orange and grapefruit sections, all without skins or seeds. Pureed, cooked dried fruits are also acceptable. Patients are urged to drink 6 to 12 glasses of tap water daily between meals, and the fluid intake with meals is generous in this diet.

Sample Menu: Bland Anticonstipation Diet

(Contains approximately 90 g protein, 100 g fat, 235 g carbohydrate, and 2200 kcal)

BREAKFAST
Canned grapefruit sections ($^1/_2$ cup)
Hot oatmeal ($^1/_2$ cup), milk, sugar
2 soft-boiled eggs
1 slice toast
Butter, apple jelly
Tomato juice ($^1/_2$ cup)
Coffee

LUNCH
Macaroni and very mild cheese (1 cup)
Sliced ripe tomatoes with hard-boiled egg
Chopped cooked spinach ($^{1}/_{2}$ cup)
Plain soda crackers, butter
Canned peaches ($^{1}/_{2}$ cup)
Coffee

DINNER
Canned pear and cottage cheese salad
Cream of tomato soup (1 cup)
Tender roast beef (4 oz)
Baked potato (do not eat skin), butter
Soft, buttered, diced carrots ($^{1}/_{2}$ cup)
White bread, butter
Custard or butterscotch pudding ($^{1}/_{2}$ cup)
Coffee

BEDTIME SNACK
Milk or chocolate-flavored milk (1 cup)
Baked apple (do not eat skin, seeds, or core)

Amoebic Enteritis

Protozoan infections of the bowel are more common than generally suspected. The most acute disease process is produced by *Endamoeba histolytica,* a true parasite which produces ulceration of the lower bowel of varying degree. In the acute state of amoebic dysentery, dietary regulation is a valuable aid in the treatment of the disease. Solids should not be given. At first, food intake is restricted to broths; this may be cautiously followed by boiled milk. As the acute symptoms subside, precooked (infant) cereals, hard-cooked eggs, and toast are added to the diet. (Some clinicians avoid milk and feed precooked cereals, hard-cooked eggs, and toast during the acute stage.) Eventually the dietary regimen grades into a bland, low-residue diet. The bland, low-residue diet is continued until the specific drug therapy has been successful and all evidence of intestinal irritation has subsided.

Bacillary Dysentery

Acute infections of the bowel by *Shigella* and *Salmonella* organisms are characterized by frequent passage of loose stools containing fluid and mucus and, in many cases, blood and pus. As the number of stools increases, dehydration and weight loss may become severe. In infants the mortality rate is high, and thus any adjunct to the primary drug therapy is of importance.

It may be necessary to administer fluids parenterally to counteract the rapid dehydration. Provided they are not vomiting, dehydrated infants should be given liberal quantities of water, dilute sugar and saline solutions, or cold bouillon, which tends to restore some of the lost electrolytes. As nausea decreases, boiled milk (without any added carbohydrate) may be given. To counteract the diarrhea, scraped ripe apple pulp may also be given every 2 to 4 hours as tolerated. Eventually, as the acute symptoms subside, the infant's regular feedings may be gradually readopted.

In the case of adults, clear fluids should be taken liberally as tolerated (water, saline, bouillon, strained juices). This is followed by boiled milk and later by a very dilute boiled milk–infant cereal mixture. As the acute symptoms subside, the patient's dietary regimen grades into a bland, low-residue diet, which is continued until recovery is complete.

Regional Enteritis

Regional enteritis (or Crohn's disease) is a progressive disease of nonspecific etiology characterized by inflammatory, hyperplastic, and granulomatous changes in the walls of the intestine. The condition commonly affects the lower ileum. Eventually, with diffuse granuloma formation, the wall of the bowel becomes markedly thickened and indurated, the lumen narrows, and stenosis may result. Although progressive, the condition is not continuous; diseased areas of the gut may alternate with healthy ones—thus the term *regional*. Early, acute cases may subside spontaneously. Chronic cases tend to progress until arrested by surgical intervention. Dietary regulation is a good palliative until surgery is done, and if for some reason an operation is not done, dietary palliation should continue. The diet should be of the bland, low-residue type. Patients who are acutely ill should start on small feedings of precooked infant rice cereal, hard-boiled eggs (to be well chewed), and tender, scraped meat; this is gradually expanded to a full, bland, low-residue diet, as tolerated. In addition to mechanical palliation, the major consideration of dietary treatment is correction of malnutrition. In the long term the diet should be high in protein and calories (but still low in fiber). Multiple feedings (six small meals per day) are indicated. Multiple-vitamin supplementation should be given. The intestinal absorption of fats and fat-soluble vitamins may be aided by the inclusion of a wetting agent in the diet (i.e., the polyoxyethylene derivative of sorbitan monooleate, 1.5 g per meal). Medium-chain triglycerides (see Chap. 26) have been employed and appear to have merit. Nutrients which are normally not well absorbed in this condition—vitamin B_{12}, vitamin K, iron—should be given parenterally, intermittently, when indicated by low blood values.

Tuberculous Enteritis

Tuberculous enteritis is the most common complication of pulmonary tuberculosis. Tubercle bacilli swallowed with sputum from the tuberculous lungs are largely responsible. The ileocecal region is most commonly involved. The condition may be ulcerative or hypertrophic, and the symptomatology may resemble ulcerative colitis or regional enteritis. The diet in this condition should be smooth, bland, high in protein, and low in residue. Orange juice and tomato juice should be given in liberal amounts between meals. Vitamin supplementation is necessary, and wetting agents are helpful in augmenting the absorption of fats and of the fat-soluble vitamins.

Chronic Ulcerative Colitis

This disease is a chronic, inflammatory, and ulcerative disorder of the colon, with nonspecific etiology. Remissions and exacerbations are not uncommon. The condition may produce extensive systemic symptomatology such as marked weight loss, weakness, anorexia, and nutritional deficiencies with anemia and hypoproteinemia.

Inasmuch as the specific etiology is unknown (psychogenic, allergic, and secondary microbial factors are implicated), the foremost objective is to support the patient's strength and nutritional status and to afford the inflamed and ulcerated bowel maximal rest. Current medical treatment centers on topical application (retention enemas) of corticosteroid preparations. Diet treatment supports the medical treatment.

Dietary Treatment

The dietary treatment of ulcerative colitis should be accompanied initially by prolonged bed rest and adequate psychotherapy. Elimination diets (Chap. 39) may be employed if true food allergy with lower bowel symptomatology is suspected. The diet for chronic ulcerative colitis should be high in calories, high in protein, rich in vitamins and minerals, bland, and low in residue. In the beginning the problem may be one of creating appetite, and when symptoms are acute, the patient may be able to take only small quantities of food, which should then be of a very concentrated nature.

High-quality proteins should be given liberally since nitrogen losses, in the form of exudates and hemorrhages from the affected bowel mucosa, may be of considerable magnitude. In addition there is increased tissue protein catabolism during fever and, especially in cases of long standing, failure of synthesis of protein as a result of impaired hepatic function.

Contrary to a widespread assumption, milk is not a low-residue food; it leaves a bulky residue in the colon. Also, many patients do not tolerate it well, and a true allergy or lactase deficiency (see Chap. 26) may be involved in these cases. Thus emphasis is on *other* sources of protein, such as tender meats, fish, fowl, liver, and eggs. Protein concentrates may also be used, and *when tolerated,* dry skim milk may be added to increase the protein level of the diet.

Vitamin and mineral supplements, particularly iron, should be given. Severe dehydration because of acute diarrheal fluid loss calls for supportive intravenous solutions.

Many patients are hospitalized when they first present themselves for treatment. Most hospitals adhere to a very definite dietary program in which the patient initially receives a restricted basic diet. This diet is used until the physician orders specific additions, one at a time. Additions and increases in the size of portions are made as quickly as tolerated to increase the caloric and nutritional content of the diet. Eventually a "full" diet is arrived at, but it is still a somewhat liberalized bland diet. In the long run, the diet in patients with chronic ulcerative colitis will vary with the extent and severity of the disease and the residual, individual psychologic and allergic factors.

Diverticulosis and Diverticulitis

Intestinal diverticula are herniations of the mucous inner lining through gaps or weak spots in the circular muscle of the gut. These outpouchings protrude through the intestinal wall, and their presence is termed *diverticulosis*. They may appear in the lower small intestine, but are more common in the distal portions of the colon. Diverticula may be single or multiple. They occur most often in the elderly, in whom they have traditionally been attributed to a general muscle tissue weakness. More recently attention has been focused on spastic colon diverticulosis, which appears in predisposed individuals, beginning with the third decade in life, as the result of unusually high intraluminal pressures. "Spastic colon" or the "irritable bowel syndrome" may indeed be a forerunner of colonic diverticulosis.

In diverticulitis, the intestinal herniations become infected and inflamed and this may result in ulceration and perforations. The symptoms resemble those of appendicitis, and surgery is indicated when perforation has occurred.

In the past, the dietary treatment of chronic diverticulosis consisted of a low-residue regimen. In recent years a growing body of evidence has been amassed and appears to indicate the advantage of supplying bulk to the large intestine. The presence of adequate bulk in the lower gut presumably increases the intestinal bore and prevents the segmentation of individual portions of the colon, which leads to highly increased, local intraluminal pressure. The currently emerging school of thought points out that a low-residue diet only serves to perpetuate a vicious cycle in colonic diverticulosis and advocates institution of a diet which supplies adequate bulk (i.e., contains sufficient vegetables, fruit, bran, and the like) to the lower intestine. An 85 percent effectiveness rate in relieving pain and bowel irregularities is being claimed for a high-residue diet. In the current absence of well-controlled studies, additional clinical evidence for the "adequate-bulk hypothesis" is desirable and should give definite indications for a rational dietary regimen in diverticulosis.

Chapter 26

Nutrition and Diet in Malabsorption Disorders

The Malabsorption Syndrome

There exist a number of disorders which share a somewhat similar picture of nutritional deficiencies after the disease has run a prolonged course. These disease entities interfere with adequate intestinal absorption of food elements which are essential for proper nutrition and normal life processes. Among these disorders may be counted:

Celiac disease
Sprue
Idiopathic steatorrhea

Certain disturbances of the pancreas, such as:

Cystic fibrosis of the pancreas (the pancreatic manifestation of systemic mucoviscidosis)
Chronic pancreatitis
Carcinoma of the head of the pancreas
Stones in the duct of Wirsung

In all these conditions the dried stools may contain 25 percent or more of fat, and fat absorption is considerably decreased from the usual 90 to 95 percent. Carbohydrate and protein absorption are variable, and carbohydrate absorption is usually impaired. In sprue, idiopathic steatorrhea, and celiac disease the pancreatic enzymes trypsin and lipase are present in normal amounts in the small intestine. In the enumerated pancreatic disorders the pancreatic digestive enzymes are either absent from the duodenum or severely reduced. In both disease groups the stools are commonly bulky, runny, pale, and greasy, and the fermentation of nonabsorbed carbohydrates makes them frothy. The clinical picture includes the signs and symptoms of severe multiple nutritional deficiencies, with or without the stigmata of chronic lack of folic acid or vitamin B_{12}.

Clinical thinking in many quarters links the first three diseases together under one name, *primary malabsorption syndrome.* These disorders are considered by some to be variations of the same genetically transmitted metabolic derangement. Other workers feel that only celiac disease in children and idiopathic steatorrhea in adults are manifestations of the same disorder, the basic etiology of which is a specific intolerance to protein-bound glutamine or a genetically conditioned inability to metabolize certain peptide configurations.

Celiac Disease

Celiac disease is a chronic intestinal disorder found in children, usually between the ages of 6 months and 6 years. It is characterized by anorexia, steatorrhea, diarrhea, arrest of growth, protuberant abdomen, and multiple nutritional deficiency symptoms. The stools in celiac disease are bulky, loose, pale, fatty, and frothy because of fermentation of unabsorbed carbohydrates. The amount of pancreatic digestive enzymes in the duodenum is normal, but there is a characteristic atrophy of intestinal villi which is demonstrated in peroral biopsies of the jejunum. The absorption of fat and fat-soluble substances and of carbohydrates is impaired. Remissions and exacerbations are characteristic for the disorder. The condition usually improves gradually after the age of 6; however, recurrences may occasionally be found in later life.

Within the last few years, hypersensitivity to two protein fractions of wheat, rye, barley, and oats (gluten and gliadin) has been implicated as the causative factor in childhood celiac disease. More recently it has been demonstrated that in predisposed individuals it is the quantity of protein-bound glutamine in any given protein which is responsible for the symptoms of the disease. Presumably, the malabsorption of nutrients from the intestinal tract is the result of the reaction of the small intestine to the presence of protein-bound glutamine. Oats, barley, rye, and wheat contain large quantities of the offending substance and must be eliminated from the diet of the hypersensitive child. Rice, corn, and buckwheat protein contain a smaller proportion of protein-bound glutamine and are usually tolerated. This is also true of beef, fish, milk, egg, potato, and some of the legume proteins, all of which are inoffensive.

Dietary Treatment

Management of the disease is based on a diet which contains little or no protein-bound glutamine. Since wheat, rye, oats, and barley are especially rich in the offending gluten and gliadin, these cereals are excluded. Rice and corn, which contain little gluten and gliadin, may be used eventually, if tolerated. Pure cornstarch may be used as a thickener; wheat starch should be avoided lest it contain traces of the protein fraction of wheat.

If the diagnosis is made early and the condition is in its beginning stages, the exclusion of all gluten- and gliadin-containing foods (see below) suffices, as the condition usually improves rapidly. If the disorder is of long standing and the child is ill, an additional modification is introduced: the amount of fat in the diet is restricted while the protein content is increased. Vitamin and mineral supplementation (see section on sprue) is always advisable initially.

The child's appetite is usually poor at first, but it should soon improve once the diet is started. Within 2 to 4 weeks the stools usually become normal and clinical symptoms subside. Foods containing gluten or gliadin should not be given for $1/2$ to 1 year. After this period, some pure wheat starch may be added, but the subsequent stools must be carefully watched for signs of a relapse. As the child grows up, usually after the sixth year the intolerance to protein-bound glutamine gradually disappears. Cautious reintroduction of wheat, rye, oats, and barley may be attempted at that time; such attempts should be abandoned if untoward symptoms reappear.

A word should be added concerning the duration of a trial on a gluten-gliadin-free diet to evaluate the patient's response (as shown by weight gain, improvement in the character of the stools, and increased fat absorption). It has been shown repeatedly that it may take as long as 6 to 8 weeks to obtain a clear-cut improvement after institution of the diet. Conversely, it may require a similar length of time to obtain an adverse response to the reintroduction of dietary gluten and gliadin. The frequently used 4-day dietary test period is thus much too brief and should *not* be relied upon to yield significant information.

THE GLUTEN-GLIADIN-RESTRICTED DIET FOR CELIAC DISEASE

All products containing wheat, rye, oatmeal, and barley or their derivatives must be excluded. Labels on all commercially prepared or packaged foods must be read carefully. Food items which contain the offending substances or their derivatives or by-products must not be used; it is important to look for wheat-containing ingredients like farina, "starch" (unless designated as cornstarch), noodles (including all the varieties such as spaghetti, etc.), dumplings, cracker meal, bread crumbs, matzo meal, etc. Adults must avoid malted beverages like beer and ale.

Permissible foods	*Foods excluded*
Skim milk, whole milk (as tolerated), soft drinks, cocoa and chocolate drinks which do not contain cereal thickeners, coffee made from ground coffee beans, tea	Cereal beverages (Postum, Ovaltine, malted milk), drinks containing cereal fillers or thickeners, beer and ale
Precooked infant cereal made from rice; refined cereals and cereal products made solely from rice or corn, if tolerated	All other cereal products
Bread or rolls made from potato flour, or rice, corn, and soy, if tolerated	All other breads, rolls, biscuits, or cereal products
Meat, fish, fowl prepared as desired, but no gravies thickened with flour; no stuffing; no "breaded" cuts; no batter on the fowl	All other meats, meat loaves, luncheon meats, sausages, or any meat product or dish which contains cereal or flour
Eggs, cheese	
Potatoes, rice	Noodles, spaghetti, macaroni, or other flour-derived dishes
Butter, margarine, oils, and other fats, as tolerated	Salad dressings or mayonnaise made with flour thickeners
All pure vegetables (not creamed)	Creamed or breaded vegetables
All fruits and fruit juices	
Clear broths and vegetable soups, cream soups if thickened with cornstarch, cream, or potato flour	All soups containing "flour" (since this is usually wheat flour), noodles, or other cereal derivatives
Jello, sherbet; homemade ice cream, rice or cornstarch puddings (to ensure that wheat flour thickeners are not used)	Pastry, cakes, cookies, prepared mixes; most commercial puddings and ice cream; ice cream cones
Honey, jelly, jam, sugar, chocolate, homemade candy prepared without cereal derivatives	All candy which contains cereal derivatives

Sample Menu: Gluten-Gliadin-Restricted Diet for Celiac Disease

(Contains approximately 110 g protein, 70 g fat, 215 g carbohydrate, and 1930 kcal)

BREAKFAST
Orange juice (1/2 cup)
2 eggs, any style
Precooked rice cereal, sugar

Skim milk (1 cup)
Ripe banana
Beverage

LUNCH
Lean ground beef patty (4 oz)
Carrots and peas ($^1/_2$ cup)
Potato, any style
1 pat butter (use with potato)
Skim milk (1 cup)
Sherbet ($^1/_3$ cup)
Beverage

DINNER
Broiled chicken (5 oz)
Chopped spinach ($^1/_2$ cup)
Squash ($^1/_2$ cup)
Mashed potatoes ($^1/_2$ cup)
2 pats butter (for vegetables)
Skim milk (1 cup)
Fruit cocktail ($^1/_2$ cup)

BEDTIME SNACK
Skim milk flavored with pure cocoa and sugar (1 cup)

Sprue

Sprue is a chronic deficiency disease of unknown etiology characterized, when of long standing, by impaired absorption of glucose, fats, and fat-soluble nutrients, steatorrhea, diarrhea, weight loss, weakness, hypocarotenemia, glossitis, hyperpigmentation of the skin, and a macrocytic anemia with megaloblastic arrest of the bone marrow. The classic sprue patient lives in a tropical or subtropical area where the disease is endemic; has a history of diarrhea, weight loss and weakness; shows laboratory evidence of malabsorption; has an abnormal histologic picture of his jejunal mucosa, macrocytic anemia, and a puzzling absence of other disorders associated with malabsorption such as celiac disease. Fully developed, classic sprue is associated with a folic acid deficiency. Calcium and iron deficiencies may also be present. Because of the megaloblastic macrocytic anemia common to both, sprue and pernicious anemia have certain similar clinical features. However, the gastrointestinal absorptive defect and stool picture is characteristic of sprue, while lack of intrinsic factor and a degree of achlorhydria (Chaps. 11 and 33) are the distinguishing marks of the patient with true pernicious anemia. Subacute combined degeneration of the sensory and motor neural pathways of the cord, a frequent complication of pernicious anemia, is rarely encountered in sprue. Because of impaired intestinal absorption a concomitant vitamin B_{12} deficiency may be found in patients with severe sprue, which has led to suggestions that tropical sprue is best treated with both folic acid and vitamin B_{12}.

Both folic acid and vitamin B_{12} exert a beneficial effect on most of the clinical symptoms; they are specific for relief of the megaloblastic anemia and usually result in a dramatic early improvement. The adrenocortical steroids have also proved very beneficial and may be lifesaving in very severe forms of the disease. Deficiency of folic acid alone is insufficient to explain the many abnormalities in small intestinal structure and function in tropical sprue. The response of patients to certain antibiotics and the occasional epidemic nature of the disease have led to the suggestion that an infectious factor may be operative. Thus optimal therapy for classic tropical sprue now also includes the long-term use of broad-spectrum antibiotics which at times leads to a dramatic improvement.

Dietary Treatment

Recent studies have shown that a large number of sprue patients in temperate climates ("nontropical sprue") respond specifically to the gluten-gliadin-restricted diet described in the section on celiac disease. Once the blood picture has returned to normal with the aid of folic acid therapy, these patients may remain asymptomatic on this diet, without further relapses. (It may require several months on the gluten-free diet before a response is obtained.) A long-term trial with the gluten-gliadin-restricted diet should be instituted in all patients with adult celiac disease, or "sprue" in adults in nontropical locations. A majority of the latter cases will respond since they tend to be adults with celiac disease for which the diet is specifically therapeutic. If the diet does not prove effective in amelioration of the gastrointestinal symptoms and steatorrhea, a trial with the conventional diet for tropical sprue is indicated.

The conventional diet used heretofore in the treatment of sprue is low in fat and high in protein, carbohydrate, and calories. Initially this diet is bland and the amount of residue is preferably restricted. A large proportion of the carbohydrates should be easily absorbed fructose. (Experience has shown that glucose and sucrose often cause gaseous discomfort in sprue patients.) The patient should receive vitamin supplementation (at least one therapeutic multivitamin capsule per day, conforming to the U.S.P. Hexavitamin Capsule strength) and 3 level teaspoons of calcium lactate daily, as well as 4 mg of water-soluble vitamin K twice weekly. The intestinal absorption of fats and fat-soluble vitamins may be aided by the use of edible wetting agents (polyoxyethylene derivative of sorbitan monooleate, 1.5 g with each meal), or by substitution with medium-chain triglycerides (described later in this chapter).

The diet will vary with the individual, depending on the extent of the absorption defect and the response of the patient. It is best to start with a restricted basic diet, which is used until the physician orders specific additions, one at a time. Eventually a "full" diet may be reached, which, however, is still a low-fat, liberalized bland diet. In favorable cases, appetite and weight are regained rapidly and the diarrhea soon ceases and improvement of the various absorptive defects occurs progressively. However, relapses are not infrequent. While some patients regain their full absorptive powers, this may not be possible in all cases, and frequently a defect in fat absorption remains.

Basic Diet for Sprue

Permissible foods	*Foods excluded*
Skim milk, tea, coffee, soft drinks (in most cases)	Whole milk and chocolate-flavored drinks
Toasted white bread	Fresh breads or rolls, crackers, breads containing bran, seeds, or whole-grain flour
	All cereals
Lean meat, fish, fowl, or dry, nonfat cottage cheese, 6–10 oz daily; 2 eggs daily	Luncheon meats, sausages, fat or fried meat, fish, fowl; fried egg, any other cheese
Potatoes	Fried potatoes, potato chips, macaroni, spaghetti, noodles, rice, hominy
Fat-free broths, soups made of strained vegetables and skim milk	All other soups
2 pats butter or margarine	All other fats
Ripe banana, soft-cooked, canned or baked apples, apricots, peaches, pears, cherries, without seeds or skins, fruit juices (except prune juice)	All other fruits
Soft-cooked or canned carrots, peas, pumpkins, squash, beets, strained lima beans	All other vegetables
Custards, jello, puddings, angel food or sponge cake, plain cookies, without nuts, seeds, or fruits	Desserts made with whole milk or cream or high in fat content
Honey, jelly, corn syrup; sugar as tolerated	Hard candy, jam, marmalade, syrups other than corn syrup
Salt, small amounts of spices, vinegar	Strong spices and condiments, alcohol, chocolate, gravies, nuts, olives, pickles, popcorn

Additions to Basic Diet in Transition to a Full Sprue Diet

The enumerated additions are made one at a time and in the order given. Omit all foods which the patient does not tolerate. (In certain cases raw fruits and vegetables will remain permanently contraindicated.)

1. Precooked infant cereals, cereal products, untoasted white or light rye bread
2. Raw fruits and vegetables, but only as tolerated; skins and seeds not permitted
3. Whole milk; eventually more butter or margarine if fat is well tolerated

Full Diet for Sprue

Permissible foods	*Foods excluded*
Whole or skim milk, tea, coffee, soft drinks	Chocolate-flavored drinks
White or light rye bread, rolls, plain crackers	Bread or rolls containing whole-grain flour, bran, or seeds
Precooked infant cereals, other refined cereals	Whole-grain or bran cereals
Lean meat, fish, fowl, or dry cottage cheese, 6–10 oz daily	Luncheon meats, sausages, fat or fried meat, fish, fowl; fried egg; any other cheese
2 eggs daily	
Potatoes, spaghetti, macaroni, noodles, rice (no bran)	Fried potatoes, potato chips, hominy
Fat-free broths or fat-free soups made from permissible foods	All other soups
2 or more pats butter or margarine, as tolerated	All other fats
All fruits except those listed on the right	Fruits with indigestible skins, fibers, or seeds; fruit not tolerated by the individual
All vegetables except those listed on the right	Vegetables with indigestible fibers, skins, or seeds; brussels sprouts, cauliflower, cabbage, cucumber, onions, dried peas, lentils, and beans, radishes, turnips, broccoli if not well tolerated by the individual
Desserts which are high in fat content only occasionally; custards, jello, puddings, angel food or sponge cake, ice cream, plain cookies, all without nuts, seeds, or tough fruits	All other desserts
Honey, jelly; sugar as tolerated	Hard "chewy" candy, jam, marmalade; strong spices and condiments, alcohol, chocolate, gravies, nuts, olives, pickles, popcorn

Sample Menus: Basic Diet for Sprue

(Contains approximately 150 g protein, 40 g fat, 280 g carbohydrate, and 2080 kcal)

BREAKFAST
2 soft-boiled eggs

2 slices white toast
Honey (2 full tsp)
Orange juice ($^1/_2$ cup)
Skim milk ($^1/_2$ cup)

LUNCH
Broiled lean fish (5 oz)
Mashed potatoes ($^1/_2$ cup)
Soft-boiled peas ($^1/_2$ cup)
2 slices white toast
1 pat butter
Honey (1 full tsp)
Skim milk (1 cup)
Sliced ripe banana
Tea
Dry skim milk (4 tbsp; stir into the tea or milk)

DINNER
Lean, trimmed ham (5 oz)
Baked potato (no skin)
Soft-boiled sliced carrots ($^1/_2$ cup)
2 slices white toast
1 pat butter
Honey (1 full tsp)
Sherbet ($^1/_3$ cup)
Skim milk (1 cup)
Tea

BEDTIME SNACK
Skim milk (1 cup)
Plain cookie

Full Diet for Sprue

(Contains approximately 150 g protein, 80 g fat, 315 g carbohydrate, and 2580 kcal)

BREAKFAST
Sliced orange (1)
Precooked rice cereal ($^1/_2$ cup)
Glucose (1 tbsp; use with cereal)
Milk ($^1/_2$ cup)
2 soft-boiled eggs
2 slices white toast
1 pat butter
Honey (2 full tsp)
Tea

LUNCH
Broiled lean fish (5 oz)
Mashed potatoes ($\frac{1}{2}$ cup)
Soft-boiled peas ($\frac{1}{2}$ cup)
$\frac{1}{2}$ canned peach
2 slices white bread
1 pat butter
Sliced ripe banana
Milk (1 cup)
Coffee
Dry skim milk (4 tbsp; stir into the coffee or whole milk)

DINNER
Sweetened grapefruit juice ($\frac{1}{2}$ cup)
Lean roast beef (6 oz)
Baked potato (no skin)
Soft-boiled sliced carrots ($\frac{1}{2}$ cup)
Asparagus tips (4)
2 slices white bread
1 pat butter
Honey (1 full tsp)
Ice cream ($\frac{1}{3}$ cup)
Milk (1 cup)

BEDTIME SNACK
Skim milk (1 cup)
Plain cookie

Idiopathic Steatorrhea in Adults

When adult patients exhibit only the gastrointestinal symptoms of "sprue," but not the complete symptomatology of the sprue syndrome, including the megaloblastic anemia, the trend has been to label the disorder *idiopathic steatorrhea,* after pancreatic disorders, intestinal lipodystrophy, lymphomata of the small intestine, amyloidosis, and chronic inflammatory disease of the small intestine have been ruled out. In many cases of idiopathic steatorrhea the course of the disorder is unpredictable. Some patients have a family history of the disease. In some patients the disease is of a constant, low-grade nature; other patients exhibit discrete exacerbations and remissions.

Present-day thinking links a majority of cases of idiopathic steatorrhea in the adult to the basic defect underlying celiac disease of childhood. The therapeutic approach is to exclude foods rich in protein-bound glutamine from the patient's diet. The recommended diet is that described above for celiac disease. Some patients will get along well on a normal diet with folic acid and/or vitamin B_{12} supplementation.

Pancreatic Disorders

In pancreatic insufficiency with steatorrhea and malabsorption, the pancreatic digestive enzymes are absent from the duodenum. The stools exhibit an increase not only in fat (and a variable increase in carbohydrates) but also in nitrogen, attesting to malabsorption of undigested protein as well as of fat and some starch. In obstructive disorders, where possible, surgical treatment attempts to reestablish the flow of pancreatic digestive enzymes into the small intestine. Before surgery an attempt should be made to improve the nutritional state of the patient by giving pancreatic extracts (Pancreatin, U.S.P., 3 to 6 tablets after each meal, or equivalent preparations), by administering wetting agents with each meal to enhance the absorption of fats and fat-soluble nutrients, by the use of medium-chain triglycerides (see below), and by intensive multivitamin supplementation.

Cystic Fibrosis

In this familial disease abnormal thick mucus is secreted by the epithelial lining of the interior of certain glands and organs and viscid mucous deposits obstruct, among other passageways, the pancreatic ducts. As a result, in about 80 percent of patients the duodenum contains little or no pancreatic trypsin, amylase, or lipase, and malabsorption and subsequent severe multiple nutritional deficiencies are part of the disease picture. In addition, these children secrete abnormally large quantities of sodium and chloride in their sweat, which may result in salt depletion and collapse under conditions of excessive sweating.

The condition is present at birth. It may be fatal during the first week of life because of intestinal obstruction caused by viscous masses of meconium. Steatorrhea appears very early, and the clinical picture resembles celiac disease, except that it develops almost from birth. Later in life, because of the viscid exudate of the bronchial tree, recurrent severe respiratory infections tend to shorten the life of the patient. A program of continuously administered antibiotics or chemotherapy improves the prognosis considerably, but to date a large proportion of afflicted children still fail to reach adulthood.

Clinical expressions of the disorder are being found increasingly among adults who apparently have a partial hereditary endowment for the disease. In such cases, the *full* clinical picture is rarely seen, and the disorder is manifested by unexplained chronic respiratory infections, intestinal malabsorption, or abnormal sweat composition.

Dietary Regimen

The gluten and gliadin in wheat, rye, and other cereals play no part in this condition. Pancreatin or similar substitutes for the missing pancreatic enzymes must be given with each meal. A complete, well-balanced diet should be given in generous amounts to satisfy the patient's appetite. In fact, since much of the food is undigested and lost in the stools, extra quantities must be allowed if the child does not gain weight satisfactorily. Emphasis must be placed on a high-calorie, high-protein content in the diet. Protein is as inefficiently absorbed by cystic fibrosis patients as fat. However, they tolerate a greatly increased dietary intake of protein and will maintain themselves in positive nitrogen balance under such a regimen.

These children usually have an excellent appetite, which should be a guide to their intake. If additional food is given, it is advisable to limit the amount of fat in the diet since the smell of stools is more offensive when large amounts of fat are being excreted. The orally administered antibiotics, a routine prophylactic procedure to check the onset of respiratory infections in such children, is also of value in reducing intestinal fermentation. Pancreatic preparations should be given routinely, except in the 20 percent of patients with generalized cystic fibrosis who do not suffer from pancreatic achylia. Because of the impairment in absorption of the fat-soluble vitamins, these must be given in liberal amounts.

During hot weather, because of the dangers of excessive salt depletion due to the characteristic, abnormally high salt content of the perspiration of these patients, additional, unrestricted salt should be given. Two grams of salt is added in each day's formula for infants, and free use of the saltshaker by older patients should be encouraged.

When pancreatic achylia is present, the function of this organ will never improve because of the eventual destruction of the exocrine glands of the pancreas. Therefore, dietary precautions will have to be observed throughout life. Fortunately, fewer restrictions seem to be needed with advancing age.

Chronic Interstitial Pancreatitis and Carcinoma of the Head of the Pancreas

In these diseases the character of the stools and the malabsorption are similar to the picture in cystic fibrosis, since there is an insufficiency of digestive pancreatic enzymes. The dietary regimen is similar, except that the diet is adapted for use by adults.

Use of Medium-Chain Triglycerides in Malabsorption

In recent years a mixture of medium-chain triglycerides (MCT) has become available which is composed of glycerides of octanoic and decanoic acids (C_8 and C_{10} fatty acids, respectively). The commercial source of this material is coconut oil which is hydrolyzed, fractionated, and reesterified with glycerol. The resulting oil contains approximately 74 percent octanoic and 26 percent decanoic acid glycerides, has a relatively low melting point, and is more readily miscible with water than the conventional edible fats composed of long-chain fatty acids, but still has a desirable high caloric density, supplying 8.3 cal/g.

Because of the differences in chemical composition, molecular size, and physical properties, MCT is more rapidly hydrolyzed and absorbed in the gastrointestinal tract than other edible fats and oils. MCT can be largely absorbed without prior hydrolysis; it is hydrolyzed by pancreatic lipase extremely rapidly and requires little if any bile for solubilization in the intestine. In contrast to long-chain fatty acids, medium-chain fatty acids are not reesterified in the mucosal cells, but are carried from the intestine as free fatty acids in the portal vein. They are readily, and almost quantitatively, metabolized in the liver as they are absorbed; they are not esterified in the liver or incorporated into blood lipoproteins, and do not affect blood triglyceride levels appreciably. Also, there is little incorporation of these fatty acids into liver lipids or extrahepatic tissues.

Because they are digested, absorbed, transported, and metabolized differently and because of their unique properties, medium-chain triglycerides have been found extremely useful as substitutes for conventional edible fats and oils in the nutritional management of patients with a wide variety of conditions characterized by impaired fat digestion, absorption, and metabolism. In these disorders substitution of MCT for ordinary dietary fats results in reduction (or cessation) of steatorrhea and is usually followed by weight gain and general improvement of nutritional status. Among the conditions in which a trial substitution of MCT for conventional fats should be tried are: pancreatic insufficiencies of varied etiology, cystic fibrosis, bile salt deficiencies and cirrhosis of the liver with steatorrhea, massive surgical intestinal resections (when the absorptive area of the small bowel has been excessively reduced), the blind-loop syndrome, regional enteritis, chyluria, chylothorax, and other forms of abnormal chylous fistulas, tropical sprue, celiac disease, congenital β-lipoprotein deficiency, and diabetic steatorrhea. In familial hyperchylomicronemia (dietary, fat-induced hypertriglyceridemia)—a lipid disorder due to defective lipoprotein lipase activity—substitution of MCt for conventional fats frequently leads to a marked reduction in the serum triglyceride level, just as a fat-free diet does.

There have been remarkably few side effects from the use of MCT. Crampy abdominal pain is an occasional occurrence when MCT is used in liquid formulas, but this may well be related to the high osmotic load characteristic of such formula diets.

DISACCHARIDASE DEFICIENCY AND SACCHARIDE MALABSORPTION

The polysaccharides in food, largely starch and glycogen, are hydrolyzed by pancreatic amylase to the disaccharides maltose and isomaltose. These disaccharides together with the disaccharides contributed as such by foods, primarily sucrose and lactose, are then split by specific disaccharidases into monosac-charides in the small intestine. The disaccharidases are not released into the lumen of the small intestine but are located in the brush border of mucosal cells where they split disaccharides into monosaccharides. These traverse the mucosal cell into the capillaries of the portal circulation.

Deficiency of one or more intestinal disaccharidases results in impaired hydrolysis and malabsorption of specific sugars. Such a deficiency may be inherited or may be secondary to a serious gastrointestinal disorder with damage to the mucosa, parasitosis, or severe malnutrition.

The main symptoms in sugar malabsorption are diarrhea, intestinal cramps, and flatulence, and in most instances the patient—or in the case of infants, the parents—eventually recognize a dietary intolerance to certain foods (those which contain the nonhydrolyzable, malabsorbed sugars). Treat-ment consists chiefly of elimination from the diet of the specific sugar involved. In most cases, the gastrointestinal symptoms respond readily to this diet therapy.

A number of specific disaccharidase deficiencies have been recognized; the most important and widespread of these malabsorption syndromes is *lactase deficiency,* sometimes also referred to as lactose intolerance.

Lactose Malabsorption (Lactase Deficiency)

In recent years it has been recognized that there exists a wide variation in the ability of individuals of different ages and racial backgrounds to digest lactose, the principal carbohydrate in milk. A specific intestinal disaccharidase, lactase, is essential for the digestion of lactose into its components glucose and galactose and thus for its ultimate absorption. In all mammals, including man, lactase activity is maximal at birth and will remain high as long as milk is the mainstay of the diet. Once weaning has occurred, in most animals the enzyme is no longer needed and its activity declines. In man, the extent to which lactose activity decreases (with subsequent inability to digest and utilize lactose) is apparently governed by a combination of hereditary, dietary, and adaptive factors.

In some races, lactase levels remain consistently high throughout life; in others, levels decline gradually to the point of deficiency at some time during later childhood and the adult may have impaired or no residual lactase activity. Populations in which the majority of adults are lactase-deficient include most African Negroes (and many of their American descendants), Indians of North and South America, Chinese, Filipinos, Thais, Eskimos, natives of New Guinea, and Australian aborigines. Populations exhibiting low rates of lactase deficiencies include European whites and their descendants throughout the world, those African Negroes who have traditionally been herdsmen, like the Masai, and possibly (research in this area is as yet incomplete) Asian population groups who have traditionally been herdsmen or have kept milk-yielding domestic animals (buffaloes, goats). The degree of lactose intolerance of adults in different cultures appears, indeed, to parallel the historic dependence of population groups on foods of high lactose content.

Pathogenesis and Diagnosis of Lactose Intolerance

When mucosal lactase is deficient, lactose is not hydrolyzed and is absorbed poorly from the intestinal lumen. Its osmotic activity results in a significant influx of water from the intestinal wall into the lactose-holding lumen followed by abdominal bloating, crampy discomfort, and watery diarrhea. Bacterial fermentation of the unabsorbed lactose in the colon results in the formation of carbon dioxide and irritating short-chain organic acids; the latter interfere with the normal resorption, in the colon, of water from the intestinal contents, contributing further to the symptoms.

So-called milk allergy plays no role in this syndrome; the patients usually do not have other allergic proclivities, do not develop antibodies to milk proteins (the sine qua non of a true hypersensitivity reaction), and are able to tolerate *small* quantities of milk without symptoms.

The presence of lactase deficiency–lactose intolerance should be suspected on the basis of the following criteria: (1) Symptoms develop within 1 to 3 hours after the ingestion of known lactose-containing foods. (2) Symptoms occur only after the consumption of milk or lactose-containing food products, and the patient is symptom-free on a lactose-free diet. (3) The intensity of symptoms is related to the quantity of lactose consumed.

A clinical diagnosis of impaired lactase activity can be established by means of a lactose tolerance test. The subject is given a loading dose of 50 to 100 g of lactose in aqueous suspension; malabsorption of lactose is suggested if the venous or capillary blood glucose level does not increase by more than 20 mg percent within a 2-hour period following lactose loading (because lactose is not hydrolyzed normally to glucose and galactose). In addition, the subject is observed for the development of the typical gastrointestinal symptoms of lactose intolerance following this test. Final confirmation can be obtained if upon biopsy the jejunal mucosa is found histologically normal but deficient in lactase activity.

Lactose intolerance should be suspected whenever otherwise unexplainable bloating, cramps, and diarrhea regularly occur, particularly in the United States in individuals of Negro or Oriental ancestry. A relationship to the consumption of lactose-containing foods should be elicited by careful questioning.

Dietary Treatment

Treatment of the condition is based on the elimination of the offending lactose from the individual's diet, and is followed by prompt disappearance of the symptoms. Since the severity of symptomatology is generally related to the *quantity* of lactose ingested by the patient, dietary treatment is usually highly successful since even the inadvertent presence of small amounts of lactose still remaining in the diet does not give rise to major reactions.

The dietary adjustment is simple since with few exceptions the only foods containing lactose are milk and milk derivatives and compounded food products to which milk or its derivatives have been added. A careful reading of the list of ingredients on the label of compounded foods is recommended since whey solids or dried milk are nowadays being added to the most unsuspected foods, such as frankfurters and cold cuts. Dairy products from which lactose has been removed by fermentation, such as yogurt and fermented and aged cheeses (see below), may be used.

Diet for Lactase Deficiency–Lactose Intolerance

Permissible foods	*Foods excluded*
All foods not excluded on the right Yogurt	Whole milk, skim milk, cream, milk shakes
	Baked goods which contain milk, whey, or "milk solids"
Fermented and aged cheeses (Swiss, cheddar, blue cheese, Parmesan, etc.)	Sausages and cold cuts containing whey or "milk solids," cottage cheese, "cheese food products," creamed, milk-containing soups
	Ice cream, ice milk, and candy containing milk or milk solids

Dietary Policy Considerations

Since the elucidation of the lactase deficiency–lactose intolerance syndrome, the question has been raised whether it is advisable to supply underdeveloped countries in Africa, Southeast Asia, and elsewhere with milk products to improve the nutritional status of their undernourished populations. Before arriving at inflexible judgments on this issue it should be recognized that many persons with indicated low lactase activity may be able to consume the equivalent of one or even two glasses of milk a day at meals or in divided doses. This has been found in studies of children in India where *small* quantities of milk, or milk given in divided doses, did not give rise to symptoms in a large proportion of children judged to be lactose-intolerant on the basis of standard clinical tests. It appears advisable at present, until more is known about the precise prevalence of lactase deficiency in older population groups and in different countries, to avoid generalizations concerning the principle of using milk products as nutritional aids in underdeveloped countries, and to let the *actual* experience in each particular country, racial group, and age group be the guide for a general inclusion or exclusion of milk products.

Chapter 27

Nutrition and Diet in Diseases of the Liver

Nutritional Aspects of Liver Function

Any discussion of special diets for liver disease is best preceded by a consideration of the vital functions of this organ with regard to systemic nutrition. The liver plays a central role in protein metabolism. It receives and stores the greater part of the freshly absorbed dietary amino acids; it synthesizes them into body proteins, and it attends to their deamination and breakdown if there is no need for amino acids for anabolic purposes. The liver holds a considerable protein reserve which is drawn upon to indirectly replenish serum proteins as the need arises.

The liver plays a vital role in carbohydrate metabolism. It helps to regulate blood glucose through conversion of excess glucose into liver glycogen, and it serves as a storehouse of this readily mobilized carbohydrate reserve.

The liver exerts a similar controlling influence on lipid metabolism; it converts absorbed dietary fatty acids into circulating phospholipids; it synthesizes cholesterol, and it converts cholesterol into bile salts and secretes these; it oxidizes fatty acids to obtain energy; it interconverts proteins, carbohydrates, and fats, and it constitutes the body's most mobilizable fat store.

If one considers, in addition to the above, the elaboration of bile salts (essential for proper digestion and absorption of fats and fat-soluble vitamins), the detoxication of indole, skatole, and other substances, the conversion of β-carotene to physiologically active vitamin A, the synthesis of prothrombin, the storage of vitamins A and D and of essential minerals, and a host of other vital functions, it becomes clear why a normal nutritional status depends on a healthy liver and why dietary therapy is important for the recovery of the diseased organ.

Nutritional Aspects of Liver Disease

Liver diseases have a variety of causes: infectious, parasitic, nutritional or metabolic, obstructive, toxic, and malignant. Among these, nutritional and metabolic causes play an unusually prominent part. Hepatic injury may be the result of inadequate protein intake or of an improperly balanced diet with excessive fat intake; it may be caused by ingestion of toxic substances, or it may result from a combination of toxic agents and dietary neglect; it may even result from the excessive intake of a nutrient in the face of an underlying metabolic disorder (hemochromatosis).

The pathologic features of the various destructive or degenerative processes which involve the liver parenchyma are quite similar regardless of the etiology of the disease. Basic changes include fatty infiltration, atrophy, fibrosis, or focal necrosis. The protection of the parenchymal cells involves similar principles, and dietary means are in the foreground.

In liver disease the diet should be formulated to permit the disabled liver to function as efficiently as possible, and it should protect the liver against metabolic stress. To counteract fatty infiltration and degeneration of the parenchyma, proteins of high biologic quality and rich in the lipotropic factors, which mobilize liver fat, should be supplied in generous quantities; simultaneously, the fat intake should be limited to a variable degree, depending on the disease. The diet should be high in carbohydrates since the resultant accumulation of glycogen in the liver cells, together with adequate protein storage, exerts a protective action and counteracts tendencies to fatty metamorphosis or toxic injury in the parenchyma. (One exception to the generalization regarding a high protein intake is hepatic coma, which is dealt with below.)

Infectious Hepatitis (Hepatitis A)

Infectious hepatitis is a not uncommon acute virus infection of the liver. The causative virus is spread by the oral-intestinal route. The disease may appear sporadically or in epidemic proportions; it is common among young people and in military establishments where crowding serves as a predisposing factor. Patients whose diet is generally inadequate, whose protein intake is low, or who consume alcohol while ill are prone to complications, prolonged convalescence, relapses, or a fatal outcome. The treatment consists primarily of bed rest, diet, and avoidance of further injury to the liver.

Dietary Treatment

The diet should be high in calories, with emphasis on good-quality proteins and carbohydrates rather than fat. The fat content should be reduced, but still compatible with attractive palatable meals. The physician should explain to the patient the importance of his diet as a therapeutic measure and warn him against the possible prolongation of recovery and relapses which may follow an inadequate and unbalanced food intake. Patients are likely to have very poor appetites, and it is up to the physician or hospital staff to make sure that the prescribed diet is actually consumed. Thiamin (10 mg daily) may be given to counteract the anorexia.

The diet should contribute 45 cal/kg body weight per day. The protein intake should be about 1.5 g/kg daily. The protein may be of both animal and vegetable origin, but should be mostly of high biologic quality; thus generous quantities of meat, fish, fowl, eggs, and skim milk are indicated. Special lipotropic supplements or amino acids are not needed if this rule is observed. "Milk shakes" made from dry skim milk powder, some fluid skim milk, eggs, and sugar and flavored with chocolate or any other desirable flavor are a great help in supplying a patient who lacks appetite with generous quantities of protein. They may be given between meals, or they may be used during meals to compensate for the patient's rejection of other proteinaceous foods.

The fat content should be held to about 25 percent of the total calories, which is actually only a moderate restriction. It is best to provide the fat through dairy products, margarine, salad dressing, and eggs rather than through fried foods or gravies.

Carbohydrates are given liberally to complete the caloric requirement. The following will exemplify the composition of the desired diet for the average adult case: 100 to 120 g protein; 60 to 75 g fat; 275 to 335 g carbohydrate.

Multivitamin therapy is not specifically needed if the diet is well balanced, but it may be helpful in malnourished patients. Because of disturbed liver function (and—sometimes—biliary insufficiency with consequent lowered absorption of dietary vitamin K) low plasma prothrombin levels are not uncommon in infectious hepatitis. Patients with hemorrhagic tendencies should receive a supplement of vitamin K (5 to 10 mg of menadione, daily, by mouth). Consumption of alcohol should not be permitted during the course of the illness and preferably for 4 to 6 months thereafter.

Homologous Serum Hepatitis (Transfusion or Injection Hepatitis, Hepatitis B)

This acute hepatitis is caused by a virus similar to that responsible for infectious hepatitis. Transmission is primarily by injection or inoculation procedures in which improperly sterilized needles are used or by transfusions with pooled plasma which contains material from a donor who carries the virus. The disease is not uncommon. Except for a very prolonged incubation period, the pathologic changes and clinical picture resemble those of infectious hepatitis and the dietary treatment is identical.

Hepatic Coma

This is a syndrome of progressive confusion, apathy, personality changes, muscle contractions, spasticity, loss of consciousness, and eventual death. It is occasionally seen in patients with severely impaired liver function, particularly in those with cirrhotic livers and natural or surgically produced vascular shunts between the intestinal veins and the systemic circulation owing to portal obstruction (see below). In hepatic coma, toxic nitrogenous materials from the bowel, primarily ammonia, presumably the result of bacterial action on protein foods, enter the systemic circulation and reach the central nervous system without prior detoxification by a normally functioning liver; this is aided by obliteration of the portal circulation and direct circulatory shunts from the intestine to the arterial systemic circulation (and thus to the brain).

The blood ammonium ion levels are characteristically increased in hepatic coma. A major feature of hepatic coma is ammonia intoxication of the central nervous system caused by failure of the liver to convert ammonia to nontoxic urea. This ammonia is primarily derived from microbial breakdown of proteins in the intestine (and apparently some of it is the result of nonmicrobial deamination of amino acids in the intestine and in the liver). Impaired ability of the liver to convert ammonia to urea, which is excreted by the kidneys, is the primary cause of hepatic coma.

Since the traditional diet in liver disease is high in protein, there is ample opportunity for the elaboration of relatively large quantities of ammonia. If liver function is adequate, the resulting ammonium ions are concurrently utilized in the synthesis of urea and do not accumulate. On the other hand, a buildup of ammonium ions in the systemic circulation takes place in extreme failure of liver function, particularly if there is considerable shunting of portal vein blood through collateral channels or a portacaval anastamosis. The withholding of dietary protein, and thus amino acids, prevents such a buildup.

Dietary Considerations

Though consumption of generous quantities of protein is a recognized part of liver therapy, excessive amounts should not be given since in selected cases hepatic coma might be precipitated. Thus the diet is limited to 2 g protein per kilogram of body weight. The attending physician must be on the alert for the first signs of impending coma. If mental confusion or the characteristic "flapping" tremor (on extension forward of arms, hands, and fingers) is noted, the diet must immediately be reversed. A low-protein, moderately fat-restricted diet is given which contains less than 30 g of protein, practically all of it in the form of animal protein. Many physicians recommend institution at this point of the Giordano-Giovanetti diet (originally devised for the treatment of uremia; Chap. 30) since it supplies only minimal amounts of new sources of ammonia production (it is limited to 20 g of high biologic quality animal protein) while actively promoting the sequestration and reutilization of any available ammonia and urea for endogenous protein synthesis. In acute hepatic coma, in addition to this diet or complete withholding of protein, the intestinal flora should be suppressed with neomycin or other antibiotics to prevent further microbial protein and amino acid breakdown in the gut with ammonia formation. Once the signs and symptoms of hepatic coma have subsided, protein may be reintroduced to the diet in small progressive increments.

Fatty Degeneration of the Liver

Fatty infiltration of the liver may be seen in overly obese persons when the diet is unbalanced by an excessive fat intake. Fatty liver is also caused by exposure to toxic agents (chloroform, carbon tetrachloride) and by a diet severely deficient in protein. Fatty degeneration of the liver is also found in prolonged starvation, nonspecific malnutrition states, and ulcerative colitis (where, again, the lack of dietary lipotropic factors and low protein intake are implicated) and in metabolic disorders (lipoid dystrophy, diabetes mellitus), chronic infections (tuberculosis), and alcoholism.

Dietary Treatment

Except for treatment of any underlying disease process and avoidance of the responsible toxic agent, the treatment is by diet. The principles are the same as in other cases of liver disease; the recommended diet is high in good-quality proteins, high in carbohydrates, and moderate in fat. The limited quantity of fat taken should be derived preferably from milk, margarine, salad oils, or eggs.

Cirrhosis

In long-standing cases of fatty degeneration or after cellular necrosis (without fatty degeneration), the liver parenchyma is gradually destroyed and fibrous elements replace the liver cells. This process is prolonged and gradual in the case of fatty degeneration and more rapid if it is the result of acute infectious or toxic damage. In either case, the end result is a liver which contains little active parenchymal tissue and consists primarily of fibrous tissue. Following fibrosis, local contraction of the fibrous tissue distorts the liver morphology and interferes with its normal circulation by obliterating the portal venous system. In contrast to the swollen, enlarged fatty liver, the cirrhotic liver is a contracted and irregularly distorted organ which has lost most of its function.

Alcoholic Cirrhosis (Portal, or Laennec's, Cirrhosis)

This form of cirrhosis, probably the most common type in North America and Europe, is the end result of long-standing toxic damage by alcohol to the hepatic parenchyma, coupled, perhaps, with the contributory effects of prolonged dietary neglect. Individuals who have taken excessive amounts of alcohol for many years develop fatty degeneration; cirrhosis will result eventually if the alcohol intake is not reduced (see Chap. 36; Nutrition and Alcohol).

Dietary Regimen

If fatty infiltration is present, regeneration of liver parenchyma will take place if alcohol is strictly withheld and a dietary regimen is started which is high in protein and carbohydrate and moderately low in fat. The diet is that previously mentioned for other liver disorders and should contain at least 100 g of high-quality protein daily. Multivitamin supplementation is helpful initially and may be discontinued after 4 weeks. If the patient's appetite is small and capricious, the milk shakes mentioned in a previous section will be helpful.

Even if cirrhosis is present, some fatty liver parenchyma will still have remained and the dietary regimen coupled with strict interdiction of alcohol will bring about some improvement. Many cirrhotics may thus be restored to a semblance of good health provided they consume no alcohol and adhere to their liberal diet.

The prognosis is not good when cirrhosis is very advanced; nevertheless, diet therapy is a major factor in successful maintenance of the patient. Hepatic coma (see above) must be watched for in advanced cirrhosis.

Sodium Restriction in Edema and Ascites with Cirrhosis

One of the complications of advanced cirrhosis is water retention in the tissues due to hypoalbuminemia (secondary to liver failure) and accumulation of fluid in the abdominal cavity (ascites) due to raised portal pressure (which is secondary to the obstructed portal venous system). Restriction of dietary sodium has a salutary effect on the generalized edema and on the accumulation of ascitic fluid.

The desired sodium limitation varies with the individual case. Generally, a diet containing between 1.15 and 2.3 g of salt (20 to 40 meq of sodium) per day will keep the cirrhotic patient "dry" after paracentesis. The sodium intake of the "dry" patient may be cautiously liberalized until the point is reached where a rapid weight gain indicates water retention. The patient should be weighed daily, and the abdomen palpated for ascitic fluid. A very slow, steady gain in weight should be expected as the clinical and nutritional picture improves and the total body tissue mass is built up again. A rapid weight gain from one day to the next indicates water retention and constitutes a signal to lower the sodium intake.

The average patient has no difficulty consuming a low-sodium diet which provides a liberal caloric allowance (50 to 100 percent over the basal caloric requirement), 2 g of protein per kilogram of body weight, 25 percent of the calories in the form of fat, and the remainder of calories as carbohydrates. Eventually, as the fluid retention subsides, the patient may be permitted moderate or even normal amounts of salt.

A detailed discussion of sodium restriction and low sodium diets is found in Chap. 29, Nutrition and Diet in Cardiovascular Diseases.

Chapter 28

Nutrition and Diet in Diseases of the Biliary Tract

Biliary Function and Dysfunction

In the healthy individual, the elaboration and release into the intestine of adequate quantities of bile are essential to normal digestion and absorption of fats and fat-soluble nutrients (Chap. 9) and of a number of metabolites and hormones which course through the enterohepatic circulation during the digestion of foods. Between meals the gallbladder concentrates the dilute bile which is elaborated by the liver and serves as an inactive reservoir. Diets high in protein tend to increase hepatic bile production. High carbohydrate diets and dehydration decrease bile formation. Before meals the gallbladder is ordinarily full and relaxed and the sphincter of the common bile duct (the sphincter of Oddi) is normally closed. As food is ingested, the presence of cholagogues like fats or fatty acids in the duodenum stimulates the sphincter of Oddi to relax and initiates contraction of the gallbladder. This ensures the release of the stored bile into the duodenum at the most propitious time for the digestion and absorption of fats and fat-soluble nutrients.

Biliary dyskinesia, gallstones, acute cholecystitis, chronic gallbladder inflammation, and cholangiohepatitis constitute different types of biliary tract disorders. Nevertheless, they are best looked upon not as separate disease entities, but as phases of pathologic evolution which may occur in succession or simultaneously.

Biliary Dyskinesia and Postcholecystectomy Syndrome

This disorder of biliary function and flow is caused by abnormal pressure relationships in the biliary tract. In hypertonic dyskinesia there is contraction of the gallbladder and peristalsis of the filled common duct in the face of concomitant spasm of the common duct sphincter, which prevents release of the bile into the duodenum. In atonic dyskinesia, the sphincter of Oddi is contracted against a passively distended, toneless gallbladder. After cholecystectomy, abnormal spasm of the sphincter may result in an increase in intraductal pressure in the absence of the gallbladder.

Dietary Regimen

The dietary treatment is aimed at prevention of the painful colic. Because they are powerful cholagogues, fats are contraindicated in hypertonic dyskinesia, and the low-fat diet (see below) is a time-honored adjunct in the treatment of this disorder. In the patient who has just been cholecystectomized, fats are also strictly limited, while a high-protein diet is given to stimulate the flow of bile and bile salts. (In addition, pure bile salts may be given to alleviate dyspepsia after cholecystectomy.)

Many patients with biliary disorders find that certain foods tend to precipitate dyspeptic symptoms. The implicated group includes some of the strongly flavored or gas-producing vegetables like onions, garlic, cabbage, radishes, sauerkraut, cucumbers, turnips, brussels sprouts, dried beans and peas, and some spicy foods like curries and peppers. Some patients have distress after coffee, fruit juices, candy, or concentrated sweets. If not tolerated well, such foods must be excluded from the diet of the patient with biliary disorders.

Gallstones (Cholelithiasis) and Biliary Calculi (Choledocholithiasis)

In the United States, gallstones are found in about 10 percent of adults who come to autopsy. They are much more common in females than in males, are more frequent among fair, obese, parous women, and usually become troublesome during the forties. Though obesity and pregnancy are predisposing factors, other contributing factors may be sought, perhaps, among nutritional abnormalities, disturbed cholesterol metabolism, biliary stasis, and genetic makeup. The incidence varies from country to country and appears to be higher among individuals who favor a high-calorie, high-fat intake. There are some indications that the predisposition to the disorders runs in families.

The presence of stones in the gallbladder is usually discovered when they obstruct the ampulla of the bladder or its duct—ordinarily a temporary occurrence which leads to a painful colicky episode, the gallbladder attack. The attacks usually subside spontaneously within a few hours when the stone drops back into the body of the gallbladder.

When a stone has passed into the common duct and obstructs it, similar, more prolonged attacks occur. Here the obstruction, though not always absolute, will be prolonged until relieved by surgical intervention. (Small stones may pass into the duodenum with a spontaneous clearing of the disorder.) In choledocholithiasis the passage of bile into the duodenum is interrupted, transient jaundice may be seen, absorption of fats and fat-soluble nutrients is impaired, and the stools will be light-colored because of the absence of bile pigments. If the condition is unrelieved over prolonged periods, biliary back pressure and stasis may damage the liver parenchyma. Repeated attacks may lead to acute or chronic cholecystitis with its complications. (If the obstruction is low enough, biliary back pressure may lead to episodes of acute pancreatitis or, eventually, chronic pancreatitis.)

Diet and Prevention of Cholesterol Gallstones

The predominant type of gallstone in the United States is that composed of cholesterol concretions. Recent studies suggest that the formation of cholesterol gallstones is due to three factors: an abnormally high biliary cholesterol concentration, a relatively small pool of bile salts (which, if larger, would prevent precipitation of excessive cholesterol), and an increased intake of calories irrespective of dietary composition. Until more is known concerning any possible effect of the nature of the diet on biliary composition, a general caloric restraint appears to be the most rational dietary prophylaxis, especially since the incidence of gallstones is considerably higher among the obese.

Principles of Dietary Regimen in Symptomatic Cholelithiasis

Antispasmodies and analgesics are used to help the patient weather the colicky episode. Between attacks, and before and after corrective surgery, a low-fat, low-calorie, high-protein, high-carbohydrate diet is employed. This diet is designed to decrease the stimulus for gallbladder and bile duct contraction and to lessen the likelihood of repeated attacks, by excluding the most powerful cholagogues, fats. Fats are also severely limited since as long as bile does not enter the duodenum, lipids will be poorly absorbed, the patient may suffer "indigestion," and the stools are apt to be very offensive if much fat is present in the large intestine. Between attacks, when dietary fats are absorbed, it is also of importance to keep fat in the diet to a minimum in order to spare the liver, which is in a precarious position because of repeated chemical trauma from biliary backwash.

The daily protein intake is best set at from 1.5 to 2 g/kg; little is gained by a higher protein consumption. Because of its high protein content, the diet presumably exerts a lipotropic and protective effect on the liver and thus decreases the eventual surgical risk. The caloric contribution of the diet varies with the individual. Since the majority of gallbladder patients are obese, the caloric intake is usually restricted with a view to weight reduction.

Foods which are known to cause dyspepsia in the individual (see section on biliary dyskinesia) should be excluded from the diet. However, these items may be eaten if they are tolerated well. The purpose of the diet is to aid the patient, not to restrict him unnecessarily.

Supplementation with the fat-soluble vitamins is indicated. This is particularly important in the case of vitamin K. Patients with biliary obstruction usually have a low blood prothrombin level because of diminished absorption of this vitamin. The resultant bleeding tendency increases the surgical risk and should be corrected by parenteral supplementation before surgical intervention (2 to 4 mg menadione daily for three successive days before the operation).

Low-Fat Diet for Gallbladder Disorders

Permissible foods	*Foods excluded*
Skim milk, tea, coffee only if tolerated, soft drinks	Whole milk, cream
Any enriched breads, crackers, nonfat rolls	Butter rolls
Any nonfat cereal foods (preferably enriched)	Griddle cakes, waffles, doughnuts
Butter, margarine, or salad oil, limited to 3 tsp/day	All other butter, margarine, cooking fats, oils, salad dressing, mayonnaise
Lean meat, fish, fowl; cottage cheese; 1 egg daily (not fried)	Fatty or fried meat, fish, fowl; bacon, luncheon meats, sausages, all other cheeses, fried egg, gravies
Potatoes, noodles, spaghetti, rice	Fried potatoes, potato chips
Any vegetables except those excluded on the right	*Depending on the individual, and if not well tolerated,* any or all of the following; onions, cabbage, brussels sprouts, cauliflower, cucumber, peppers, dried beans and peas, radishes, turnips, sauerkraut
Any fruits except those excluded on the right	Avocados; *if not well tolerated:* melons, raw apples, berries
Any low-fat soups	Fatty soups

Angel food cake, plain vanilla wafers, fruit whips, gelatin desserts, sherbet, puddings made with skim milk

Only if tolerated: honey, jam, jelly, sugar, syrups, sugar candy

Rich pastries, pie, ice cream, whipped cream, cookies, cakes

Chocolate, chocolate candy (pure cocoa may be used for flavoring purposes); candy containing nuts, fat, or lecithin

Olives, nuts, peanut butter, buttered popcorn; *if not well tolerated:* spices, spiced dishes, condiments, pickles

Sample Menu: Low-Fat Diet for Gallbladder Disorders

(Contains approximately 110 g protein, 35 g fat, 175 g carbohydrate, and 1450 kcal. The lunch is planned as an ambulatory meal which may be carried to work or purchased at a lunch counter. In the hospital or home, a cooked lunch based on lean meat, fish, or fowl and cooked vegetables may be substituted.)

BREAKFAST
Orange juice ($\frac{1}{2}$ cup)
Cereal, sugar
Skim milk (1 cup)
1 soft-boiled or poached egg
1 slice toast, jelly
Coffee or tea, sugar

LUNCH
1 sandwich made with:
    2 slices bread
    1 pat butter
    Lean meat or fowl (3 oz)
1 sliced tomato (or 1 bowl of tomato soup)
Skim milk (1 cup)
Angel food cake (small slice)
Coffee or tea, sugar

DINNER
Cottage cheese ($\frac{1}{3}$ cup) on lettuce, with carrot sticks
Lean roast beef (6 oz)
Chopped spinach ($\frac{1}{2}$ cup)
Mashed potatoes ($\frac{1}{2}$ cup)
1 pat butter (used on vegetables)
Skim milk (1 cup)
Fruit
Coffee or tea, sugar

BEDTIME SNACK
Skim milk flavored with pure cocoa and sugar (1 cup)

Chronic Obstructive Jaundice

Chronic obstruction of the biliary tract with consequent jaundice is commonly the result of undetected, impacted stones, posttraumatic stricture, malignancy or cysts in the head of the pancreas, or biliary cirrhosis. In this condition the nutritional status of the body is disturbed by chronic failure of bile flow; there is chronic malabsorption of fat-soluble nutrients, and steatorrhea is common. Often a caloric deficit occurs, with consequent endogenous energy production through tissue breakdown, leading to protein depletion. The stigmata of deficiencies in vitamins A, D, and K develop gradually, anemia of multiple etiology is not uncommon, and liver damage due to biliary stasis is bound to occur.

Dietary Regimen

Before and after surgical intervention, or if conservative treatment is decided upon, the patient is placed on the diet described in the previous section. Parenteral vitamin supplementation is of great importance in chronic biliary obstruction. If bone lesions exist because of vitamin D deficiency, generous quantities of skim milk or skim milk powder should be given, concurrent with parenteral vitamin D therapy. In severe cases 4 to 10 g of Calcium Gluconate, U.S.P., may be given daily. The anemia of long-standing obstructive jaundice may respond to parenteral vitamin B_{12} and folic acid therapy but may also require supplementation with parenteral iron.

Acute and Chronic Cholecystitis

Acute inflammation of the gallbladder, with varying involvement of the adjacent biliary passages, is commonly considered to be precipitated by obstruction of the ampulla or of the cystic duct. If symptoms do not subside quickly, the treatment, after brief observation, is usually surgical. If symptoms subside spontaneously, the patient may be maintained on conservative treatment, namely, a low-fat, low-calorie, high-protein, high-carbohydrate diet.

Chronic inflammation of the gallbladder is a common sequel to repeated attacks of acute cholecystitis. The disorder is often clinically indistinguishable from cholelithiasis. Conservative therapy with a low-fat, low-calorie, high-protein, high-carbohydrate diet is indicated unless operative measures are decided upon.

Chapter 29

Nutrition and Diet in Cardiovascular Diseases

Atherosclerosis

Atherosclerosis is a chronic, usually progressive vascular disease characterized by thickening, induration, and loss of elasticity of arterial walls, followed by secondary degenerative changes. The changes brought about by the disorder may be generalized or may be more prominent in certain organs or locations—heart, kidney, brain, lungs, extremities—where they induce specific clinical syndromes. The cause of the disease is as yet unknown. It has been variously attributed to abnormal fat transport or metabolism, dietary habits, disorders of blood flow and blood clotting, hormonal disturbances, extensive or long-term use of nicotine, obesity, a sedentary mode of life characterized by habitual physical inactivity, and stress-seeking personality type. In different geographic regions a negative correlation has been observed between hardness of the drinking water and a positive correlation between softness of the water and cardiovascular disease. Heredity appears to be a factor in individual susceptibility. Long-standing hypertension and diabetes constitute predisposing factors. The disease is more common in males and among obese individuals. The onset usually takes place gradually during the early adult years; progressive clinical pathology and specific secondary illness are usually observed in the fifth and sixth decades of life.

Primary Pathology

Since disordered fat metabolism has been implicated as a possible causative factor, a brief description of the pathologic changes is indicated. Atherosclerosis is basically a disease of the intima (the inner lining) of the artery. The intima thickens gradually and loses its elasticity. At the same time the medial layer of the vessel loses its normal structure and intima and media become infiltrated with lipids. Free cholesterol and cholesterol esters, triglycerides, ceroid (a lipid pigment), iron, and calcium are gradually deposited in the involved areas, and fibrous elements invade the growing plaque. The vessel may show discrete rough, barklike plaques, or the lesion may be diffuse. Early lesions appear to the naked eye as fatty streaks in the inner surface of the blood vessel. Old lesions are prominent through deposition of calcium in the areas of fatty degeneration and infiltration. Plaques may form anywhere in a vessel but are usually more frequent near branches or orifices. The roughened areas constitute ideal locations for the attachment of blood platelets and subsequent formation of thrombi which, if large enough, may occlude the lumen of the vessel. If this occurs in a coronary artery or cerebral vessel, it may lead to a near-fatal, or fatal, occlusion.

In general, atherosclerosis is the underlying cause of coronary heart disease, stroke, aortic aneurism (ballooning of the aorta), and gangrene of the extremities. It may narrow the lumen of arteries, thereby impairing blood and oxygen supply to dependent tissues and organs (which if severe enough may cause gangrene in the extremities). Such narrowing and the abnormal roughening of the inner lining of the vessel also set the stage for the formation of thrombi with gradual or sudden occlusion of the vessel and consequent death of the dependent tissue, be it the heart wall (myocardial infarction) or a portion of the brain (stroke). Atherosclerotic lesions in a major vessel and the consequent weakening of its wall may give rise to a local ballooning or dissective rupture of the vessel (aortic aneurism) or may be the source of emboli when blood clots break away and are swept to other portions of the body where they may lodge in and occlude smaller vessels and cause local infarctions.

Dietary Fat, Plasma Lipids, and Atherogenesis

A body of suggestive evidence indicates that the nature and extent of fat intake, as well as fat transport and metabolism, are involved in some fashion, yet unclarified, in atherogenesis. Patients with known advanced atherosclerosis or with established coronary heart disease very often exhibit elevated plasma cholesterol levels. It has been suggested that an altered pattern of blood phospholipids plays a role in atherogenesis. In hyperlipemia the β-lipoproteins carry most of the excess fat and cholesterol. It has been demonstrated that the β-lipoprotein level is higher in older people than in young ones, in males than in females, and in a number of diseases associated with a higher incidence of atherosclerosis. It has also been shown that there is a good statistical correlation between levels of β-lipoproteins, triglycerides, and cholesterol and atherosclerosis and its complications (coronary heart disease and local impairment of blood circulation), but a direct causal relationship has not been demonstrated and there exist a number of specific departures from this general correlation.

A relationship exists between the quantity of dietary fat and its qualitative makeup and the blood lipids (Chap. 9). A high dietary cholesterol intake is reflected in high blood cholesterol levels. Moreover, the nature of the dietary fat, primarily the degree of unsaturation of its component fatty acids, has a significant effect on plasma cholesterol and β-lipoprotein levels. Lauric (C_{12}), myristic (C_{14}), and palmitic (C_{16}) acids strongly enhance blood cholesterol levels. Fatty acids containing fewer than 12 carbon atoms and stearic acid (C_{18}) do not affect serum cholesterol but they produce elevations of serum triglycerides. The isocaloric substitution of saturated fats in the diet with unsaturated fats results in a marked lowering of the previously elevated plasma cholesterol levels. Even more striking results are obtained if pure polyunsaturated fatty acid esters are administered. Conversely, plasma lipids rise when a diet rich in saturated fats is given. The mechanisms by which polyunsaturated fatty acids lower serum cholesterol are as yet poorly understood. It has been shown that consumption of polyunsaturated fatty acids causes an increase in the excretion of neutral sterols and bile acids in the feces. Bile acids, formed in the liver, are the principal end products of cholesterol metabolism. The blood cholesterol–lowering action of polyunsaturated fatty acids may be the result of increased degradation of cholesterol in the liver with increased excretion of the resulting bile acids into the gastrointestinal tract; or it may be the result of decreased reabsorption of bile acids from the gut, mediated, possibly, through a change in the intestinal flora (with a concomitant increase of bile acid formation in the liver at the expense of blood cholesterol); or both mechanisms may be involved.

The ingestion of cholesterol per se also has an influence on plasma cholesterol levels, and thus the cholesterol content of a diet (in addition to the nature of the triglycerides which it contains) is another major factor in its atherogenic potential.

Ingestion of a diet which contains calories in excess of the daily requirements for maintenance and physical activity in the form of refined carbohydrates leads to elevated cholesterol and blood triglyceride levels which have also been implicated in setting the stage for prematurely enhanced atherosclerosis. Recent experimental evidence has shown that the ingestion of sucrose by itself or in large quantities when mixed with other food components may lead to a sustained elevation of blood triglycerides. Intestinal synthesis of triglycerides in the presence of a surfeit of dietary sucrose appears to play a role in this process, in addition to a highly enhanced lipogenic effort on the part of the liver and of the adipose tissues of the body.

Many studies of diets in relation to mortality from degenerative heart disease have shown that populations with high rates of coronary artery disease also have high mean serum cholesterol values, high β-lipoprotein concentrations, and/or high blood triglyceride levels, and consume diets rich in animal proteins, saturated fats, and calories. While it has been clearly demonstrated that dietary fat and other dietary components influence the serum lipid picture, abundant evidence also exists that factors other than diet influence serum lipid levels and may play influential roles, directly or indirectly, in atherogenesis and thrombosis. Among these are heredity, age, sex, stress, obesity, hypertension, cigarette smoking, endocrine factors, and physical exercise. There exists a considerable body of suggestive evidence to the effect that the role of physical activity in maintaining a low serum cholesterol level and low cardiovascular mortality may be as significant as dietary factors.

The exact relationship between dietary fat, blood lipids, and atherogenesis is still unclear. A correlation between dietary fat and certain features of the blood lipid picture has been established. A relationship between high blood cholesterol, β-lipoprotein, and triglyceride levels and atherosclerosis is strongly suggested. To date there is not enough direct experimental evidence to establish that the three factors are sequentially involved, i.e., that the dietary fat pattern leads through elevation of β-lipoprotein or cholesterol blood levels to the development of atherosclerosis. On the other hand experimental evidence has been emerging during the last decade which seems to establish that maintaining a low serum cholesterol level with fat-controlled diets for 5 to 10 years or more results in a reduced incidence of deaths from coronary artery disease.

Dietary Considerations

The evidence linking the kind and amount of dietary fat to atherogenesis is as yet too circumstantial to justify the recommendation of definite, major changes in the dietary pattern of *all* healthy individuals. However, it has been adequately shown that obesity is associated with a greater incidence of coronary atherosclerosis, and avoidance of caloric excess should be generally recommended. In the control of obesity, some limitation of fat intake is usually indicated. There is no doubt that in the United States, Canada, and some European countries the fat intake is very liberal. In the United States, dietary fat, both visible and invisible, accounts for about 44 percent of the total caloric intake. Some reduction in the use of fat need not interfere with the nutritional value or palatability of the diet. How far such a reduction should go is still a matter of opinion. A reduction in intake of the more saturated fats or a substitution by more unsaturated fats may ultimately prove desirable from the standpoint of prophylaxis, but currently available evidence is as yet too inconclusive to indicate whether, or to what degree, a change should be made in the diet of the average *healthy* individual.

However, in the light of present knowledge, it appears logical to attempt to reduce high serum concentrations of cholesterol and β-lipoproteins as an experimental therapeutic procedure in the case of patients with known coronary artery disease or with other frank clinical manifestations of atherosclerosis—especially persons who have had one or more myocardial infarctions or cerebrovascular accidents, or patients who exhibit abnormally high blood cholesterol or β-lipoprotein levels—particularly if there is a family history of cardiovascular disease, or the patient manifests an elevated blood pressure and/or overweight coupled with a sedentary mode of life. In this group of atherosclerotic accident-prone individuals, the physician should seriously consider the institution of prophylactic dietary measures aimed at a lowering of abnormally high blood cholesterol, triglyceride, β-lipoprotein, and chylomicron levels.

Types of Hyperlipidemia

Hyperlipidemia may be classified as a symptom or sign of five different clinical types of hyperlipoproteinemia, most of which are genetically determined. Clinical classification can be based on a determination of plasma cholesterol and triglyceride levels and on the lipoprotein electrophoretic pattern. Hypercholesterolemia without elevation of triglycerides is the most common and gives the type II pattern; in the other four patterns hypertriglyceridemia predominates. Treatment of hyperlipoproteinemia is usually undertaken for one of three reasons. Most commonly it is used because certain types of hyperlipoproteinemia (II, III, and IV) are associated with a high risk of premature atherosclerosis. Another much less common reason is to relieve recurrent abdominal pain and the risk of acute pancreatitis that attends severe hyperlipidemia (types I and V). Also, unsightly skin lesions—xanthomas—may be due to hyperlipoproteinemia and frequently disappear on proper treatment.

Dietary intervention alone or diet in conjunction with specific drugs is utilized in the treatment. Dietary therapy for hyperlipidemia includes manipulation of the *total number of calories* in the diet, the *cholesterol* content, and both the specific *kind* (saturated fats versus unsaturated ones; unrefined carbohydrates versus sucrose) and *amount* of calories coming from carbohydrate and fat. Table 37 summarizes the dietary treatment for the five basic types of hyperlipidemia. As can be seen from this table, patients with types III, IV, and V hyperlipidemia respond very favorably to caloric restriction and

Table 37 Dietary Prescription for Different Types of Hyperlipoproteinemia

	Type I	Type II	Type III	Type IV	Type V
Type of diet	Low fat, 25 to 35 g	Low cholesterol, polyunsaturated fat increased	Low cholesterol approximately: 20% cal protein 40% cal fat 40% cal CHO	Controlled CHO (approximately 40 to 45% cal); moderately restricted cholesterol	Restricted fat (30% cal), controlled CHO (50% cal), moderately restricted cholesterol
Calories	Not restricted	Not restricted, except in type IIb where weight reduction is often indicated	Achieve and maintain "ideal" weight—reduction diet if necessary	Achieve and maintain "ideal" weight—reduction diet if necessary	Achieve and maintain "ideal" weight—reduction diet if necessary
Protein	Total protein intake not limited	Total protein intake not limited	High protein	Not limited other than control of patient's weight	High protein
Fat	Restricted to 25 to 35 g; kind of fat not important	Saturated fat intake limited; polyunsaturated intake increased	Controlled to 40 to 45% cal (polyunsaturated fats recommended in preference to saturated fats)	Not limited other than control of patient's weight (polyunsaturated fats recommended in preference to saturated fats)	Restricted to 30% cal (polyunsaturated fats recommended in preference to saturated fats)
Cholesterol	Not restricted	Less than 300 mg or as low as possible; only source of cholesterol is meat	Less than 300 mg, only source of cholesterol is meat	Moderately restricted to 300 to 500 mg	Moderately restricted to 300 to 500 mg
Carbohydrates	Not restricted	Not restricted (may be controlled in type IIb)	Controlled; most concentrated sweets eliminated	Controlled; most concentrated sweets eliminated	Controlled; most concentrated sweets eliminated

weight reduction to ideal body weight. In contrast, in type I, weight reduction and calorie restriction have little effect on the abnormal pattern. Diets high in carbohydrate and low in fat are helpful to patients of type I. Diets balanced in fat and carbohydrate and restricted in cholesterol are effective in the treatment of patients with type III. The patient with type V does best with a fat-restricted diet. In type II, the amount of dietary cholesterol and polyunsaturated fats is of primary importance. It is this latter group which is the most common, for which the largest body of experimental evidence exists that suggests that the coronary attack rate in middle age can be reduced by dietary manipulation, and for which dietary prophylaxis and treatment are described below in greater detail.

Prophylactic Diet in Atherosclerosis

The permanent prophylactic maintenance diet for the patient with known atherosclerotic manifestations, or the individual with an abnormally elevated blood cholesterol level, combines a desirable caloric level, conforming to the needs of the particular individual, with as complete a substitution as possible of saturated fats with polyunsaturated fats and avoidance of cholesterol. No attempt is made to administer supplements of polyunsaturated fats in addition to the regular diet. This would lead to a gain in body weight and does not depress blood β-lipoprotein levels as effectively as a severe curtailment of saturated fats coupled with an isocaloric substitution with polyunsaturated fats. No attempt is made to reduce *drastically* the overall fat content of the diet below 35 percent; high-carbohydrate, low-fat diets tend to produce high serum triglyceride levels and are harder to adhere to when they embody a caloric restriction to prevent obesity. While the overall fat content of the diet might range between 30 and 35 percent, the primary feature of the regimen consists of the substitution of saturated fats with polyunsaturated fats and avoidance of dietary cholesterol. Reducing calories from fats tends to increase somewhat the proportion, but not necessarily the amount, of calories from carbohydrates to close to half the total. Deriving these from complex carbohydrates (grains, fruits, vegetables) is preferable to consuming simple sugars, particularly sucrose. Because of the implication of a long-term high salt intake in the etiology of idiopathic hypertension (see below), a lowering of the salt intake, especially avoidance of the use of the saltshaker at the table, is another prudent dietary recommendation.

The principal reduction of fat in the diet must come from two main food groups which contribute most of the saturated fat—dairy products and meats. Only lean meats are used and all visible fat must be trimmed off. Lean fowl and fish are favored and substituted for meats which are inherently rich in fat (pork, lamb). Variety meats, cold cuts, bacon, and sausages are eliminated. Only skim milk is used, and cream, butter, ice cream, cheeses (except nonfat cottage cheese), and chocolate are avoided. Because of their high cholesterol content, eggs are limited to three per week. Commercial bakery goods (pies, doughnuts, cookies, cakes, etc.) other than bread contain significant amounts of saturated fats (shortening, butter) and should be avoided. Whenever possible, foods are baked or broiled in preference to frying; when frying, vegetable oils are used. Unsaturated oils like corn, soy, safflower, and cottonseed oils are rich sources of linoleic acid and are used as extensively as possible. These oils are used in frying, cooking, and baking, to replace the saturated shortenings and butter. Special margarines distinguished by a high ratio of polyunsaturated to saturated fats and a high linoleic acid content should be used on bread and vegetables, instead of butter, and in cooking.

Such general dietary instruction in selected patients should be followed and evaluated carefully, using clinical and laboratory observations. It may not result in a visible slowdown or arrest of the atherosclerotic process, and in some cases it may even fail to lower elevated blood lipid levels; however, it represents a positive approach of potential benefit, which is just about all that can be offered at this point.

Prophylactic Diet for Atherosclerotic, Accident-prone Individuals[1]

Permissible foods	*Foods excluded*
Skim milk, coffee and tea (in moderation, and depending on physician's judgment), cocoa (in moderation) made with skim milk, soft drinks	Whole milk, cream
Enriched breads, nonfatty rolls, biscuits and crackers	Butter rolls, fatty crackers, or biscuits
Nonfat cereal foods (preferably enriched), griddle cakes and waffles prepared with permissible oil or margarines (see below)	Doughnuts, ordinary griddle cakes and waffles
Polyunsaturated oils: safflower, corn, soy, cottonseed, sesame; mayonnaise and salad dressing made from these, "special" margarines (see text)	Butter, lard, shortening, other fats, olive oil, ordinary margarines
Well-trimmed lean meat, fish, fowl; 3 eggs per week, nonfat cottage cheese	Fatty meat, fish, fowl; gravies, bacon, sausages, cold cuts, variety meats, all
Potatoes, noodles, spaghetti, rice	other cheeses
Any fruits and vegetables	Avocados except sparingly
Gelatin desserts, fruit whips, sherbet, puddings made with skim milk, homemade pastries with permissible fats	Ice cream, commercial cakes, pastries, cookies and pies, whipped cream
Sugar, honey, jams, jellies, and candy in moderate quantities only	Sugar-containing foods except with moderation

[1]The American Heart Association (44 East 23d Street, New York, New York 10010) has published a series of descriptive booklets on fat-controlled diets. These very well-organized brochures permit the average layman to plan fat-controlled meals with ease. Booklets may also be obtained from local chapters through a physician's prescription.

Herbs and spices (as tolerated), popcorn   Olives, nuts, and peanut butter except
   (with special margarines)   sparingly

The fat content and major fatty acid composition of commonly used sources of fat are given in Table 38 in decreasing order of linoleic acid content (used as an index of desirable degree of unsaturation) within each food group. The approximate amounts of cholesterol in servings of selected foods are given in Table 39. Also, note Table 8B, Fatty Acid Content of Food Fats, in Chap. 9.

Coronary Heart Disease

Coronary artery disease is the result of narrowing of the lumen or complete occlusion of coronary arteries, usually due to atherosclerotic changes. The condition is characterized by an inadequate coronary circulation. On occasions of increased cardiac effort, the deficient coronary blood supply may result in temporary myocardial ischemia accompanied by a characteristic thoracic pain, angina pectoris.

Dietary Consideration

The patient with coronary insufficiency will be asymptomatic as long as his coronary blood flow is not sufficiently embarrassed to cause myocardial anoxia. However, an anginal attack may be initiated by any condition which places too great a burden on his circulation, and thus his heart. This may be physical exercise, excitement, or the digestion of a heavy meal. The food intake is best divided equally throughout the day, and heavy meals must be avoided. Dinner is traditionally the meal which places the greatest digestive and circulatory burden on the consumer. A moderate amount of alcohol (such as is found in a glass of wine or 1 or $1^{1}/_{2}$ ounces of brandy) taken half an hour before dinner exerts a vasodilatory action on the remaining functional coronary vessels and may represent a wise prophylactic measure for the patient with chronic coronary insufficiency.

    If the patient is overweight, the caloric intake should be decreased and his weight reduced in order to decrease the work load of the heart, in addition to favoring the metabolic balance with respect to lipid metabolism. The prognosis of the cardiac patient is definitely better when he is slightly underweight. Not only is the heart spared the burden of an overweight body which must be supported when moving on a horizontal plane and lifted when moving vertically; a general decrease in superfluous tissue mass favors a reduction in circulating blood volume and thus constitutes a reduced internal work load. In addition to weight reduction, the physican should consider the prophylactic dietary changes outlined in the previous section on atherosclerosis.

Table 38   Fat Content and Major Fatty Acid Composition of Selected Foods

Food	Total fat, %	Saturated,[b] %	Unsaturated, % Oleic[c]	Unsaturated, % Linoleic[d]
Salad and cooking oils:				
Safflower	100	10	13	74
Sunflower	100	11	14	70
Corn	100	13	26	55
Cottonseed	100	23	17	54
Soybean[e]	100	14	25	50
Sesame	100	14	38	42
Soybean, specially processed[f]	100	11	29	31
Peanut	100	18	47	29
Olive	100	11	76	7
Coconut	100	80	5	1
Vegetable fats—shortening	100	23	23	6–23
Table spreads:				
Margarine, first ingredient on label:[g]				
Safflower (liquid)—tub	80	11	18	48
Corn oil (liquid)—tub	80	14	26	38
Corn oil (liquid)—stick	80	15	33	29
Partially hydrogenated or				
hardened fat	80	17	44	14
Butter	81	46	27	2
Animal fats:				
Poultry	100	30	40	20
Beef, lamb, pork	100	45	44	2–6
Fish, raw:[h]				
Salmon	9	2	2	4
Mackerel	13	5	3	4
Herring, Pacific	13	4	2	3
Tuna	5	2	1	2
Nuts:				
Walnuts, English	64	4	10	40
Walnuts, black	60	4	21	28
Brazil	67	13	32	17
Peanuts or peanut butter	51	9	25	14
Pecan	65	4–6	33–48	9–24
Egg yolk	31	10	13	2
Avocado	16	3	7	2

[a] Total is not expected to equal "total fat."
[b] Includes fatty acids with chains from 8 through 18 carbon atoms.
[c] Monounsaturated.
[d] Polyunsaturated.
[e] Suitable as salad oil; not recommended as cooking oil.
[f] Does not include the isomers of oleic or linoleic acid for which nutritional significance has not been established.
[g] Does not include small amounts of monounsaturated and diunsaturated fatty acids that are not oleic or linoleic.
[h] Linoleic acid includes higher polyunsaturated fatty acids.
   Source: U.S. Department of Agriculture Information Bulletin No. 361.

Table 39 Cholesterol Content of Common Measures of Selected Foods

Food	Amount	Cholesterol, mg
Milk, skim, fluid, or reconstituted dry	1 cup	5
Cottage cheese, uncreamed	½ cup	7
Lard	1 tbsp	12
Cream, light table	1 fl oz	20
Cottage cheese, creamed	½ cup	24
Cream, half and half	¼ cup	26
Ice cream, regular, approximately 10% fat	½ cup	27
Cheese, cheddar	1 oz	28
Milk, whole	1 cup	34
Butter	1 tbsp	35
Oysters, salmon	3 oz, cooked	40
Clams, halibut, tuna	3 oz, cooked	55
Chicken, turkey, light meat	3 oz, cooked	67
Beef, pork, lobster, chicken, turkey, dark meat	3 oz, cooked	75
Lamb, veal, crab	3 oz, cooked	85
Shrimp	3 oz, cooked	130
Heart, beef	3 oz, cooked	230
Egg	1 yolk or 1 egg	250
Liver, beef, calf, hog, lamb	3 oz, cooked	370
Kidney	3 oz, cooked	680
Brains	3 oz, raw	More than 1700

Source: U.S. Department of Agriculture Information Bulletin No. 361.

Myocardial Infarction

Myocardial infarction is a syndrome caused by permanent damage to a portion of the heart musculature due to sudden, overwhelming myocardial ischemia, secondary to insufficient blood supply. It usually results from the thrombotic occlusion of one of the larger branches of an atherosclerotic coronary artery and is accompanied by severe pain, shock, cardiac dysfunction, and often abrupt death.

The thrombus occurs most commonly in an atherosclerotic vessel with a narrowed lumen. The clot often starts on a roughened calcified plaque or ulcerated atheroma, and it may form gradually or rapidly.

The contributory role which fats may play in the clotting process has recently been under increased experimental scrutiny. It has been shown that postprandial hyperlipemia may aid in clot formation, either through decreased flow rate of the blood or increased coagulability. After a meal rich in butter, lard, or hydrogenated vegetable fats, the clotting time is markedly shorter than the normal interprandial fasting value. Other experimental work points at a lag in blood clot dissolution in hyperlipemia. Thus the makeup of the diet may, perhaps, play a double role in coronary heart disease: it may influence the course of the underlying atherosclerotic process (see section above), and it may conceivably constitute a precipitating or aggravating factor in permanent thrombus formation through encouragement of rapid clotting and interference with fibrinolysis whenever blood lipids are elevated.

Dietary Regimen

The type of diet given the hospitalized patient after the myocardial infarction depends on the severity of the damage and the patient's condition. During the first days, when symptoms are usually severe, fluids alone will suffice; a volume of 1,000 to 1,500 ml per day is indicated. When milk is tolerated without abdominal distention, the Karell diet may be employed; it consists of 200 ml of milk given four times per day. Following these first days, a semiliquid diet contributing about 800 cal may be given. This is gradually changed to a soft diet of 1200 cal as the patient improves. Feedings should be small and given at fairly frequent intervals. The sodium intake must be restricted to 250 to 500 mg daily until the danger of congestive failure can be ruled out (see below for sodium-restricted diets).

After the acute phase has passed, the patient may receive a bland diet with a caloric content adjusted to his needs. Care should be taken to avoid any foods which are likely to cause abdominal distention. The pattern of five to six small meals per day may now be changed gradually to three normal meals, provided there are no symptoms of anginal pain or dyspnea after a meal. With continued improvement, a regular, solid, sodium-restricted diet (containing 250 to 500 mg of sodium) may be given.

Vitamin supplementation may be advisable until the patient's food intake becomes normal. Sodium restriction may be lifted if the signs and symptoms of congestive failure are absent.

After the myocardial infarct is healed, the patient's diet depends on the peculiarities of the individual case. If cardiac insufficiency keeps the patient on the brink of congestive failure, some measure of sodium restriction should be continued. The extent of sodium limitation will depend on the capacity of the damaged heart and must be adjusted on the basis of clinical experience and trial and error.

The dietary recommendations concerning weight reduction, avoidance of heavy meals, and prophylactic judgment in fat intake, as outlined in the section on coronary insufficiency, apply even more strongly to the patient who has weathered a myocardial infarction.

Congestive Heart Failure

In congestive cardiac failure the heart fails in forcing the normal quantity of blood through the circulatory system. As a result of decreased arterial output, venous return is retarded and stasis results; consequently fluid diffuses from the vascular tree through the capillary walls into the tissue spaces, and the extracellular fluid compartment becomes engorged.

Progressive heart failure may result from a number of etiologic factors such as hypertension, atherosclerotic coronary disease, cardiac arrhythmias, rheumatic valvular disease, syphilitic aortic valvular damage, hyperthyroidism, and others. If it persists, cardiac decompensation from any cause will eventually result in a congestive state; the vascular engorgement may start in the pulmonary circulation (left heart failure) or in the systemic circulation (right heart failure). Of primary importance in the chain of events leading to the congestive state is decrease in renal blood flow secondary to a reduced cardiac output; the decrease in renal circulation leads to decreased glomerular filtration and excretion of sodium, with consequent retention of sodium and water in the body. (Probably an increase in secretion of aldosterone also aids sodium retention.) The excess of sodium and water is stored in the interstitial tissue spaces as edema fluid.

Sodium Economy and Hydration

The basic aim in the management of a failing heart is to reduce its work load, decrease the semistagnant circulatory blood volume, and reduce the patient's edema. Stringent exclusion of additional dietary sodium will permit a gradual excretion of the excess body sodium via the kidney. As sodium is excreted, extracellular water follows and diuresis sets in until the edema has receded. At any time when the sodium intake exceeds the impaired excretory capacity of the kidney (which in turn depends on the capacity of the ailing heart to maintain proper renal blood flow), sodium will again be retained by the individual; in accordance with the osmotic forces at play, water will also be retained in proportion to the sodium buildup and the patient will again become edematous. Reduction of the sodium intake to below the impaired excretory capacity of the kidney will reverse the process. The extent of edema depends primarily on the amount of excessive sodium in the body, not on the fluid intake of the individual. If the patient is on a limited sodium intake which is within his renal excretory capacity, he may be permitted fluids freely since water is readily excreted from the blood or extracellular fluid compartment of the body in the absence of osmotic forces set up by retained sodium.

Dietary Regimen

The use of a diet low in sodium (see below) is a definite aid in mobilizing excess extracellular fluid from the edematous patient with congestive failure; it also serves as prophylaxis against future resumption of fluid collection. Normally, the average individual ingests from 7 to 15 g of salt (2.8 to 6 g of sodium) per day. In congestive failure, the sodium intake should be limited to 250 to 800 mg daily initially until clinical experience permits establishment of the excretory capacity of the individual under balanced conditions. A stringent sodium deprivation is best managed when the individual is institutionalized and his dietary intake is under strict supervision. However, an intelligent and cooperative patient who has been well instructed can maintain a strict low-sodium regimen in the home.

Body weight is the best index of fluid retention, and the decompensated patient should be weighed daily to establish the progress of his fluid loss or to recognize a trend toward fluid retention. If the patient's sodium intake is well controlled, water may be given freely; in some cases forcing fluids while the sodium intake is negligible may actually aid in mobilization and excretion of sodium through the process of dilution.

Once medical treatment, bed rest, diuretics, and sodium deprivation have stabilized the patient, he may, in a few selected cases, be permitted to return to a normal diet. Usually, however, considering the impaired functional capacity of his heart, some measure of sodium limitation will be retained. The patient's permanent maintenance diet may thus be a strict 250- to 500-mg sodium regimen, a more moderate 1,000-mg diet, or a mildly restricted meal plan which permits 2,400 to 4,500 mg of sodium (see below).

As in most other cardiac conditions, the patient fares best if he is on the lean side of normal, and his caloric intake should be adjusted to permit a weight reduction, if this is indicated, and maintenance at the desired body weight. In many cases five or six small meals are better tolerated than three larger ones. Foods which tend to produce flatulence, fried or greasy foods which are not easily digested, and large meals should be discouraged; the patient's semi-incapacitated heart should not be needlessly burdened by mechanical displacement and spatial encroachment by distended infradiaphragmatic viscera.

Hypertension

Hypertension per se is not a disease; it is a symptom which may be the manifestation of different underlying disease processes. It may appear in the course of glomerulonephritis, polycystic renal disease, pyelonephritis, tumors of the brain or the adrenal glands (pheochromocytoma), hyperthyroidism, and other disorders. If hyptertension is secondary to a known primary disease, its treatment is essentially that of the basic disorder.

Essential Hypertension

Another type of elevated blood pressure is essential hypertension, a disorder characterized by an abnormal increase in systolic, diastolic, and mean arterial pressure due to increased resistance to blood circulation exhibited by the arterioles. The exact cause is unknown and has been variously ascribed to renal humoral factors, autonomic nervous system or adrenocortical dysfunction, and disturbed sodium chloride metabolism.

The disorder affects about 5 percent of the adult population of the United States; it is somewhat more common in women and among individuals with a short, stocky, and obese body type. Hereditary predisposition appears to play a role in this disease. Essential hypertension induces permanent damage to arterioles, primarily in the kidneys and other organs, and accelerates the generalized or localized degenerative processes of atherosclerosis. The disease may have a prolonged, relatively benign duration, or it may run a relatively brief, malignant clinical course. The ultimate outcome is usually cardiac failure, a cerebrovascular accident, or renal insufficiency with uremia.

Dietary Considerations

Obesity is very common among those suffering from essential hypertension. Considering that the heart labors under a compounded load, that of hypertension and that of obesity, the best interests of the patient are served by the adjustment of the caloric intake to bring about a normal weight. In most cases weight reduction influences the blood pressure but mildly; however, in a minority of patients the drop in blood pressure is surprisingly marked. Even among those whose blood pressure is unaffected there is usually an improvement of subjective symptoms (difficulty in breathing, fatigue) proportionate to the loss of excess weight—which justifies the dietary weight reduction program.

Clinical evidence does not warrant the rigid restriction of dietary proteins which has been advocated in the past; the ingestion of moderate amounts of protein does not elevate the blood pressure or aggravate existing hypertension. (See Chap. 30 for protein restriction when the kidney's ability to excrete nitrogen has become impaired.) Similarly, there appears no adequate reason for forcing fluids in general or for restricting them. As to specific beverages, coffee or tea in moderation is not detrimental and may be permitted for those patients who do not suffer unduly from nervousness or insomnia. The use of small amounts of alcohol by those who do not find it objectionable may be advantageous because of its vasodilating effect.

In recent years, experimental and epidemiologic evidence has been obtained which indicates that normally both genetic and environmental factors regulate blood pressure. Among the environmental factors, dietary sodium appears to be an important element in setting the mean blood pressure level of population groups. Epidemiologic research has implicated the very high daily salt intake in the extremely high rate of hypertension (and the associated high incidence of death from cerebrovascular accidents) in northern Japan, where a daily salt intake of 20 g is part of the traditional diet. Introduction of Western style foods, which supply considerably less salt, in northern Japanese school-children and subsequent long-term follow-up have demonstrated that the expected, traditional rise of blood pressure with increasing age is considerably reduced. Direct evidence in experimental animals and circumstantial, and not yet unequivocally established, indirect evidence in man have brought to the fore the role which the level of dietary salt intake may play in entire population groups and particularly in genetically predisposed individuals, and a reduced general level of sodium intake and sodium restriction in individuals afflicted with hypertension has become widely recommended.

Most advocates of sodium deprivation emphasize that halfway measures will not work; they maintain—and clinical experience appears to bear this out—that a regimen which permits more than 250 mg of sodium per day will not be efficacious, while a limitation to 200 to 250 mg will frequently accomplish a lowering of blood pressure for the duration of the strict diet. Many clinicians feel that even a stringent control of sodium intake is not too effective in reducing blood pressure in many patients who suffer from severe essential hypertension, and most prefer medical antihypertensive therapy to a sodium-restricted diet—especially since nowadays a broad array of effective blood pressure–lowering drugs is available.

When congestive heart failure appears as a secondary complication of hypertension, the dietary treatment is that outlined in the previous section of congestive failure. (Attention should, however, be paid to a possible concomi-tant lowered renal reserve since severe sodium restriction may be dangerous in the case of renal insufficiency where the kidneys cannot conserve sodium.) The dietary regimen in the case of hypertensive arteriolar nephrosclerosis is outlined in Chap. 30.

Sodium-restricted Diets

Sodium-restricted diets are described at this point, though their use is by no means limited to the management of cardiovascular disorders. These diets also serve in the management of nephritis with edema, cirrhosis of the liver with ascites and edema, the toxemias of pregnancy, and when treatment with adrenocorticotropic hormone, cortisone, or similar steroid hormones makes limitation of sodium intake desirable.

In the preparation of sodium-restricted diets salt and other sodium compounds are avoided and foods are chosen for their low natural sodium content. Water treated in most water softening equipment cannot be used for drinking or preparation of meals since many water softeners contribute additional sodium to the water in exchange for the removal of calcium and magnesium ions. In certain communities the water supply may contain more sodium than is compatible with a 250-mg sodium diet. The patient must avoid not only certain foods, but also sodium-containing drugs and sodium compounds used in food manufacture. Chief among these are "antiacid" or "alkalizing" proprietary preparations, saline cathartics, sodium-containing sulfonamides, salicylates, barbiturates, and bromides, as well as baking powder, sodium bicarbonate, sodium benzoate and propionate, sodium alginate (found in chocolate milk drinks and ice cream), sodium cyclamate (an artificial sweetener), and monosodium glutamate.

It is important for the patient to read the label and ingredient list on commercially prepared foods to acquaint himself with their composition. Special low-sodium dietetic foods intended for use in low-sodium diets must declare the amount of sodium contained in 100 g or in an average serving of the food; scrutiny of the label will easily establish whether a particular dietetic food fits the needs of the sodium-restricted diet.

In general, animal foods rich in high-quality proteins also contain more sodium than most other foods, and a definite relationship exists between the protein content of a diet and the degree of sodium limitation which it permits. Thus ordinary milk, meat, poultry, fish and seafoods, and eggs are used in measured amounts. Most cheeses contain excessive amounts of salt, as most other milk products do. On the other hand, most fresh vegetables and fruits and unprocessed cereals contain only insignificant amounts of sodium and may be used freely. The following are exceptional vegetables, characterized by a high sodium content, which should be avoided: beets, beet greens, carrots, celery, kale, dandelion, mustard greens, spinach, sauerkraut.

Generally speaking, all processed meats, meat products, fish, and canned vegetables (and many frozen foods) contain more salt than is compatible with low-sodium diets. Canned, dried, or frozen fruit and fruit juices may be used freely unless the label specifies that salt or sodium compounds have been added.

The sodium content of fresh meats and fish can be reduced by boiling in water and discarding the liquid. Low-sodium milk is now commercially available in most localities in the United States. Low-sodium cottage cheese may be found in the larger cities or may be made at home from low-sodium milk. Salt-free bread, salt-free butter and margarine, and low-sodium plain Passover biscuits (matzos) are usually available in larger cities.

A low-sodium diet is admittedly insipid-tasting and leaves much to be desired from a gourmet's viewpoint. There are a number of sodium-free salt substitutes available in drug and food stores which may be sprinkled over the cooked food. Sodium-free calcium glutamate and ammonium glutamate are also used to add zest to the diet. These and spices, herbs, and lemon juice may be used freely to lift the sodium-restricted diet out of what may otherwise be gustatory doldrums.

The 500-mg Sodium Diet

Permissible foods	*Foods excluded*
Coffee, whole or skim milk (2 cups daily), tea, cocoa (made from the milk allowance)	"Dutch process" cocoa, carbonated beverages, any other drinks
Low-sodium bread, rolls and breads made with sodium-free baking powder or potassium bicarbonate, yeast rolls and breads made without salt	Commercial breads and baked goods, biscuit, pancake or waffle mixes, self-rising flours, crackers, pretzels, any baked goods made with regular baking powder
Cooked farina, grits, oatmeal, rolled wheat or wheat meal; puffed rice or wheat and other cereals whose label does not indicate the presence of salt or sodium compounds	All other cereals
Unsalted butter or margarine, vegetable oils and shortening, dietetic salad dressings or mayonnaise	Salted butter or margarine, bacon fat, regular commercial salad dressings or mayonnaise, cream, except as part of the permitted milk quota
Fresh meat, fish, fowl (4 oz daily) prepared without salt, fresh oysters (if thoroughly washed), dietetic canned fish and meat, 1 egg per day, low-sodium cottage cheese, and dietetic cheeses. (*Note:* Orthodox Jews must not salt cuts of fresh meat in preparation for cooking.)	Salted, smoked, canned, or frozen (unless unsalted) meats, fish, or fowl, organ meats (except liver and heart once a week), sausage, luncheon meats, shellfish (except fresh oysters), all other cheeses
Unsalted potatoes, rice, homemade (salt-free) or dietetic spaghetti, macaroni, and noodles	Regular commercial spaghetti, macaroni, or noodles, hominy, potato chips
Fresh or unsalted, frozen (read the label carefully), or dietetic canned vegetables	All regular canned or frozen vegetables; the following vegetables in any form: beets, beet greens, carrots, celery, dandelion, kale, mustard greens, spinach, sauerkraut, Swiss chard. Susceptible cardiac patients should avoid the following gas-producing vegetables: dried beans and peas, broccoli, brussels sprouts, cabbage, cauliflower, cucumber, onions, garlic, green pepper, radishes, rutabaga, turnip
Fresh, frozen, canned, and dried fruits except as noted on the right	Any processed fruit which lists salt or sodium compounds on the label; maraschino cherries; cardiac patients susceptible to distention should

Unsalted vegetable soups or dietetic canned soups

Gelatin desserts made with plain pure gelatin, unsalted fruit desserts, homemade puddings, custards, and ice cream using the egg or milk allowance (do not use sodium-containing prepared mixes), cakes and cookies made without salt and baking powder

Sugar, pure sugar candy, honey, jams and jellies (if free of sodium benzoate), chocolate (except if "Dutch process" cocoa or salt is listed on the label)

Herbs, spices, and vinegar (as tolerated), unsalted nuts, dietetic peanut butter, unsalted popcorn

avoid raw apples, cantaloupes, watermelons, other melon varieties, and berries

All other soups

All other desserts

Molasses, syrups, brown sugar, "Dutch process" cocoa and candy or foods made from it, commercial candy

Salt, catsup, chili sauce, pickles, olives, relishes, meat flavorings such as Worcestershire sauce and others, soy sauce, tabasco sauce, bouillon cubes, vegetable salts, mustard, horseradish, salted nuts, potato or corn chips, popcorn, peanut butter, instant cocoa mixes, prepared beverage mixes, baking powder, rennet tablets, chemically softened water, sodium cyclamate (sugar substitute), monosodium glutamate, and other sodium compounds used in food preparation

Sample Menu:[1] 500-mg Sodium Diet

(Contains approximately 60 g protein, 35 g fat, 175 g carbohydrate, and 1255 kcal)

BREAKFAST
Orange juice (½ cup)
Puffed rice, sugar (½ cup)
Skim milk (1 cup)
1 soft-boiled egg
1 slice unsalted bread or toast, jelly
Coffee or tea, sugar

[1]The American Heart Association (44 East 23d Street, New York 10010) has published a series of descriptive booklets on sodium-restricted diets. These very well-organized brochures permit the average layman to plan low-sodium menus with ease on the basis of exchange lists. Booklets may be obtained from local chapters through a physician's prescription.

LUNCH
Open sandwich made with:
  1 slice unsalted bread
  2 oz dietetic pack tuna
  2 lettuce leaves
Dietetic salad dressing
1 sliced tomato
$^1/_2$ canned peach
Coffee or tea, sugar

DINNER
Broiled steak (3 oz)
Mushrooms
Mashed potatoes ($^1/_2$ cup)
Summer squash ($^1/_2$ cup)
1 pat unsalted butter
1 unsalted roll, jelly
Fruit cocktail ($^1/_2$ cup)
Coffee or tea, sugar

BEDTIME SNACK
Hot chocolate (1 cup) made with pure cocoa, sugar, and skim milk
3 apricots or unsalted cookies

The 250-mg Sodium Diet

The 250-mg sodium diet is identical with the 500-mg sodium diet described above except for a substitution of dialyzed low-sodium whole or nonfat milk for the regular whole or skim milk. No other quantitative or qualitative adjustments need to be made, except that the attending physician or dietitian should be consulted concerning the sodium content of the local water supply.

The 1,000-mg Sodium Diet

The 1,000-mg sodium diet is identical with the 500-mg sodium diet except that the patient is permitted the use of $^1/_4$ teaspoon of salt, either at the table or in cooking. This $^1/_4$ teaspoon of salt contains about 570 mg of sodium; instead of using this allowance in cooking or for flavoring at the table, the patient may eat regular yeast bread (200 mg of sodium per slice) and salted butter or margarine (50 mg of sodium per teaspoon). The allowance of $^1/_4$ teaspoon of salt may thus be used up in the form of bread and butter or (provided the calories are permissible) in the form of salted butter or margarine melted over the vegetables or meat to give them a gustatory lift.

The Mild Sodium-restricted Diet

This diet supplies from 2,400 to 4,500 mg of sodium. Such a mild limitation of sodium is primarily designed for patients who have recovered from an episode of congestive heart failure, in cases where the physician prefers to maintain some control of sodium intake. The basic qualitative and quantitative guiding principles of the 500-mg sodium diet apply here with the following exceptions:

All fresh and canned vegetables are permitted except sauerkraut and, in the case of the susceptible cardiac patient, the gas-producing vegetables listed previously.
Regular commercial baked goods are permitted, except those with salt toppings like pretzels, salt rolls, etc.
Organ meats, shellfish, plain canned or frozen meats and fish are permitted.
Regular butter, margarine, salad dressing, and mayonnaise may be used.
Commercial pudding mixes and nonsalty candy may be used.

The patient is not permitted to use salt at the table; however, he may use it lightly in cooking.

Precautions with Sodium Restriction

Prolonged, severe sodium restriction may not always be without hazard, since deficiency of sodium or chloride may occur in cases where impaired renal resorptive capacity prevents the conservation of salt. It is thus important to test renal function before embarking on permanent or prolonged sodium restriction.

Even with normal kidney function, sodium and chloride depletion are a possibility in severely sodium-restricted patients in congestive cardiac failure if diuretic drugs are extensively used and bring about a massive diuresis; also, the sodium-restricted cirrhotic patient who has undergone repeated paracenteses or massive drug-induced diuresis may become depleted with respect to sodium and chloride.

The low-salt syndrome is characterized by progressive weakness and lethargy, loss of appetite, nausea and vomiting, mental confusion, abdominal and general muscular cramps and pain, possible convulsions, and an eventual uremic demise. Salt-deprived patients who are suspected of pathological salt depletion should immediately receive *hypertonic* saline infusions (1.5 to 2 liters of 3 percent saline intravenously, very slowly) in an effort to restore their sodium and chloride balance.

The attending physician should be on the lookout for suspicious symptoms, especially in elderly patients who have been on severely sodium-restricted diets for long periods. Special attention should be paid to such patients in hot climates and in the summer when large quantities of salt may be lost through profuse perspiration.

Chapter 30

Nutrition and Diet in Diseases of the Kidney and Urinary Tract

The majority of nonsurgical conditions in the realm of renal disease are not amenable to permanent cure. Thus medical therapy aims at prolonged control of the disorder and amelioration of the systemic abnormalities which result from disturbed kidney function. A well-planned dietary regimen is part of a long-range control program in renal disease. The diet in renal disease is not static; as the clinical situation changes with different stages of the disease, dietary adjustments may be called for. The continued well-being of the patient requires a major degree of unwavering cooperation in adhering to a diet which is often difficult and depends on the physician's alertness in prescribing a dietary regimen which must be adjusted to the kidney's diminishing function.

General Principles of Dietary Control in Renal Disease

The kidney's chief functions are excretory, regulatory, and endocrine. The kidney excretes the end products of protein metabolism—urea, uric acid, sulfate, creatinine, and organic acids; it adjusts the electrolyte balance of the

355

body by excretion and selective reabsorption of sodium, chloride, potassium, and other ions. It maintains the body's water balance and helps to maintain acid-base equilibrium through selective excretion of excess acid. In addition, the kidney produces a substance—renin—which, through its action on angiotensin, profoundly affects systemic blood pressure once released into the circulation; it probably also produces a hormone, erythropoietin, which regulates red blood cell production by the bone marrow. The kidney is essential for the conversion of biologically inactive vitamin D (from food or produced in the skin), after its initial hydroxylation in the liver, to the biologically active metabolite 1,25-dihydroxy-vitamin D.

The two basic objectives in the dietary treatment of renal disease are (1) to lighten the work of the diseased organ by reducing the amount of urea, uric acid, creatinine, and electrolytes (especially potassium, sodium, and phosphate) which has to be excreted, and (2) to replace substances (such as protein and sodium) which are lost to the body in abnormal amounts because of the impaired renal function.

Because of the vital role which renal function plays in preserving a normal equilibrium in the body's internal environment, despite extreme variability in food and fluid intake and in factors such as external temperature and physical exercise, kidneys have been granted a wide reserve capacity. Thus they maintain their excretory and regulatory capacity even if 60 percent of their functioning units, the nephrons, have been destroyed by various disease processes. In fact, renal excretory capacity is maintained until only about 10 percent of functioning kidney tissue remains. When this point is reached, both excretory and regulatory kidney functions are severely diminished, and the waste products of body metabolism are no longer excreted adequately. They accumulate in the tissues and blood, and uremia, the final common pathway of chronic, progressive kidney disease, develops. At this point the end of life is near unless dialysis with an artificial kidney or renal transplantation is instituted, but it can still be postponed for many months (depending on the speed with which residual renal function is destroyed) by rational dietary treatment.

Kidney Diseases Leading to Chronic Renal Failure

Chronic pyelonephritis is the result of recurrent or continuous infections of the kidney which eventually lead to loss of functional tissue, scarring, and contraction of the organ. Obstruction to a free flow of urine from the kidney (such as congenital abnormalities of the urinary tract, or prostatic hypertrophy), with consequent urinary stasis and infection, predisposes to this condition.

Chronic glomerulonephritis comprises a group of renal diseases, most with an unknown specific etiology. Their basic pathologic mechanism is progressive destruction of the glomeruli by an abnormal immunologic process.

Vascular kidney diseases, such as malignant hypertension, hypertensive arteriosclerosis and atherosclerotic nephrosclerosis are local manifestations of a generalized vascular disease. Of primary importance is the vascular renal lesion of generalized essential hypertension which results in progressive degenerative destruction of functional nephrons. The disorder may run a prolonged, benign course or a more acute, malignant one.

Certain systemic diseases have specific, grave renal manifestations. Thus collagen diseases affect the kidneys with a glomerulitis (lupus erythematosus) or destruction of internal renal vessels (periarteritis nodosa). Diabetic patients are predisposed to several types of nephropathy which gradually destroy the nephrons and may lead to a fatal outcome: intercapillary glomerulosclerosis, nephrosclerosis, pyelonephritis, papillitis, and nephrosis. In long-neglected gout, crystalline deposits of uric acid salts in the kidney lead to scarring and atrophy. In amyloidosis, a protein substance (amyloid) deposits in the kidney and destroys the organ.

Congenital abnormalities, such as polycyctic kidney disease, are characterized by a defect, present since birth, which will lead to eventual renal failure later in life.

There are several other disorders, including drug toxicity, which belong in this general group. All have in common that they cause progressive destruction of renal functional tissue resulting in an atrophied organ and death from renal failure unless dialysis or renal transplantation is initiated.

Uremic Syndrome

The syndrome which develops when the kidneys have lost their function is called the uremic syndrome or *uremia,* after the substance which accumulates in large quantities in the blood and tissues, i.e., urea. This syndrome is characterized by the retention of urea, creatinine, and other products of protein metabolism (uric acid, sulfates, phenols, guanidines, and unknown toxic substances) in the blood and tissues, by progressive acidosis, inability to excrete a water load within a brief period of time, and electrolyte disturbances—such as impaired excretion of potassium and consequent hyperkalemia which induces cardiac arrhythmia and eventually cardiac arrest. Blood phosphate is high and calcium low—a combination which leads to secondary hyperparathyroidism and eventually results in uremic osteodystrophy (demineralization of bone and, sometimes, abnormal deposition of calcium in soft tissues). An added reason for low serum calcium in uremia is an inhibition of intestinal absorption of calcium (which in turn is due to an impairment of normal vitamin D activity). Early in uremia anemia develops, owing to toxic suppression of red blood cell production in the bone marrow, toxic shortening of the life-span of erythrocytes, and impaired production of the bone marrow–stimulating hormone erythropoietin by the nonfunctioning kidney. Toxic sensory, and eventually motor, neuropathy develops in the long-standing uremic state. Uremic gastritis and enteritis are late manifestations of the uremic syndrome as is uremic pericarditis, which is an ominous development.

The clinical manifestations of the uremic syndrome include weakness; dyspnea on exertion and other cardiovascular symptoms; a yellowish discoloration and itching of the skin; anorexia, belching, nausea, vomiting, diarrhea, bone pains, and sensory disturbances ("burning feet"). The patient may become disturbed, disoriented, even psychotic, and eventually comatose.

Generally, the uremic syndrome develops in the late stages of chronic, progressive kidney disease, after 90 percent or more of renal function has been lost. It may, however, develop wholly or in part in earlier stages because of a superimposed stress, such as a severe infection or hemorrhage. An acute uremic state will also develop rapidly as a result of acute renal failure due to a sudden shutdown of previously healthy kidneys (see below).

Dietary Principles in the Treatment of Chronic Renal Failure

The dietary treatment of chronic kidney disease is based on the following principles: judicious regulation of protein intake, regulation of fluid intake to balance fluid output and insensible water loss, regulation of sodium to balance its output, restriction of potassium and phosphate, insistence on an adequate caloric intake, and supplementation with appropriate vitamins.

Protein Restriction

Urea, creatinine, uric acid, and organic acids are the major breakdown products of dietary and tissue proteins. In addition, there are small quantities of other end products of protein metabolism, some of which are believed toxic to specific tissues and organ systems if they are permitted to accumulate in the body in inordinately high concentrations. It would be perfect if proteins could be withheld entirely from the diet of patients in advanced renal failure, but in them, as in normal man, there occurs a continuous tissue protein breakdown. This endogenous protein catabolism must be compensated for by an adequate protein intake; otherwise the individual will develop a negative protein balance, and he will become progressively emaciated from breakdown of muscle protein.

The normal concentration of waste products of protein metabolism in the blood is 25 to 38 mg nonprotein nitrogen per 100 ml. The healthy kidney constantly endeavors to excrete this nonprotein nitrogen as it is formed and manages to keep its concentration in the blood within physiologic limits; any excessive buildup of nitrogen wastes in the blood and tissues is incompatible with life.

A high level of dietary protein makes for an increase in urea production and excretion and thus places a functional burden on the kidney. For this reason, and since an accumulation of metabolic protein waste products in the body is progressively toxic and eventually fatal, the dietary intake of protein is restricted in patients with renal disease where there is renal insufficiency and nitrogen retention. At the same time, carbohydrates and fat are given liberally to satisfy all caloric requirements and to prevent as much as possible the breakdown of *tissue* proteins for energy production which would necessitate the excretion of urea resulting from such endogenous protein catabolism.

The timing of the decision to intervene with diet therapy—beginning with protein restriction—in chronic renal failure is based primarily on the clinical state of the patient. With progressive deterioration of renal function, most patients develop some degree of anorexia, nausea, vomiting, and diarrhea, and these signs are the commonest indications for restriction of protein. Another more arbitrary bench mark indicating the desirability of manipulation of protein intake would be a creatinine clearance dropping below 25 ml/min or a blood urea nitrogen concentration exceeding 100 mg percent.

The daily protein intake is best adjusted to the following schedule: When the creatinine clearance is from 30 to 20 ml/min, 50 g; 20 to 15 ml/min, 40 g; 15 to 10 ml/min, 30 g; 10 to 5 ml/min, 25 g. To these amounts should be added, gram for gram, increments for urinary protein loss. Once patients are placed on chronic dialysis—usually after their creatinine clearance has fallen below 5 ml/min—they should receive daily from 0.8 to 1.0 g of protein per kilogram of body weight (see below).

Clinical experience has shown that patients may be maintained in nitrogen equilibrium for prolonged periods on as little as 37 to 40 g of protein per day provided the caloric requirement is liberally met. Such a diet requires the excretion of only about 5 to 5.4 g of nitrogen in the urine compared with 8 to 9.5 g of nitrogen excreted on a 50- to 60-g protein intake. (About 1 to 2 g of nitrogen is lost in the stool.) When the blood urea level is very high, the total protein intake may be reduced to 20 g, provided only milk and egg proteins are used, which supply primarily the essential amino acids which are needed daily for internal synthesis of tissue proteins, and do not burden the patient excessively with nonessential amino acids which do little to counteract endogenous tissue protein breakdown but make demands on the body for disposal of their nitrogenous waste products. (The Giordano-Giovanetti diet for end-stage kidney disease, which is based on such a regimen, is described in detail further on in this chapter.)

Whenever the protein intake is as small as the rigid restriction in renal insufficiency demands, practically all the dietary protein should be of the highest biologic value. The protein should thus be given in the form of milk, eggs, meat, and fish.

High Protein Intake

In the nephrotic state (see below) the kidney usually functions adequately in the excretion of urea. However, there is a constant loss of serum protein into the urine which results in hypoproteinemia and consequent edema due to loss of colloidal osmotic pressure in the blood. The prevailing clinical opinion holds that provided the kidney can excrete nitrogenous waste products satisfactorily, a diet high in protein should be given to patients in the nephrotic state in order to compensate for the constant urinary protein loss and to correct the low plasma protein levels.

Based on clinical experience, the recommendation is to allow 1 g of protein per kilogram body weight per day, and an additional quantity of protein equivalent to the amount lost in the urine. Diets containing 100 to 130 g of protein are usually prescribed for patients in the nephrotic state with depressed blood protein levels.

Water Balance and Fluid Restriction

The fluid intake of patients with kidney failure must keep pace with their ability to eliminate fluid. They should be advised to consume 2 to 3 cups of fluids more than their 24-hour urine output; this will provide for the insensible daily loss of water via the lungs and skin and for water eliminated in the feces.

A high fluid intake constitutes a serious danger in patients in acute renal failure or in anephric patients maintained on dialysis with artificial kidneys. On the other hand, a high fluid intake is *less* of a danger in kidney patients who still have urine output than an unreasonable fluid deprivation would be. Renal patients who still have a daily urine output of 1 to 1.5 liters manage to eliminate a significant proportion of metabolic wastes via this route. An overzealous fluid restriction at this point in the course of their illness cuts seriously into their excretory capacity and leads rapidly to a deterioration of their status and to uremia.

Sodium and Potassium Regulation

The desirable sodium and potassium intake of renal patients depends on individual circumstances and must be determined by repeated measurements of these electrolytes in the serum and urine (if any). The sodium intake of the patient with renal failure must be restricted to prevent sodium retention in the body and consequent generalized edema. Similarly, hyperkalemia must be avoided since it introduces the danger of cardiac arrhythmias and eventual cardiac standstill.

Significant losses of sodium and potassium may occur during severe vomiting or diarrhea or in rare cases of sodium- or potassium-losing nephropathies; this calls for judicious supplementation with these electrolytes.

The kidney of the nephrotic patient is often incapable of excreting sodium in a normal fashion, and sodium is retained with a consequent water retention and generalized edema. Therefore sodium restriction is also practiced in the nephrotic state.

High-protein diets usually contain more sodium than ordinary ones. Consequently, the final dietary prescription for the nephrotic patient is a compromise between the desire for a high protein intake needed for replacement of urinary protein losses and for increase of the depressed plasma protein levels (which is needed to combat the attendant edema) and the need to restrict the sodium intake in an effort to correct any edema resulting from sodium retention. Ordinarily, the sodium intake is restricted to 500 mg daily, which is compatible with a 100-g protein diet. Sometimes diuresis is obtained in the edematous patient only when the sodium intake is reduced to 250 mg; such a sodium restriction is possible only within the framework of a diet supplying no more than about 70 g of high-quality protein.

Phosphate Restriction

The patient in uremia exhibits hypocalcemia and hyperphosphatemia. In an effort to turn off the consequent secondary hyperparathyroidism (which, in turn, leads to uremic bone disease) through a reverse feedback mechanism, many physicians encourage a restriction of phosphate intake. Since uremic patients are generally subject to protein restriction, they are not likely to consume large quantities of phosphates. In the case of patients on chronic dialysis, however, who are permitted a moderate protein intake, it is best to limit the intake of milk and milk products—which are rich in phosphates. Many dialysis centers, in addition, administer to their patients aluminum hydroxide preparations which act as phosphate-binders in the intestinal tract. Dietary phosphate sequestered by such preparations in the gut will not be absorbed and is carried out of the intestinal tract with the feces.

Caloric Intake

The caloric intake in patients with renal disease must be adequate at all times. The patient is permitted all the carbohydrates and fats he can and will consume, since the end products of their catabolism—carbon dioxide and water—do not impose a burden on his compromised excretory ability. An inadequate caloric intake encourages tissue protein breakdown by the body which requires a source of energy to carry on its vital functions. Such gratuitous endogenous protein catabolism only serves to aggravate the existing uremia. An adequate supply of calories from carbohydrates and fats is protein-sparing and must be built into the diet of the renal patient.

Vitamin Supplementation

Supplementary vitamins become advisable in conjunction with prolonged, severe protein restriction since a diet supplying 40 g of protein does not contribute a full daily complement of all vitamins. A multivitamin tablet or capsule supplying the full spectrum of known vitamins is usually added to the diet of renal patients on protein restriction. Because of the nature of dialysis with artificial kidneys (which leads to a considerable loss of all water-soluble vitamins from the blood during treatment), all dialysis patients are given a daily multivitamin preparation with their dietary prescription.

DIET IN SPECIFIC KIDNEY DISORDERS

Acute Renal Failure

Acute renal failure denotes an acute shutdown of kidney function in a person with previously adequate renal capacity. The condition is manifested by a severely decreased urinary output, amounting usually to no more than 200 to 600 ml of urine, with a low specific gravity, per 24 hours. Oliguria lasting more than 1 to 2 days will lead to the development of the full clinical picture of uremia.

The mechanism which most commonly underlies acute renal failure is acute destruction or degeneration of the kidney tubules owing to ischemia (insufficient supply of oxygen caused by impaired blood flow) or direct toxic action of chemical substances. Prominent among nephrotoxic substances are mercury, bismuth, carbon tetrachloride, antifreeze solutions, certain insecticides, and a wide spectrum of drugs. Tubular ischemia which can lead to acute renal shutdown is usually caused by and follows severe crushing injuries and other trauma followed by shock, severe burns and burn shock, mismatched blood transfusion reactions, septic abortions, and surgical operations.

Patients in acute renal failure are severely ill and require the most attentive care. They are oliguric or even anuric and may soon be uremic and moribund. Even with the best of care, survival is about 50 percent. If they can be maintained alive during the initial oliguric phase, which may last from 8 up to 25 days, their renal tubular cells will regenerate and they will regain near-normal or normal renal function. Restoration of kidney function usually is heralded by a phase of high urinary output which follows the anuric and oliguric phase.

During the anuric phase, fluid intake is limited to 300 to 500 ml per day, which compensates for water losses from the lungs and skin. To this must be added fluid equivalent to other overt losses from the gastrointestinal tract or urine (if any). The only nourishment patients receive at this stage is glucose given intravenously to supply calories for their basal metabolism, and to diminish tissue protein breakdown. With the patient's cooperation, feedings of sugar and fat ("butterballs") should be given. Prolonged oliguria without adequate provision of calories can cause serious wasting and hyperkalemia (from muscle breakdown), and attempts to increase caloric intake, orally or intravenously, should be made as soon as possible. Palatable and well-tolerated carbohydrate concentrates can be prepared while using only small volumes of fluid. A recent development adds the eight essential amino acids and histidine, and vitamins, to the intravenous glucose infusion—with a resulting greatly diminished mortality. Presumably this intravenous application of the basic Giordano-Giovanetti diet (see below) significantly enhances renal tubular regeneration while counteracting the existing uremia. The patient is also treated by hemodialysis or peritoneal dialysis, where available, to diminish toxic effects of his uremia. If patients are treated by dialysis, protein and appropriate vitamin supplements should be given to compensate for nutrient losses during the treatment.

Once the diuretic or polyuric phase has been reached, it is important to match the increasing daily urine output with a corresponding increase in fluid intake. Simultaneously, the patient is permitted from 20 to 40 g of protein daily. Once urine output persists and the abnormally high blood urea nitrogen concentration begins to fall, a gradual increase in the daily protein intake is initiated, culminating, eventually, in a normal diet. During the diuretic phase the blood sodium and potassium levels must be closely monitored because large amounts of these minerals are lost in the urine. Ordinarily, during this phase, for each liter of urine passed about 3 g of salt and 2 g of sodium bicarbonate are given and high-potassium fruits and fruit juices are fed.

Acute Glomerulonephritis

Acute glomerulonephritis is a disorder of the kidney characterized by diffuse inflammatory changes in glomeruli and an acute onset with albuminuria, hematuria, edema, hypertension, and a varying degree of nitrogen retention. The clinical course of the disease varies. Acute glomerulonephritis may heal completely, or it may grade into a terminal outcome; in many instances the disease enters a latent stage, or it may turn gradually into chronic glomerulonephritis.

Dietary Regimen

The fluid intake must be manipulated according to the volume of urine. In severe oliguria the fluid intake must be restricted in order not to enhance the edema. It is customary to allow 500 to 1,000 ml more fluid per day than the total urinary output of the previous day.

Because of the acute illness with attendant anorexia and nausea, the diet is best limited to fruit juices during the first days after onset. About 2 to 3 ounces may be given each hour, the total not to exceed the fluid allowance mentioned above. Two hundred and fifty grams of sugar, or more, is added to any fluids given in order to contribute to the caloric requirement of the patient and to spare his tissue proteins. Once the nausea has subsided, a low-protein, low-salt, medium-fat, high-carbohydrate diet is given which contributes no more than 40 g of protein and 500 mg of sodium per day. This diet is gradually liberalized with respect to protein during the following 10 to 15 days. If there is nitrogen retention on a liberalized protein intake (i.e., if the blood nonprotein nitrogen level rises above 40 mg per 100 ml), protein limitation is reimposed until the kidney's urea-excreting function has improved to permit a normal protein intake.

Sodium restriction is maintained until the edema has subsided. Daily weighing of the patient will indicate the extent to which his sodium intake may be liberalized; any rapid increase in weight will indicate water retention and the need for further sodium limitation.

Chronic Glomerulonephritis

Chronic glomerulonephritis is a chronic inflammatory process in the kidney characterized by gradual fibrosis of glomeruli and degeneration of tubules accompanied by progressive renal insufficiency. The clinical course of the disease may show a prolonged latent stage, followed by a nephrotic stage (see below), before renal insufficiency with nitrogen retention becomes severe and uremia sets in.

Dietary Regimen

During the latent stage there is no need for special dietary regulation unless signs of edema and urinary protein loss appear.

The dietary regimen during the nephrotic stage is discussed below in the section on the nephrotic syndrome.

In the next stage of early renal failure with nitrogen retention, the high protein intake maintained during the preceding nephrotic stage must be reduced sharply lest the patient be forced into early uremia. A kidney which is able to excrete 8 g of nitrogen daily may fail badly when required to excrete 16 to 20 g. As the blood urea nitrogen level begins to rise, dietary protein is restricted to 45 to 64 g of protein per day. Carbohydrates and fats are given liberally to meet caloric requirements. The daily protein allowance is decreased further to 35 to 40 g in accordance with the blood nitrogen picture.

At this stage, the sodium restriction which was practiced during the nephrotic state is *lifted* since the failing kidney is incapable of conserving sodium and chloride and a gradual depletion takes place without the help of dietary regulation. The fluid intake should be comparatively high, between 2,500 and 3,500 ml daily, to aid in renal clearance of nitrogenous waste products. The extra fluid will not be retained in the blood and tissues as long as the failing kidney leaks salt from the body and as long as cardiac function is not impaired. If dependent edema indicates the onset of cardiac failure, the latter condition should be treated with appropriate measures. The fluid intake should not be reduced except in extremis since it is important to maintain whatever kidney action is left.

The Nephrotic Syndrome

The term *nephrotic syndrome,* or *nephrotic state,* applies to those cases of renal disease (or stages thereof) which, regardless of underlying etiology, exhibit albuminuria, hypoalbuminemia, hypercholesterolemia, and often massive edema. There is no concomitant hypertension or nitrogen retention. This syndrome may be seen during the nephrotic stage of chronic glomerulonephritis, in lupus nephritis, lipoid nephrosis, renal amyloidosis, and other disorders.

In this condition large amounts of protein (4 to 40 g) may be lost daily in the urine. The kidney is able to retain plasma globulins to some extent, but plasma albumins leak out passively. The total blood proteins may be reduced from 7 to 4.5 g per 100 ml or less because of the massive albumin loss. When the blood albumin concentration falls below 2 g per 100 ml, the colloidal pressure of the blood decreases to a point where clinical edema usually appears.

In the nephrotic syndrome the kidney is also often unable to excrete salt normally, and salt retention and consequent edema compound the effects of the prevailing hypoalbuminemia.

Dietary Regimen

A high protein intake and sodium limitation are the primary therapeutic measures. The diet should contain 100 g of protein or more in order to compensate for the urinary loss and to encourage synthesis of new plasma albumin. Depending on the patient's weight and protein loss, the daily intake may vary from 95 to 130 g. Simultaneously, the sodium intake is restricted to 500 mg, or less, to diminish available food sodium in the face of the patient's sodium retention. With salt rigidly restricted, the fluid intake is not critical and the patient may be allowed fluids ad libitum.

Nephrosclerosis (Arteriolar Nephrosclerosis)

Nephrosclerosis is a vascular renal lesion which appears in conjunction with generalized essential hypertension and is characterized by sclerosis of the afferent arterioles, followed by eventual degenerative destruction of functional nephrons. The disorder may run a prolonged, benign course or an acute, malignant one.

The dietary regimen in benign arteriolar nephrosclerosis is that of essential hypertension (Chap. 29); the dietary program in the acute, malignant disorder is that of chronic glomerulonephritis.

Sample Menus in Renal Disease: Sodium-restricted Low-Protein Diet

(Contains approximately 500 mg sodium, 40 g protein, 100 g fat, 250 g carbohydrate, and 2060 kcal. No salt is permitted in preparation of meals or at the table.)

BREAKFAST
1 sliced orange, sugar
Cooked, salt-free cereal ($^1/_2$ cup), sugar
1 slice salt-free bread
1 pat salt-free butter
Jelly
Coffee, cream, sugar

LUNCH
Sandwich made with:
  1 hard-boiled egg
  2 slices salt-free bread
  Dietetic mayonnaise ($^1/_2$ tbsp)
1 sliced large tomato on lettuce
Milk (1 cup)
1 medium banana

DINNER
Salt-free cream of tomato soup (1 cup)
Cooked rice (3 oz)
2 pats salt-free butter
Buttered, salt-free string beans ($^1/_2$ cup)
Tea

BEDTIME SNACK
Milk ($^1/_2$ cup)
$^1/_2$ grapefruit, sugar

Sodium-restricted Moderate-Protein Diet

(Contains approximately 500 mg sodium, 70 g protein, 110 g fat, 220 g carbohydrate, and 2150 kcal. No salt is permitted in preparation of meals or at the table.)

BREAKFAST
1 sliced orange, sugar
Cooked, salt-free cereal ($^1/_2$ cup), sugar
1 soft-boiled egg
1 slice salt-free bread
1 pat salt-free butter
Jelly
Coffee, cream, sugar

LUNCH
Sandwich made with:
  Lean, unsalted ground beef (2 oz)

2 slices salt-free bread
Dietetic mayonnaise ($^1/_2$ tbsp)
1 sliced large tomato on lettuce
Milk (1 cup)
1 medium banana

DINNER
Sliced unsalted chicken (2 oz)
Cooked rice (3 oz)
2 pats salt-free butter
Buttered, salt-free string beans ($^1/_2$ cup)
Lettuce and pear salad
3 sodium-free cookies
Tea

BEDTIME SNACK
Milk (1 cup)
$^1/_2$ grapefruit, sugar

Sodium-restricted Moderately High-Protein Diet

(Contains approximately 800 mg sodium, 100 g protein, 115 g fat, 210 g carbohydrate, and 2275 kcal. No salt is permitted in preparation of meals or at the table.)

BREAKFAST
1 sliced orange, sugar
Cooked, salt-free cereal ($^1/_2$ cup), sugar
2 soft-boiled eggs
1 slice salt-free bread
1 pat salt-free butter
Jelly
Coffee, cream, sugar

LUNCH
Sandwich made with:
   Lean, unsalted ground beef (2 oz)
   2 slices salt-free bread
   Dietetic mayonnaise (1 tbsp)
1 sliced large tomato on lettuce
Milk (1 cup)
1 medium banana

DINNER
Sliced chicken (4 oz)
Cooked rice (3 oz)
2 pats salt-free butter
Buttered, salt-free string beans ($^1/_2$ cup)
Lettuce and pear salad
Milk (1 cup)
3 sodium-free cookies

BEDTIME SNACK
Milk (1 cup)
$^1/_2$ grapefruit, sugar

Sodium-restricted High-Protein Diet

(Contains 800 mg sodium, 135 g protein, 120 g fat, 220 g carbohydrate, and 2480 kcal. No salt is permitted in preparation of meals or at the table.)

BREAKFAST
1 sliced orange, sugar
Cooked, salt-free cereal ($^1/_2$ cup), sugar
2 soft-boiled eggs
1 slice salt-free bread
1 pat salt-free butter
Jelly
Coffee, cream, sugar

LUNCH
Sandwich made with:
  Lean, unsalted ground beef (4 oz)
  2 slices salt-free bread
  Dietetic mayonnaise (1 tbsp)
1 sliced large tomato on lettuce
Milk (1 cup)
1 medium banana

DINNER
Sliced chicken (6 oz)
Cooked rice (3 oz)
2 pats salt-free butter
Buttered salt-free string beans ($^1/_2$ cup)
Lettuce, pear, and cottage cheese salad (made with 3 oz of dietetic cottage cheese)
Milk (1 cup)
3 sodium-free cookies

BEDTIME SNACK
Milk (1 cup)
$^1/_2$ grapefruit, sugar

Special Diet for Patients with Advanced Renal Failure (Giordano-Giovanetti Diet)

A very large functional margin of safety is built into man's kidneys. Thus a loss of normal functional capacity of 50 percent still leaves the patient with progressive kidney failure (or the accident victim who lost one kidney) sufficient renal excretory capacity to permit a normal existence. In fact, the patient with *gradual* progressive renal failure can adjust quite well to further losses in renal functional capacity unit a stage is reached where his glomerular filtration rate has dropped to about 10 ml/min. At this point generally the first clinical symptoms of renal failure make their appearance. If the patient's diet is not henceforth adjusted quite drastically, the retention of metabolic waste products is rapidly enhanced and leads progressively to end-stage uremia. Usually, by the time a glomerular filtration rate of 1.5 ml/min is reached, the patient's ability to excrete a urine containing metabolic wastes is so severely compromised and such a uremic state is reached that only dialysis with an artificial kidney (and if possible, eventual kidney transplantation) can save his life. A well-adhered-to special diet for patients in advanced renal failure can, in many cases, permit a patient whose renal status is between the two bench marks mentioned above, to function well and lead a moderately productive life. In fact, where there is no possibility to extend to the patient either dialysis or transplantation for further long-term maintenance of life, this diet can prolong life and eliminate the symptoms of advanced uremia (especially gastrointestinal symptoms, disorientation, and itching) for many months. The length of survival on this diet depends on retention of a minimal residual kidney function (a ml/min). Once the residual renal function falls below these limits, potassium and nitrogenous wastes other than urea accumulate, acidosis sets in, and the patient who has been maintained previously reasonably comfortably with the aid of his diet deteriorates rapidly and requires dialysis or transplantation as a lifesaving measure.

A number of such special diets exist, all of them based on the principles of the so-called Giordano-Giovanetti diet (G-G diet), named after the Italian physicians who developed it in the early 1960s. The principles of this diet, in brief, are: A minimum of protein is provided, primarily in the form of *essential* amino acids. These are used entirely in the requisite daily endogenous protein synthesis to maintain nitrogen balance. Simultaneously the body synthesizes the needed *nonessential* amino acids (which are not supplied by the diet) by cannibalizing the pathologically excessive urea in blood and tissues. The requisite daily calories are supplied in the form of unlimited amounts of carbohydrates and fats which do not require the kidney for elimination of their metabolic waste products. Thus with this diet urea accumulation is counteracted by the reuse of nitrogenous wastes while nitrogen equilibrium is maintained with a minimal allowance of essential amino acids. Since no other additional protein is permitted, there is little accumulation of toxic nitrogenous wastes while the patient's elevated blood urea level decreases. Concomitantly, there is a marked general improvement in the patient's physiologic status.

The G-G diet may be described in the following simplified terms: It supplies the entire caloric needs of the patient (which will usually vary from 2000 to 3000 cal), most of it in the form of carbohydrates and fats; in addition, there is a daily allowance of about 20 g protein of as high a biologic quality as possible. The daily allowance includes one egg, $3/4$ cup milk, and occasional substitution of an ounce or two of meat, fish, or fowl, a multivitamin preparation, and iron-containing tablets. To keep the total nitrogen intake low, only proteins of highest biologic value are used. As proteins from grains and vegetables are of lower biologic value (and would contribute to the ultimate urea load), such foods are avoided assiduously. Thus, the rest of the diet consists of equivalents of many wheat starch products (made from deglutenized wheat grain) to supply protein-free calories. Commercially available low-protein bread for phenylketonuric patients (PKU bread) can also be used. In addition, the patient is given generous equivalents of minimal-protein, low-potassium fruits and vegetables, and ad libitum quantities of sugars and fats until the daily caloric allowance is filled. Fluid intake is limited to the usual level of lung, skin, and stool losses and volume of daily urine (if any). The effectiveness of this life-maintaining diet depends on strict adherence to this admittedly monotonous and restrictive diet and on consumption of the *full* daily complement of calories to prevent the catabolism of tissue proteins as sources of energy. Success therefore depends on careful selection of well-motivated and cooperative patients, intensive dietary indoctrination and instruction, and careful follow-up.

Dietary Management of the Dialysis Patient

Long-term dialysis is an effective, lifesaving maintenance treatment in end-stage renal failure. It is beset, however, with unpredictable and uneven results and complications unless personalized and careful dietary management is combined with a regular pattern of multiple (usually three) weekly dialyses. Nitrogenous end products of dietary and tissue protein metabolism and excess fluid accumulate between dialyses and are removed during dialysis. At the same time sodium and potassium are maintained at desirable levels (if the patient adheres to his diet). A picture of alternatingly fluctuating blood levels of these substances before and after dialysis results, and the well-being of the patient between dialyses depends to a large extent on a low amplitude of these up-and-down fluctuations. In an otherwise stable patient, biochemical control of his status depends on duration and frequency of dialysis, residual native kidney function, and—very important—the patient's diet. As most patients lose all renal function soon after initiation of maintenance dialysis, *diet* becomes the determining factor of biochemical control in any systematic dialysis treatment.

The basic objectives of the individually tailored diet of the dialysis patient are: (1) to maintain protein and caloric equilibrium, (2) to maintain a near-normal potassium and sodium level, and (3) to prevent fluid overload or dehydration.

A *protein allowance* of 1 g of protein per kilogram of ideal body weight will not result in the buildup of excessive nitrogenous wastes, will maintain a positive nitrogen balance, and will replace the quantities of amino acids lost during each dialysis treatment. At least three-quarters of the daily protein allowance should consist of proteins of the highest biologic quality—eggs, meat, fowl, white fish, and milk. (Milk is given fairly sparingly because it contributes fluid and because of its high potassium, sodium, and phosphate content.)

Carbohydrates and fats are supplied generously to provide the energy for daily activities and to spare tissue protein breakdown. Thirty-five to forty-five calories per kilogram of ideal body weight is usually prescribed; tissue building and weight gain are achieved with an allowance of 45 cal/kg. Care should be taken that the quantities of the carbohydrate foods chosen do not contribute much protein of *low* biologic quality (beans, legumes, cereals).

The choice of "bulk" carbohydrates like bread, spaghetti, and other noodles is critical since they may contribute significant amounts of less desirable proteins of low biologic quality. A minimum of 150 g of salt-free bread daily is suggested. It may be used as the carrier of large quantities of butter, jam, or honey, all of which will markedly increase the total caloric intake. Cookies and other pastries should be made without eggs but with a high proportion of fats and sugar. Rice may be used freely as its protein and electrolyte content is low. Sugar, marmalade and jams, honey, hard candies, and other sugar-based foods are desirable since they contribute needed calories while being virtually free of protein and containing few electrolytes. For the same reasons, patients are permitted liberal quantities of salt-free butter and margarine, oils, lard, and heavy cream.

Hyperkalemia can become a serious problem for the dialysis patient; an unsuspected potassium accumulation may result in cardiac arrhythmias or arrest without warning. A daily dietary restriction to 52 meq is usually invoked if the dialyzate bath contains 2.6 meq of potassium. Potassium limitation is difficult since varying amounts are found in meats, fruits, and vegetables.

Fruits and vegetables are distinguished by a low protein and calorie content and fairly high potassium and fluid contribution. Thus they must be selected carefully, the size of servings must be controlled, and their method of preparation may be critical. For instance, potatoes are rich in potassium and do not fit into a low-potassium regimen. They may be included quite freely, however, if they are prepared by first slicing them and parboiling them in a large volume of water which is discarded after a prolonged leaching period (overnight); they are again cooked in a large volume of water, which is discarded. Such potatoes may now be used for preparation of different dishes since 50 percent or more of the potassium has been leached out (together with other electrolytes). Fruits and vegetables, even if they are potassium-rich, may be used in *small* quantities to provide variety to the diet. Whenever possible, additional sugar or whipped cream should be added to fruits, and (unsalted) butter or margarine and cream sauces to carbohydrate foods and vegetables, to enhance the caloric contributions of these foods. Vegetables high in protein of low biologic value, like peas, corn, beans, and lentils, are completely excluded, as are celery and kale, which are high in sodium content.

Sodium intake should be limited to between 65 and 87 meq daily to control body fluid retention and hypertension, which may precipitate pulmonary edema and congestive heart failure. A restriction to 87 meq will still permit the patient regular bread and butter or margarine and a small amount of salt in his cooked food (but no additional salt at the table). This is an adequate limitation for most dialysis patients; a greater restriction may interfere with the patient's appetite and may consequently result in tissue loss.

Patients should not eat freely in restaurants or other people's homes where salt-free cooking cannot be assured. In such locations only truly innocuous food items should be consumed. Patients should read all food labels carefully and avoid commercially prepared foods to which salt has been added. On the other hand, many salt substitutes and "salt-free" dietetic products contain potassium chloride instead and should be avoided.

Fluid restriction is one of the most important aspects of the diet of dialysis patients. They are usually permitted 300 to 500 ml plus an amount equal to urine output (if any). Considering additional fluids contained in the foods consumed and water derived from the catabolism of foods, on one hand, and insensible and fecal fluid losses on the other, such a regimen usually results in mild fluid retention and a daily weight gain of 1 pound between dialyses.

Because of significant losses during dialysis, and during preparation of the food, empirically one multivitamin tablet daily is prescribed and iron supplements are given. Vitamin C and folic acid are particularly prone to be lost during dialysis.

Sample Menus[1] for Patients on Maintenance Dialysis: Sodium- and Potassium-restricted Moderate-Protein Diet

(Contains approximately 1,000 mg sodium, 1,500 mg potassium, and 60 g protein. No salt is permitted in preparation of meals or at the table.)

BREAKFAST
Applesauce or apple juice (¹/₂ cup)
Cooked, salt-free cereal (¹/₂ cup), cream, cinnamon, sugar
1 scrambled egg
1 slice regular bread
3 pats unsalted butter

---

[1]The Artificial Kidney Program, National Institute of Arthritis, Metabolism, and Digestive Diseases (National Institutes of Health, Bethesda, Md. 20014) has published a special diet booklet for patients on maintenance dialysis, complete with "exchange lists" for food items where protein, potassium, and sodium are critical, meal plans, and other helpful hints. This booklet permits the dialysis patient to plan a multitude of proper menus on the basis of his dietary prescription; it is available from the Institute upon request.

Jam
Coffee, cream, sugar (within fluid limitation)

LUNCH
Sandwich made with:
  Lean, unsalted meat or chicken (2 oz)
  2 slices regular bread
  Unsalted butter or dietetic mayonnaise (2–3 tsp)
1/2 sliced small tomato on lettuce
1/2 canned peach
Milk (1/2 cup)
Hard candy

DINNER
Beef, unsalted (3 oz)
Rice, butter (unsalted, 2 pats)
Corn (1/2 cup)
Lettuce and pear salad
Roll
Butter (unsalted, 1 pat)
Tea, cream (within fluid allowance)

BEDTIME SNACK
Apple juice (1/4 cup or within fluid allowance)
Hard candy

Sodium- and Potassium-limited Moderate-Protein Diet

(Contains approximately 2,000 mg sodium, 2,000 mg potassium, and 80 g protein. No salt is permitted in preparation of meals or at the table.)

BREAKFAST
Applesauce or apple juice (1/2 cup)
Cooked, salt-free cereal (1/2 cup), cream, cinnamon, sugar
2 scrambled eggs
2 slices bread or rolls, regular
3 pats unsalted butter
Jam
Coffee, cream, sugar (within fluid allowance)

LUNCH
Sandwich made with:
  Lean, unsalted meat or chicken (4 oz)
  2 slices regular bread
  Unsalted butter or dietetic mayonnaise (3 tsp)
1/2 sliced small tomato on lettuce
1/2 canned peach

Milk ($^1/_2$ cup)
Hard candy

DINNER
Beef, unsalted (4 oz)
Rice, butter (unsalted, 2 pats)
Corn ($^1/_2$ cup)
Lettuce and pear salad
Roll
Butter (unsalted, 1 pat)
1 slice sponge cake
Tea, cream (within fluid allowance)

BEDTIME SNACK
Apple juice ($^1/_2$ cup or within fluid allowance)
Raisin toast (buttered, 1 slice)

Caloric Requirements of Children on Maintenance Dialysis

Growth failure is commonly seen in children with chronic renal failure treated with dialysis and is one of the chief drawbacks of this treatment modality for the younger age group. Because of small body size, the intake of potassium, sodium, and nitrogen must be more rigorously controlled in the child than in adults on dialysis. The dietary restrictions imposed on such youngsters combined with the malaise and anorexia caused by their disease and the attendant emotional disturbance and psychologic maladaptation to long-term treatment with an artificial kidney result in a profound lack of appetite and prevent consumption of sufficient calories to support normal growth. The consequent growth failure is a strong indication against long-term dialysis treatment for children unless it can be overcome.

It has been shown that children on maintenance dialysis will normally consume between 45 and 80 percent of their recommended caloric intake. No growth occurs at the lower end of this range, and normal growth is achieved at the upper extreme; insistence on a full consumption of the caloric prescription results in normal growth in most instances.

A preoccupation with the underlying renal disease and the sustained effort required to maintain children on dialysis in a tolerable state of health make it all too easy to accept growth failure as an inevitable consequence of renal insufficiency. On dialysis, growth failure of a large proportion of such children apparently is due primarily to undernutrition, and catch-up growth is possible if an adequate caloric intake (with additional supplementation) is successfully introduced and permanently accepted by the child.

URINARY STONES

Stones may be found anywhere along the urinary tract, in the kidney, ureters, bladder, and urethra. They usually originate in the kidney where supersaturated urinary salts precipitate around small foci (consisting usually of a mucoid matrix) to form crystalline concretions which serve as nuclei for further growth. Precipitation and calculus formation are enhanced in infection, during urinary stasis, by high urinary concentration, and in hyperexcretion of calcium, phosphorus, oxalate, uric acid, and cystine.

Dietary Considerations

The role of diet has been inextricably linked with speculations as to the etiology of calculi. Actually, diets containing an excess of calcium, phosphate, oxalate, or purines have never been established as causative factors in stone formation, except in patients with recognized predisposing systemic diseases. On the other hand, there is evidence linking some form of single or multiple dietary deficiency to a high incidence of urinary calculi, especially bladder stones in young boys and men in certain areas of southern China, Thailand, Pakistan, Iran, and certain other countries. This type of bladder stone was quite common among the poorer population strata in England and Western Europe 100 to 200 years ago. The subsequent decline in incidence of vesical stones in these developed countries during a period of improving nutrition, and its preponderance in underdeveloped countries in the poor countryside where most people subsist on diets primarily of vegetable origin, suggest a dietary cause. A marginal diet, based largely on rice, almost devoid of animal protein, and low in phosphate, has been implicated in the bladder stones endemic in Southeast Asia, but the specific deficiency and the mechanisms of action have remained unknown, to date. Pyridoxine (vitamin B_6) deficiency has been shown to produce oxalate stones in rats; its role, if any, in human calculi has not been elucidated.

In the United States, dietary considerations apply primarily to the retardation of stone growth and to prevention of a recurrence after spontaneous passage or surgical removal of stones whose composition has been ascertained. In predisposed individuals the fluid intake should exceed 3,000 ml in order to ensure a dilute urine in which potential calculus-forming salts cannot reach concentrations at which they may readily precipitate out of solution. The acidity of the urine may also be regulated by dietary means in an effort to prevent precipitation. Foods which contribute ingredients or precursors of ingredients for renal calculi may be excluded, though there is no convincing evidence that dietary surfeit (without nutritional deficiency) is a major factor in stone formation. The efficacy of dietary means in the prophylaxis of most urinary stones is not well documented; however, for the sake of thoroughness, some methods of approach relating to the major classes of stones have been enumerated.

Cystine Stones

Cystinuria, an inborn error of metabolism, is responsible for about 3 percent of urinary calculi. In the past, a low-protein diet has been suggested for prophylaxis of cystine stones; however, there is little evidence that in this disorder the amount of cystine in the urine can be sufficiently reduced by dietary restrictions to be of value. Effective measures, commonly employed, are (1) alkalization of the patient's urine with alkalizing agents like sodium citrate (alkalizing agents are simpler and more effective than dietary manipulation), and (2) an increase in the fluid intake in order to obtain a very dilute urine in which the urinary cystine is held in solution until it is voided.

Uric Acid Stones

The measures recommended in the prophylaxis of uric acid calculi, which include about 10 percent of all urinary stones, are (1) alkalization of the urine in an effort to keep the urinary uric acid in solution (free uric acid is less soluble than alkaline urates which are formed in the alkalized urine); (2) an increase of the fluid intake in order to reduce the concentration of uric acid in the urine and to enhance its solubility; and (3) a low-purine diet as described for gout (Chap. 31).

The rationale of this diet is based on the fact that ingested purine compounds are metabolized to uric acid in the body. However, avoidance of dietary purines alone does not suffice since there is a considerable independent endogenous synthesis of uric acid from ingested nitrogen compounds other than purines. In view of this, many clinicians favor a general reduction of protein intake, in addition to the selective features of the low-purine diet, for refractory individuals who have a higher than normal urinary uric acid excretion. A protein intake of 1 g/kg body weight is normally considered optimal; the reduction of the protein intake to half this level, in addition to avoidance of dietary purines, reduces uric acid production appreciably and is considered an effective prophylaxis against recurrent uric acid stone formation. Where these measures are ineffective, allopurinol (200 to 800 mg daily) may be given. This drug inhibits xanthine oxidase and blocks the formation of uric acid from xanthine, thus reducing blood and urinary uric acid.

Hypercalcinuria

High levels of urinary calcium predispose to the precipitation of calcium-containing crystalloids and the formation of calcium oxalate and calcium phosphate stones. Hypercalcinuria is met in a number of conditions, the most common of which are (1) a high calcium intake, (2) hypervitaminosis D, (3) prolonged skeletal immobilization with disuse demineralization of bone, (4) prolonged acidosis, (5) postmenopausal osteoporosis, and (5) hyperparathyroidism.

The most common, avoidable instances of hypercalcinuria are found among individuals who habitually consume more than 1 quart of milk per day. Ulcer patients who have been kept on a Sippy diet far too long, or continue to ingest large quantities of milk and cream, or consume excessive amounts of proprietary antacids which contain calcium salts are particularly prone to develop calcium stones.

Calcium Oxalate Stones

The measures recommended in the prophylaxis of calcium oxalate stones, which include about 70 percent of all urinary calculi, are (1) an increase in the fluid intake in order to reduce the concentration of calcium and oxalate ions in the urine, (2) acidification of the urine by means of administration of acidifying agents in order to keep the urinary calcium and oxalate ions in solution (2 to 3 of sodium acid phosphate daily, in divided doses), and (3) avoidance of an excessive calcium intake (quantities in excess of 1.0 per day). The latter involves a limitation in the intake of the following calcium-rich foods: milk, cheese, and other milk products and canned sardines and salmon (with bones). In some persons the risk of calcium oxalate stones may be further decreased by diets high in pyridoxine and magnesium (or by the daily administration of 250 mg magnesium in the form of a magnesium oxide tablet).

In the past the exclusion of dietary oxalates has been advocated in the hope of reducing the amount of urinary oxalic acid. Clinical experience has shown that oxalate calculi may recur even after strict elimination of dietary sources of oxalate. This may be based on the fact that endogenous production of oxalate takes place in the human body, independent of an exogenous dietary supply.

Calcium Phosphate Stones

The measures recommended in the prophylaxis of calcium phosphate stones are (1) an increase in the fluid intake, acidification of the urine, and limitation of calcium intake, all as described in the previous section on calcium oxalate stones, and (2) avoidance of excessive dietary phosphate. The latter involves a limitation in the intake of the following phosphate-rich foods: milk, cheese, and other milk products, whole-grain cereals, bran, oatmeal, eggs, organ meats, nuts, soybeans, meats, and cereal products. Orally administered Aluminum Hydroxide Gel, U.S.P., is very helpful in depressing phosphaturia; it acts as a phosphate-binder in the intestine, preventing the absorption of dietary phosphate.

Chapter 31

Nutrition and Diet in Gout and Osteoarthritis

Gout

Gout is a disorder of purine metabolism characterized by abnormally high uric acid levels in the blood, deposits of sodium urate in selected tissues, and recurrent attacks of acute arthritis. The hyperuricemia of gout may be due to overproduction of uric acid or inadequate excretion of the compound by the kidney. Deposits of sodium urate occur in both soft and bony tissues and are commonly found in cartilage and bone and near and in joints, bursae, ligaments, and tendons. The condition is found predominantly among males. Though it may begin at any age, it occurs most frequently in middle life. Hyperuricemia appears to be genetically conditioned, but only a portion of individuals who are heterozygotes with respect to the inherited tendency will develop clinical gout.

Uric acid is a normal end product of the breakdown of purine compounds like nucleic acids, xanthines, and others. At one time it was thought that in man the only sources of uric acid were preformed purines, such as the individual's own tissue nucleoproteins and purines ingested with foods. However, it has been conclusively proved that the metabolic precursors of urates in man are not restricted to endogenous or exogenous preformed purines, and that the human body can synthesize uric acid from relatively simple carbon and nitrogen compounds which are abundantly present in its metabolic pool, such as glycine, carbon dioxide, and ammonia. Thus the characteristic hyperuricemia of the gouty patient is not necessarily the result of an excessive supply of preformed dietary purines or of an abnormally large breakdown of tissue nucleoproteins.

The level of serum uric acid in gouty individuals may be 6 mg or more per 100 ml; the normal level is 3 to 5 mg. The characteristic acute attack of gouty arthritis is not necessarily accompanied or preceded by a rise in blood uric acid levels, and uric acid may be injected into a gouty patient in relatively large amounts during a quiescent interlude without setting off an acute attack. Many persons who exhibit hyperuricemia never suffer the clinical symptoms of gout. Therefore some investigators feel that mechanisms other than uric acid are also etiologically involved and that the last word on gout remains to be said.

Dietary Considerations

Present-day concepts of the desirable diet in gout have been somewhat altered by the recognition that uric acid is derived not only from preformed purine compounds but also from simple and readily available carbon and nitrogen precursors. Once it was believed that the outright exclusion of dietary purines would effectively depress uric acid formation and thus control the metabolic circumstances which lead to clinical symptomatology. Many clinicians feel, nevertheless, that the diet should not contribute more purines than are unavoidable. Some limitation of purines is certainly advisable in an effort to prevent a needless increase in the uric acid pool.

Some clinicians feel that a permanent decrease in protein intake is helpful in the prophylaxis of acute episodes in known patients with gout. The rationale of this proposed low-protein regimen in conjunction with a low purine intake is based on the desire to decrease the concentration and availability of amino acids in the metabolic pool, which may be potential precursors for endogenous purine synthesis.

Nucleoproteins (which yield uric acid when catabolized) are found in most animal foods in varying quantities and also in the germ of seeds and in some vegetables. The following foods contain high concentrations of purines (150 to 1,000 mg per 100 g).

Group A	
Liver	Anchovies
Kidney	Sardines
Sweetbreads	Meat extracts, consommé
Brains	Gravies
Heart	Fish roes
Mussels	Herring

The following foods contain moderate amounts of purines (50 to 150 mg per 100 g).

Group B

Meats	Beans
Fowl	Peas
Fish (except as noted above	Asparagus
Other seafoods	Cauliflower
Lentils	Mushrooms
Yeast	Spinach
Whole-grain cereals	

The following foods contain negligible amounts of purines and are not subject to limitation in the diet of gouty individuals.

Vegetables (except as noted above)	Refined cereals and cereal products
Fruits	Butter and fats (but these should be taken
Milk	with moderation for reasons given
Cheese	below)
Eggs	Sugars and sweets
	Vegetable soups

Coffee, tea, and chocolate, at one time excluded from the diet of gouty patients, contain methyl xanthines which are metabolized to methyl urates, which apparently are not deposited in tissues. Thus the elimination of these beverages only imposes an unnecessary hardship on the patient.

Experience has shown that a diet high in fat interferes with the excretion of urates, whereas a high-carbohydrate diet enhances urate clearance from the blood. It is also desirable to maintain the gout patient at a normal weight and to give him abundant fluids at all times, the latter in order to decrease the precipitation of urates in his kidneys.

Dietary Regimen during Acute Attacks

During acute attacks of gout the diet should not contribute exogenous purines which, once metabolized, would add to the existing high uric acid load. Consequently a diet is given which does not contain foods listed above as containing high or moderate amounts of purine (see Purine-free Diet, below). An abundant fluid intake, up to 3,500 ml, is encouraged with the dual purpose of preventing urate precipitation in the kidney and combating dehydration of the febrile patient. The purine-free diet given should emphasize a relatively high carbohydrate intake and a moderate protein level and should be low in fat.

Dietary Regimen for Quiescent Intervals

Between attacks the diet should correct any overweight of the patient and should adjust his weight to normal. The desired diet is low in purine content, moderate in protein, and relatively low in fat (see Low-Purine Diet, below). The fluid input should be such that a minimum urinary output of 2,000 ml results. This less restrictive diet is considered a permanent maintenance diet and, being nutritionally adequate, requires no special vitamin supplementation.

The efficacy of such a regimen should be judged only after sustained, long-continued effort and on an individual basis. This limitation of purine input and promotion of uric acid output is a salutary adjunct to specific colchicine therapy during acute episodes and to continuous systematic administration of uricosuric agents and antiuricogenic drugs during the intercritical period, which are the mainstay of modern medical management of gout.

Purine-free Diet

This diet is characterized by the complete exclusion of foods in Groups A and B (see above). Protein, fat, and carbohydrate levels reflect the principles outlined for the dietary regimen in gout.

Sample Menu

(Contains approximately 70 g protein, 50 g fat, 285 g carbohydrate, and 1870 kcal)

BREAKFAST
Orange juice ($^1/_2$ cup)
Enriched breakfast cereal ($^3/_4$ cup, dry), sugar
Skim milk (1 cup, used with cereal)
1 soft-boiled egg
2 slices white toast, jam
1 pat butter
Coffee, sugar

LUNCH
Cream of tomato soup (1 cup)
Cottage cheese (3 oz) with pear and lettuce salad
2 hot rolls, jelly
1 pat butter
Skim milk (1 cup)
1 banana

DINNER
Lettuce and tomato ($^1/_2$) salad
Cheese soufflé (1 cup)

1 medium baked potato
1 pat butter
Yellow squash (½ cup)
2 hot biscuits, jam
Canned peaches (2 halves)
Beverage

BEDTIME SNACK
Skim milk (1 cup)
Cake or cookies

Low-Purine Diet

This diet is characterized by the exclusion of foods in Group A (see above) and limitation of foods in Group B to one serving per day. Protein, fat, and carbohydrate levels reflect the principles outlined for the dietary regimen in gout.

Sample Menu

(Contains approximately 75 g protein, 60 g fat, 290 g carbohydrate, and 2000 kcal)

BREAKFAST
1 sliced orange, sugar
Enriched breakfast cereal (¾ cup, dry) sugar
Skim milk (1 cup, used with cereal)
1 soft-boiled egg
2 slices white toast, jam
1 pat butter
Coffee, sugar

LUNCH
Cream of tomato soup (1 cup)
Sandwich made with:
　2 slices white bread
　2 slices cheddar cheese
　Mayonnaise (2 tsp)
　Lettuce
4 carrot sticks
Skim milk (1 cup)
1 banana

DINNER
Lettuce and tomato (½) salad
Lean ground steak (3 oz)
1 medium baked potato

1 pat butter
Buttered string beans ($^1/_2$ cup)
2 hot biscuits, jam
Canned peaches (2 halves)
Beverage

BEDTIME SNACK
Skim milk (1 cup)
Cake or cookies

Osteoarthritis (Degenerative Arthritis)

Degenerative arthritis is a chronic progressive disorder which involves primarily the weight-bearing joints and is the result of wear and tear of long duration. It is common in individuals in the fifth and sixth decades, particularly in obese persons. The degenerative joint changes are particularly pronounced in the parts exposed to major weight-bearing trauma—the knees, the hips, and the lumbar and cervical spine.

When the first symptoms of osteoarthritis become evident, the weight of the individual should be evaluated and a program of dietary weight reduction instituted (Chap. 21) in order to take any excessive load off the damaged joints. A reduction in weight, not only of the grossly obese but also of those who are only moderately overweight, is the most effective single step toward alleviation of symptoms, preservation of the impaired function of the involved joints, and deceleration of future, progressive degenerative changes.

Aside from a reduction of gravitational trauma on the damaged joints there is no effective dietary regimen with specific intrinsic value in the treatment of osteoarthritis or, for that matter, in the treatment of rheumatoid arthritis or other arthritides as long as the nutritional status of the individual is satisfactory.

Chapter 32

Nutrition and Diet in Congenital Metabolic Disorders

In recent years a number of more or less rare disorders with heretofore puzzling etiology have been defined as disease entities caused by the outright absence—or diminution in activity—of one or more key enzymes involved in normal body metabolism. The term *inborn error of metabolism* has been applied to these conditions though, perhaps, the designation *disorders of incomplete metabolism* might be preferable (the latter term does not allege the presence of a new aberrant metabolic pathway, but emphasizes an interruption or quantitative limitation in the normal metabolic process). Certain familial disorders of metabolism have been covered in individual chapters since they are classic, not uncommon diseases (see diabetes, gout). The less well-known disorders based on genetically determined defects in enzyme systems in which dietary therapy is an important factor are discussed in this chapter.

Phenylketonuria

Phenylketonuria is an inborn defect of phenylalanine metabolism which occurs about once in every 25,000 births and is transmitted as a simple Mendelian recessive trait on the basis of inheritance of an autosomal recessive gene. The underlying biochemical defect is a failure to convert the essential amino acid phenylalanine (derived from proteins of the diet or from the body's metabolic pool) into tyrosine, which is the normal metabolic pathway.

In phenylketonuria the liver enzyme phenylalanine hydroxylase is absent (or deficient), and consequently there exists a complete or partial block in the formation of the normal metabolite tyrosine. As a result phenylalanine accumulates and is eventually transaminated to its keto analog phenylpyruvate (some of it is also converted to phenylacetylglutamine). The excess phenylalanine and the abnormal phenylpyruvate accumulate in the blood and tissues and eventually spill over into the urine. The abnormal metabolites damage, among other tissues, the central nervous system, and progressive mental retardation is one of the clinical symptoms; nonspecific neurologic abnormalities, minor epileptic fits, an eczemalike skin eruption, and deficient skin and hair coloration are part of the clinical picture. The brain damage is cumulative and apparently irreversible and depends on the length of time during which the abnormal metabolites were permitted to act on the central nervous system. Thus early detection is essential, since mental deterioration is greatest during the early months of life. Diagnosis is established by demonstration of phenylpyruvate in the urine at levels exceeding 100 mg percent; blood phenylalanine levels of 20 mg percent or higher; blood tyrosine lower than 5 mg percent; and urinary levels of orthohydroxyphenylacetic acid exceeding 100 mg percent.

Dietary Treatment

The only known effective treatment is dietary and preventive and is directed toward decreasing the body's metabolic phenylalanine pool by stringently restricting the phenylalanine intake.

Two commercial phenylalanine-free diet preparations are now available. They consist of casein hydrolysates from which phenylalanine has been removed and which are supplemented with additional amino acids, minerals, and vitamins. In addition to these phenylalanine-free amino acid sources, the patient should receive a normal carbohydrate and fat allowance and a generous vitamin and mineral supplementation.

Initially the infant is given 5 g of the basic amino acid preparation per kilogram of body weight without any additional protein. To this are added fruit juices, vegetable oil, strained fruits, and strained low-protein vegetables. Once the (previously abnormally high) blood phenylalanine level has dropped to the normal range of 1 to 2 mg per 100 ml, foods containing small amounts of protein may be gradually added in order to contribute the minimal amount of phenylalanine which is needed for growth. (Phenylalanine is an essential amino acid.) Thus after 3 or 4 weeks the total phenylalanine intake of the afflicted infant should be adjusted to 15 to 20 mg/kg/day, in contrast to a normal intake of 90 to 200 mg. Carrots, apples, low-protein vegetables, frozen sweetened cream, and tomato juice thickened with cornstarch lend themselves well to the initial low-protein expansion of the diet. Whey protein formulas or whey solids can be used as sources of a high-quality protein which is lower in phenylalanine than that of whole milk. Eventually almost any low-protein foods may be fed to the child, subject of course to the total daily permissible phenylalanine intake. For all practical purposes one may assume that most good proteins contain 5 percent of phenylalanine; the phenylalanine content of a food is therefore readily calculated by multiplying the amount of protein which it contains by 0.05.

Results

Results of low-phenylalanine diets vary, depending on how soon in life therapy is begun and on the amount of cerebral toxic damage previously sustained. Generally the skin eruption clears, skin and hair pigmentation become normal, and epileptic seizures tend to cease. Usually motor ability improves, there is increased awareness and lengthened attention span, and the characteristic apathy and irritability disappear. The effect of the diet on mental ability varies; e.g., when the diet is instituted during the first weeks of life, the infants develop almost normally, but when the diet is instituted in children over 2 years of age only minor or no improvement can be seen. Usually improvement in behavior, motor coordination, and ease of handling is such that the dietary restriction of phenylalanine is justified even when the outlook for improvement of the mental retardation is dim.

As far as is known to date, the phenylalanine restriction must be continued at least until the child has reached the age of 5; a premature return to an uncontrolled diet reverses the improvement. Apparently the critical time for nutritional therapy is during the early phase of central nervous system development. A cautious reintroduction of a more normal diet later in life has been attempted in patients who had been maintained on a strict low-phenylalanine regimen since early infancy and reportedly has resulted in only negligible decreases in the intelligence quotient.

Because of the extremely low protein intake in the low-phenylalanine dietary regimen, the attending physician must be on the alert for any manifestations of malnutrition in the infant or child under treatment. Such a diet when applied too rigorously or faultily in early infancy can induce a modicum of mental retardation because of excessive protein restriction and consequent restricted brain development. Unless all of the four diagnostic parameters mentioned earlier are positive, it may happen that a highly restrictive and dangerous diet is unnecessarily given to children who do not suffer from classic homozygous phenylketonuria. In some infants increased blood phenylalanine levels are transitory because of immaturity of specific hepatic enzymes; others display a persistent mild hyperphenylalaninemia (8 to 12 mg percent) which is compatible with normal mental development. Recently it has been proposed that a separate gene at an independent locus has a modifying effect on what was previously considered a classic unilocular Mendelian recessive defect. Since screening tests for phenylketonuria are sometimes positive in children who may not benefit from the difficult and hazardous dietary management, an infant with a positive screening test is best referred to a medical center experienced in diagnosis and treatment of the disease. When the presence of true phenylketonuria is confirmed, dietary management should be started as soon as possible.

Pregnancy and Phenylketonuria

In recent years the pregnancies of untreated phenylketonuric mothers (of normal intelligence) and the intelligence of their offspring have been studied. All the children were mentally retarded or suffered from a variety of congenital physical defects, although none were phenylketonuric. This implicates the high maternal blood phenylalanine levels in causation of developmental defects in the otherwise normal fetuses while in utero. Therefore, if a female patient with known phenylketonuria insists on having children, it is imperative that her blood phenylalanine levels be kept low (with the aid of dietary restriction) to prevent infliction of fetal damage with her otherwise abnormally high blood phenylalanine. To date, pregnancies controlled in this fashion have resulted in normal offspring. Since the breast milk of untreated homozygous mothers presumably contains higher than normal levels of phenylalanine, avoidance of breast feeding by such mothers deserves serious consideration.

Galactosemia

Galactosemia is a congenital disorder of carbohydrate metabolism character-ized by inability to metabolize galactose. The defect is said to occur about once in 25,000 births and is transmitted as a simple Mendelian recessive trait based on inheritance of an autosomal recessive gene. The infant lacks (or is deficient in) the enzyme galactose 1-phosphate uridyl transferase which normally catalyzes the conversion of galactose 1-phosphate to glucose 1-phosphate. Thus galactose and galactose 1-phosphate accumulate in the blood and liver, and galactose is spilled in the urine. (The normal pathway for *reverse* conversion of glucose to galactose is intact, and the growing brain of the galactosemic infant seems able to procure its needed galactolipids from the endogenous conversion of glucose to galactose.)

The clinical picture is that of an infant with gastrointestinal symptoms and progressively enlarging liver who fails to thrive. Jaundice may or may not be present. Lamellar cataracts develop eventually; they may be frequently noted by the end of the second month. Affected infants usually fail to grow satisfactorily. Aminoaciduria and proteinuria appear secondarily, possibly based on competition between galactose and amino acids for renal tubular reabsorption or on renal toxicity of galactose or galactose 1-phosphate.

Epileptiform seizures may be seen in some patients. Others may eventually develop a cirrhosed liver. Mental retardation is a major complication; it is progressive and becomes more pronounced as the infant grows older without benefit of treatment.

Diagnosis of galactosemia is established by the finding of elevated blood galactose levels and by a grossly abnormal galactose tolerance curve followed by galactosuria; about 40 to 50 percent of the administered galactose can usually be recovered in the urine. The determination of the presence or absence of the enzyme galactose 1-phosphate uridyl transferase (see above) in the erythrocytes is another diagnostic test. It requires only 2 hours and avoids the metabolically less desirable galactose tolerance test.

Dietary Treatment

The only known effective treatment is preventive and consists of the rigid exclusion of all dietary sources of galactose and lactose (lactose yields galactose and glucose on digestion). Once the intake of lactose and galactose is interrupted, there is no further progression of clinical symptomatology, and often all symptoms clear up with restoration of normal health. It is not uncommon even to see established cataracts disappear. The prognosis depends, in part, on the severity of the condition, on the strictness of the diet, and particularly on the age at which the diagnosis was made and therapy was started.

Milk and milk derivatives must be completely eliminated from the infant's diet once a diagnosis of galactosemia has been confirmed. For all practical purposes, milk and milk products are the only major significant dietary source of galactose in infancy and except for them, the diet of the patient may be essentially normal. Thus instead of breast milk or cow's milk formula, the young infant should receive strained meats either by spoon or in the form of a liquid formula (with vegetable oil, sugar, water, and starch; see Chap. 39). The routine use of proprietary formulas based on soybeans—commonly used for infants allergic to cow's milk—is not advisable since soybeans contain stachyose, a tetrasaccharide which contains two molecules of galactose, and it is not precisely known how much galactose is liberated and absorbed from this source. As time goes by, the growing infant receives a diet which is essentially normal except for the careful exclusion of any milk derivative and a few other foods. Particular attention must be paid to commercially prepared foods which may contain milk products where they are not expected; the ingredient list on labels of all processed and packaged foods should therefore be carefully scrutinized. (Not the least important of such items are commercial breads, many of which are enriched with skim milk powder, and many pharmaceutical tablets which contain lactose as a filler.) The list of commercially prepared foods which contain milk derivatives is very large and includes sausages, wieners, cold meats, commercial baked goods, pudding and pie mixes, and many others that contain whey, whey powder, dry milk solids, or lactose.

Other foods which can yield galactose when digested are peas, beets, lima beans, liver, brains, sweetbreads, cocoa, and chocolate. Other quantitatively less likely dietary sources of galactose which must be eliminated are agar and gum arabic. These two vegetable gums are occasionally used as stabilizers in processed foods and may be avoided by perusal of ingredient lists on labels.

The lactose-galactose-free diet for galactosemia patients should be considered a permanent maintenance regimen and should continue throughout the child's development and possibly throughout life. Cautious reintroduction of lactose and galactose into the diet might be tried during the early adult years under painstaking clinical control, provided the galactose tolerance curve is found to be normal. Dietary treatment of galactosemia has not been practiced long enough to collect clinical data on a statistically significant number of patients raised on a galactose-free regimen who have reached adulthood.

Experience to date with this disorder and its dietary treatment has made it abundantly clear that satisfactory results may be obtained provided that a correct diagnosis is established at the earliest possible point in the infant's development and strict dietary control is instituted immediately thereafter. In recent years a body of suggestive evidence has accumulated which emphasizes the possibility that a galactosemic fetus may sustain early damage in utero, before delivery, which, once established, will remain irreversible. Knowledgeable investigators in this field have therefore proposed that all women who have produced a galactosemic child (where therefore both parents are known to harbor the galactosemic trait, and the expectation exists that one out of every four children will be galactosemic) be placed on a strict galactose-free diet immediately after the pregnancy has been established. Such a regimen would exclude the possibility of intrauterine galactosemic damage to the fetus. It has been suggested further that it would be a justified and advisable precaution to exclude galactose from the maternal diet in *all* instances where the pregnant mother is known to be heterozygous for the galactosemic trait.

Wilson's Disease (Hepatolenticular Degeneration)

Wilson's disease is a rare familial disorder of copper metabolism. The underlying biochemical lesion is a deficiency in the formation of a specific serum protein, ceruloplasmin, which normally binds the small amount of copper which is in circulation and plays a critical role in the quantitative regulation of the absorption of dietary copper (Chap. 12). The pathologic and clinical picture is the direct and indirect consequence of unregulated, constant, and unlimited absorption of dietary copper and the retention of the excessive copper in certain body tissues. The characteristic biochemical feature of the disease, on which its diagnosis is also based, is the abnormally low concentration or complete absence of ceruloplasmin. Normal blood contains 25 mg of ceruloplasmin per 100 ml, while in Wilson's disease only 0 to 5 mg is found.

The brain and liver of affected individuals contain increased amounts of copper. A progressive degeneration of the lenticular nucleus of the central nervous system occurs simultaneously with liver impairment and eventual cirrhosis. The central nervous system damage results in a characteristic neurologic picture. The amount of copper excreted in the urine is higher than normal; urinary excretion of amino acids is also increased, presumably because of a secondary renal tubular defect. Deposits of copper are present in the cornea (in the pathognomonic Kayser-Fleischer ring) and sometimes in the lunulae of the fingers. Some children may not show neurologic symptomatology, but will have the liver disease. The disorder usually becomes evident when the affected child is 5 to 7 years old and is eventually fatal unless treatment intervenes.

Since the patient with Wilson's disease absorbs too much copper, the treatment is based on avoidance of an excessive dietary copper intake and the oral administration of special agents which prevent intestinal absorption. Potassium sulfide will react with dietary copper to render it insoluble and unabsorbable; a dose of 20 mg per meal is usually administered. In addition, agents like BAL (British anti-lewisite) and penicillinamine hasten the urinary excretion of copper and even mobilize copper which has been deposited in tissues.

A combination of a low-copper diet with potassium sulfide and penicillamine instituted promptly after diagnosis of Wilson's disease and strictly adhered to thereafter is of demonstrated effectiveness in prevention of additional tissue and organ damage and, in many cases, will gradually reduce the body's abnormal copper burden. The following is a tabulation (in descending order of concentration) of foods which contain relatively large amounts of copper and should be excluded or deemphasized in the formulation of the copper-restricted diet:

Liver	Organ meat other than liver
Cherries	Nuts
Chocolate	Dried currants and peaches
Mushrooms	Dark molasses
Shrimp	Bran
Dried beans	Spinach
Lentils and peas	Beef
Shellfish	Whole-grain cereals

Other Hereditary Metabolic Disorders

In recent years more than 20 new inherited disorders of amino acid metabolism alone have been described. Most are associated with failure of orderly degradation of dietary amino acids. Maple syrup urine disease, for instance, involves blockage of the oxidative decarboxylation of the keto derivatives of the branched-chain amino acids leucine, isoleucine, and valine. Undiagnosed infants soon sustain lasting brain damage. A promptly instituted synthetic diet devoid of the implicated amino acids ameliorates the clinical symptoms and biochemical abnormalities of this rare disorder. Infants, however, will not thrive solely on a synthetic diet, and supplements of brewers' yeast must be added in small quantities. Gelatin, a protein which contains only low concentrations of the branched-chain amino acids, is used to supply half the protein requirements of the growing infant. To date, a few children have been raised in this fashion and have developed normally.

Other inborn errors of metabolism are due to inadequate conversion of ammonia to urea; still others are due to impaired activity of enzymes which synthesize vitamins or which require vitamins as coenzymes. New inborn errors are being discovered each year. A detailed description of the various experimental diet therapies attempted to date is beyond the scope of this book. There is a need to develop more effective and less expensive diets free of the various offending substrates, or modified in other ways, and for more physicians and nutritionists to become familiar with diet therapy in these fortunately rare, inherited metabolic diseases.

Chapter 33

Nutrition and the Anemias

Classification

Anemia per se should be regarded as a symptom of an underlying disorder, not a disease. It is a condition in which the total quantity of hemoglobin in the circulating blood is less than normal. This deficiency in circulating hemoglobin may be due to a decreased number of red blood cells per unit volume of blood or to a deficient hemoglobin content in the erythrocytes. The various anemias may be classified in the following simplified fashion on an etiologic basis:

I   Anemias caused by blood loss
   A   Anemia of chronic blood loss
   B   Acute posthemorrhagic anemia

II   Anemias caused by excessive destruction of erythrocytes
   A   Acute hemolysis
      1   Due to immune bodies, as in erythroblastosis or hypersplenism
      2   Due to toxic reactions to bacterial toxins or chemicals (drugs)

B Chronic hemolysis as in:
 1 Congenital disorders—sickle-cell anemia, Mediterranean anemia, congenital hemolytic jaundice
 2 Acquired disorders—paroxysmal nocturnal hemoglobinuria

III Anemias due to impaired production of erythrocytes
 A Caused by deficiency of substances essential for erythropoiesis
  1 Iron
  2 Vitamin B_{12}
  3 Folic acid
  4 Protein
  5 Vitamin C
  6 Trace minerals
  7 Other vitamins

 B Caused by congenital defects in erythropoiesis
  1 Congenital hemolytic diseases (mentioned above)
  2 Formation of abnormal hemoglobins

 C Caused by acquired impairment of erythropoiesis
  1 Infection
  2 Chronic diseases
  3 Replacement or infiltration of the bone marrow
  4 Inhibition or destruction of the marrow by noxious chemicals, drugs, or irradiation
  5 Endocrine disorders

Erythropoiesis and Anemia

The maintenance of the normal complement of erythrocytes and hemoglobin depends on a dynamic equilibrium between the formation of red blood cells and their removal. Most constituents of the erythrocytes are effectively conserved and reutilized; however, the conservation of materials which cannot be synthesized by the body de novo and must be supplied by exogenous dietary sources such as iron and essential amino acids is not always complete, and anemia due to deficiency of these components is not uncommon.

 The functional red blood cell is the end result of a complex developmental process which involves, among other phenomena, the synthesis of nucleic acids and nucleoproteins. The vitamins folic acid and vitamin B_{12} play a special essential role in this synthesis, and thus in the formation and maturation of primordial erythrocytes, when their supply is inadequate, the orderly development of many erythroblasts is impaired and arrested before maturation is reached and a qualitative and quantitative insufficiency results. The terms *megaloblastic arrest in the bone marrow* (where erythrocytes are formed) and *megaloblastic anemia* refer to the cytologic changes wrought by such a biochemical aberration.

Iron is a constituent of the hemoglobin molecule, and if the supply of iron is inadequate, there is a limitation in the amount of new hemoglobin which can be synthesized and incorporated into developing erythrocytes. In such a case, although the new erythrocytes will mature, as long as there is no intercurrent folic acid or vitamin B_{12}, deficiency, they will carry a subnormal complement of active hemoglobin.

Proteins of high biologic quality, iron, vitamin B_{12}, folic acid, and vitamin C are all dietary constituents of importance from the standpoint of deficiency anemia; in most cases, however, an insufficient dietary supply of these factors is less important in the creation of a deficiency than impaired absorption, excessive loss, or an abnormally increased requirement.

Iron-Deficiency Anemias

In this group belong a number of chronic anemias which are characterized by small pale erythrocytes. The basic causative factor in these conditions is the depletion of the individual's iron stores owing to a discrepancy between the iron intake and the iron requirement, be it normal or abnormally high. In adults, chronic blood loss is the most common cause for iron-deficiency anemia. It may be physiologic, as in excessive or prolonged menstruation or after repeated pregnancies, or pathologic, as in occult intestinal blood loss due to ulceration, parasites, or malignancy.

Disorders of the gastrointestinal tract such as achlorhydria or chronic diarrhea may also lead to iron-deficiency anemia because of impaired iron absorption. In pregnancy, a certain degree of hypochromic anemia results from the iron demands of the fetus coupled with an increase in the volume of circulating blood. Infants and children often develop iron-deficiency anemia during periods of rapid growth when their iron intake is not equal to the demands of the constantly increasing tissue mass, be it for iron for circulating hemoglobin or for fixed muscle myoglobin. A pure nutritional iron-deficiency anemia is often encountered in infants who have been kept on an exclusive milk diet too long or whose large milk intake, which contributes only negligible amounts of iron, prevents them from taking enough other iron-rich foods.

The symptoms of iron-deficiency anemia are similar to those of other types and include weakness, easy fatigability, pallor, dyspnea on exertion, and a constant feeling of tiredness. The onset is usually insidious. There may be vague gastrointestinal symptoms. Achlorhydria is not uncommon. The skin, mucous membranes, and nails are pale in proportion to the reduction in the circulating hemoglobin. A large proportion of adults with long-standing hypochromic anemia exhibit atrophy of the papillae of the tongue. There may be slight cardiac enlargement with eventual failure if the anemia becomes severe enough. Nails may be brittle, longitudinally ridged, or even concave and spoon-shaped. (The relatively uncommon clinical picture of hypochromic anemia, achlorhydria, glossitis, dysphagia, and spoon-shaped nails is referred to as the Plummer-Vinson syndrome.) Individual blood cells are pale (hypochromic) and smaller than normal (microcytic). The major defect is in the makeup of individual erythrocytes, not their total number; thus the total cell count may be normal or slightly low.

Iron-Deficiency Anemia in Infancy and Early Childhood

Whereas most instances of iron-deficiency anemia occurring in adults can be traced to current or past blood loss, the majority of cases of iron-deficiency anemia in infants and children must be regarded as dietary in nature. Exceptions are the relatively uncommon cases of blood loss in infants and children (where repeated nose bleeding can be a factor) and those regions of the world where parasitic infestation is frequent in children and leads to a chronic, occult blood loss.

It is discouraging that in the last decades, during which the incidence of most nutritional deficiencies in infants and young children has been substantially reduced, the incidence of iron-deficiency anemia appears to have decreased very little. Approximately 25 percent of infants who are being hospitalized for a variety of ills exhibit iron-deficiency anemia of moderate degree, and data obtained in ambulatory pediatric care show that subclinical or marginal states of iron deficiency are very common in the 6- to 36-month-old group in infants who are otherwise deemed healthy and normal—particularly among the poorer population.

Detection of anemia in infancy is difficult since the infant does not express complaints of feeling "run down" and being easily fatigued. Thus many a case goes unrecognized by parent and physician alike and is discovered when investigation of another nonassociated disease yields telltale laboratory data.

The high incidence of iron-deficiency anemia in the young is not surprising in view of the fact that during the first 2 years of life the requirement for iron to be incorporated into hemoglobin and into fixed muscle myoglobin and iron-containing intracellular enzymes is up to three times as great as at any other time. Whenever this iron requirement is not met by the daily dietary intake or whenever the infant is handicapped by a subnormal endowment of iron at birth, iron deficiency occurs.

In contrast to the normal adult who possesses adequate iron stores, the newborn inherits most of its iron in the form of circulating hemoglobin and has very little effective tissue stores. Prenatal factors influence the infant's total iron at birth; thus infants of anemic mothers frequently share the maternal iron deficiency. There is a greater incidence of anemia in infants of a high birth order in contrast to first and second children (presumably because of progressive iron depletion in the mother). Conversely, infants born to mothers treated with oral iron during pregnancy exhibit higher iron values than control groups. The total amount of fetal hemoglobin increases with gestational age. Therefore prematurity or a low birth weight is the most common predisposing factor to iron deficit in the newborn. As a rule twins also seem to be more predisposed. An unduly long period of feeding on milk only or an inadequate mixed diet lacking meats, eggs, or iron-enriched baby cereals, as well as repeated intercurrent infections, predisposes to the development of iron deficiency in all infants.

Dietary Considerations and Prevention in Infancy

The infant depends solely on its diet for a supply of iron to permit normal expansion of its tissue mass and blood volume. In the case of the newborn who starts life with a low endowment, a compensatory supernormal acquisition of iron is essential, and the availability of dietary iron is indeed a critical factor. Normally, given a diet which is adequate with respect to iron, an infant will overcome its relative neonatal iron deficit; on the other hand, a normal complement of body iron at birth is not adequate to prevent the development of iron-deficiency anemia later, in the face of a diet low in iron.

The average total body iron at birth is 300 mg and that in adulthood 3,000 to 5,000 mg. Even if we assume that the daily iron loss in infancy is negligible (in the adult it amounts to about 1.2 mg per day), the average infant must accumulate about 0.5 mg of iron daily for about 20 years if it is to avoid anemia. Since normally only about 10 to 15 percent of the dietary iron is absorbed, up to 5 mg of iron must be contained in the diet of the infant to prevent an iron deficit. A diet based on milk alone (as is often the case during the first semester of life) or in which the predominant role of milk excludes adequate quantities of other iron-containing foods falls far short of this goal since a quart of milk supplies only about 1.5 mg of iron.

The major sources of iron in an infant's diet are iron-enriched cereals, eggs, meat, and green leafy vegetables, and only if such food items are liberally represented in the menu will it contribute 5 mg of iron. (Liver and other organ meats are excellent iron sources, but are not usually adequately emphasized in children's diets.) For instance, 1/2 ounce (dry weight) of the average iron-enriched infant cereal contains 5 to 8 mg of iron, one egg yolk contains approximately 1.2 mg, and 2 ounces of strained beef contains approximately 1 mg of iron. Thus the inclusion in the menu of one or more servings of enriched infant cereal, one egg yolk, and one serving of meat will normally ensure an adequate dietary supply of iron for the normal infant.

The majority of *premature* infants who derive iron solely from iron-fortified and iron-containing solid foods, even when these foods are fed from an early age, will develop iron-deficiency anemia. This can be corrected effectively by the addition to the diet of a formula containing 12 mg of iron, or more, per quart. Such a formula, given from birth, affords effective prophylaxis against iron deficiency and will permit the acquisition of hemoglobin to keep pace with the rapid growth of these infants.

The iron requirement remains high throughout childhood and adolescence—as long as the individual grows rapidly—and a liberal inclusion of meat, organ meats, eggs, green leafy vegetables, and enriched cereal in the daily diet is necessary not only to meet the need for blood and tissue synthesis but also to build up iron reserves in the body for use in contingencies. Since the protein economy of the child's body is intimately connected with tissue expansion and hemoglobin synthesis and since protein deficiency is an äggravating factor in anemia, the diet should at all times supply liberal amounts of proteins, with emphasis on those of high biologic value.

Prevention in Adulthood

Just as the infant walks a tightrope with regard to its iron supply, the parous female between menarchy and menopause treads a narrow path between dietary supply and daily loss of iron. In males the daily loss of iron is estimated to be between 0.5 and 1.0 mg per day; thus the normal male adult can maintain a normal hemoglobin level on a diet containing from 5 to 10 mg of iron per day on the basis of an average 10 percent absorption of dietary iron. However, the total iron loss for women of menstrual age (averaged out over a 28-day cycle) has been estimated to be 1.5 to 2.5 mg per day. The cost of pregnancy in terms of iron is still higher; it amounts to from 300 to 500 mg of iron per pregnancy, which, when spread over the period of a year, adds another 1 to 1.5 mg to the daily requirement. Thus the average woman who is menstruating or parous requires more iron-containing foods than the male, and generally speaking, she receives less. It has been established that children and adults who are anemic or on the borderline of iron deficit absorb a higher percentage of the ingested dietary iron than normal controls, and it is quite feasible that this mechanism also serves to prevent any greater frequency of iron-deficiency anemia among women.

   In males and females alike the problem is to build up storage depots of iron to meet emergencies: hemorrhage and other blood loss, destruction of erythrocytes by infections or poisons, pregnancy in the case of women—and blood donation. Iron reserves in the form of ferritin and hemosiderin in the liver, spleen, and bone marrow are essential to meet contingencies since sudden calls for extensive erythropoiesis after hemorrhage cannot be satisfied by the small trickle of iron absorbed daily from food. Normally, once the emergency is met, the incoming dietary iron will restock the partially depleted iron stores. As long as the requirement is high, after hemorrhage, in anemia, or in pregnancy, the dietary iron is more effectively absorbed, only to be rejected to a large degree once the body reserves have been replenished.

   For ordinary needs, the dietary allowances recommended by the Food and Nutrition Board are generous and adequate (Table 22). It is possible to provide a daily intake of 10 to 18 mg of iron if the menu includes one liberal serving of meat and one egg per day; this plus enriched cereal and bread and two to three servings of vegetables (one of which should be green, leafy) and/or fruit will supply from 75 to 100 percent of the daily requirement, depending on the *size* of the servings. Thus there is relatively little trouble in providing adequate dietary iron for males, who require less iron than females and who require and consume, on the average, more food because of a generally greater energy expenditure. The picture is quite different with regard to females in their reproductive years, from adolescence to menopause.

The actual amount of food ingested by most persons in the Temperate Zone has undergone a gradual decrease. It is estimated that the average American diet provides 6 mg of iron per 1000 cal. As food is subject to greatly diminished beneficial contamination with iron owing to a significant decline in the use of iron cooking utensils in the house and iron processing equipment in food plants, and as iron water pipes are replaced with copper plumbing, it is difficult to obtain an ordinary diet with a much higher iron content per 1000 cal. With a decrease in need for calories associated with diminished physical activity and the striving for a slender figure, most women obtain from their diet approximately 9 to 10 mg per day (*including* iron which has been added to products containing enriched flour). In the menstruating female between the ages of 14 and 45 the iron balance is thus borderline, and iron-deficiency anemia may result from such normal events as heavy menses, repeated pregnancies, and blood donation. It is estimated that in the United States, iron deficiency exists in 10 percent of menstruating women, particularly in teen-agers, and in 25 percent or more of pregnant women who have not received medicinal iron supplementation.

It has been suggested that this situation can be remedied through an increase in the iron enrichment level of flour from an average of 15 mg/pound to 40 mg/pound and in baked goods from an average of 10 mg/pound to 25 mg/pound. The problem in such an iron enrichment program is that a level suitable and beneficial for vulnerable groups—women in the childbearing years, infants, and children—may provide a surplus of iron for male adults, especially for those who consume large quantities of bread and other enriched foods. Controversy has developed particularly over the hazard which enhanced iron fortification levels may pose to the one person in 10,000 in the population who is genetically incapable of controlling his intestinal iron absorption, who is as yet unaware of his predicament because symptoms of iron overload have not yet become manifest, and in whom onset of symptomatic hemachromatosis may be accelerated (see Chap. 12).

Treatment

Treatment of uncomplicated iron-deficiency anemia is by oral administration of inexpensive, simple, soluble iron salts such as ferrous sulfate, ferrous gluconate, or ferrous fumarate whenever possible. The usual dose, expressed as elemental iron, is 200 mg/day. "Shotgun" preparations containing vitamin B_{12}, folic acid, cobalt, and other additives have no advantage and are contraindicated since they may obscure the correct diagnosis as indicated by a positive response to iron alone. Vitamin C, on the other hand, will increase intestinal iron absorption. Parenteral administration of other iron compounds is chosen if there is intestinal malabsorption, in the presence of serious gastrointestinal diseases, when oral supplementation proves irritating or ineffective, or when the patient is unable or unwilling to take iron via the oral route. In all cases, the food intake should be planned with a view to providing maximal amounts of dietary iron in a diet, otherwise adequate (especially with regard to protein and vitamin C), which should obviate the need for further supplementation in the long run, barring absorption defects or abnormal blood losses. A list of common foods which contribute above-average amounts of dietary iron is found in the section on iron in Chap. 12.

Anemias Due to Deficiency of Vitamin B_{12} or Folic Acid

This group includes a series of anemias whose underlying cause is a deficiency in either vitamin B_{12} or folic acid. Vitamin C is thought to function in the conversion of folic acid to its biologically active analog tetrahydrofolic acid (Chap. 11), and a severe ascorbic acid deficiency may thus have the same effect as folic acid deprivation. Vitamin B_{12} and folic acid or its metabolically active derivative are essential for the synthesis of nucleic acids, and formation of new nucleic acids and nucleoproteins must necessarily precede any orderly cell division and the development of new erythrocytes and other cells. Thus deficiency in these factors will interfere with the normal development of erythrocytes and will lead to anemias which are characterized by megaloblastic arrest in the bone marrow and the production, in insufficient numbers, of large erythrocytes which carry a normal complement of hemoglobin (megaloblastic, macrocytic, normochromic anemias). See Chap. 11 for other anemias due to deficiency of vitamin B_{12} or folic acid not mentioned here.

Pernicious Anemia

Pernicious anemia is a chronic macrocytic anemia, found mostly in middle-aged and elderly individuals, which is characterized by atrophy of the gastric mucosa and achlorhydria. A common complication is progressive, subacute degeneration of the posterior and lateral nerve tracts of the spinal cord.

The basic defect in patients with this condition is lack of normal intrinsic factor activity (which is essential for proper intestinal absorption of vitamin B_{12}). At one time it was thought to be exclusively due to a degenerative change in the gastric mucosa which atrophies and ceases to elaborate and secrete intrinsic factor. More recently, specific antibodies to intrinsic factor have been found in the gastric juice, saliva, and blood of patients with pernicious anemia, which either precipitate the factor or block its binding of vitamin B_{12}. In such patients, although the secretion of intrinsic factor appears normal, its facilitation of vitamin B_{12} absorption is impaired. The resulting deficiency in vitamin B_{12} is responsible for the defect in erythropoiesis and for the damage to the nervous system.

Treatment is specific and consists of parenteral supplementation with vitamin B_{12}. Folic acid is contraindicated since it reverses the abnormal blood picture without preventing or ameliorating the neurologic damage, which continues progressively. Oral vitamin B_{12} with Intrinsic Factor Concentrate, U.S.P., may be used for maintenance (only) but should not be relied on exclusively. It should not be used in the initial therapy or in the treatment of patients in relapse or with spinal cord lesions. Liver, given daily in large quantities, was formerly used as specific and effective dietary therapy. The efficacy of this dietary regimen was probably based on the fact that vitamin B_{12}, when ingested in large quantities (25 mg or more), is apparently absorbed by another mechanism than that normally stipulated, that is, even in the absence of intrinsic factor.

Sprue and Other Malabsorption Anemias

The macrocytic anemia of sprue is the result of folic acid and/or vitamin B_{12} deficiency. The disorder and its treatment are discussed in detail in Chap. 16.

Malabsorption syndromes such as those found in cases of diminished absorptive surface, chronic enteric obstruction, and intestinal blind loops frequently involve the lack of both folic acid and vitamin B_{12}. In treatment, surgical correction and antibiotic therapy are usually combined with the specific supplementation.

After gastrectomy, the absence of intrinsic factor, which is normally elaborated by the gastric mucosa, impairs the absorption of vitamin B_{12} and leads to a macrocytic anemia which responds specifically to parenteral therapy with the vitamin.

Megaloblastic Anemia of Pregnancy

Megaloblastic anemia of pregnancy is due to a folic acid deficiency, and is probably precipitated by the increased physiologic requirement for the vitamin during pregnancy, especially during the last trimester. The incidence varies with the prevailing dietary adequacy with respect to folic acid. Reports from India have set the incidence of megaloblastic anemia of pregnancy as high as 12 percent, while recent figures have set the occurrence in England at 7 percent. Signs of folic acid deficiency have been seen with increasing frequency in metropolitan maternity clinics and among private obstetrical patients in the United States and Canada, and at a higher rate among those with preeclampsia and eclampsia.

The condition responds readily to supplementation with folic acid. Treatment consists of oral administration of this vitamin (5 to 15 mg/day) coupled with the introduction of a well-balanced, normal diet as described in Chap. 16. In view of the frequency of folic acid–deficiency anemia in pregnancy, the ingestion of small, physiologic supplements of folic acid (0.2 to 0.4 mg daily) is recommended during the last trimester of pregnancy.

Megaloblastic Anemia of Infancy

Megaloblastic anemia of infancy is believed to be due to inadequate formation of tetrahydrofolic acid (or its metabolically active equivalent) secondary to a deficient intake of vitamin C and/or folic acid. A higher than normal requirement for tetrahydrofolic acid may play an important role in individuals with megaloblastic anemia of infancy or pregnancy. Treatment consists of administration of liberal quantities of vitamin C and folic acid, coupled with the introduction of a well-balanced, normal diet as described in Chap. 17.

Nutritional Macrocytic Anemia

This is a term frequently applied to a macrocytic anemia associated with the long-standing consumption of marginal, protein-poor, restricted diets which are deficient in folic acid and, less frequently, in vitamin B_{12}. This disorder responds to administration of folic acid and/or vitamin B_{12}, coupled with the introduction of a normal, well-balanced diet.

Scurvy

A macrocytic anemia may be associated with severe cases of scurvy. It is thought that in such instances the vitamin C deficiency may interfere with the conversion of folic to tetrahydrofolic acid and the tetrahydrofolic acid deprivation may be responsible for the special character of the attendant anemia. Treatment with vitamin C and folic acid is recommended and should be coupled with a well-balanced diet to achieve a normal nutritional status.

Not all instances of anemia in scurvy are true macrocytic anemias which require folic acid therapy. Many cases of anemia in scurvy respond to administration of vitamin C only, while others appear to be instances of iron deficiency.

Chapter 34

Nutrition and Diet in Neurologic and Psychiatric Disorders

The integrity and normal function of all human organ systems and tissues are dependent on the nutritional status of the individual, and the peripheral and central nervous systems are no exceptions to this rule. For the purposes of the nutritionist, neurologic disorders may be classified as (1) those which are uninfluenced by diet, (2) those in which the state of the nutrition plays a secondary, contributory role, and (3) those in which dietary deficiencies or disorders of absorption, transportation, or utilization constitute the primary etiology. The latter group includes such deficiency disorders as pellagra, beriberi, combined system disease, and others.

Encephalopathy of Pellagra

The encephalopathy of pellagra (Chaps. 10 and 22) is usually slow in onset and expresses itself at first principally in the form of mild anxiety states, or neurasthenia. This neurasthenia is characterized by easy fatigability, lack of appetite, digestive disorders, insomnia, and alternating depressions and tension states. This syndrome is apparently not a specific result of niacin deficiency alone since a similar state is not uncommon in other forms of malnutrition, including severe thiamin deprivation and starvation. Irritability, headaches, and emotional instability are other central nervous system manifestations which may accompany the early signs of the disease. In later stages loss of memory may occur in some patients. If pellagra is not recognized as the underlying cause of the encephalopathy, the disorder may be considered of psychoneurotic origin and the treatment will be ineffective. In advanced cases, confusional psychosis with acute fearful hallucinations, mania, delirium, and even catatonia may be observed.

Niacin alone may dramatically relieve the early mental syndrome in the pellagrous state, but it is not necessarily effective in treatment of the neurologic damage in long-standing cases. It is important to ameliorate any other associated deficiency states concurrently; thus large but balanced multivitamin supplementation must also be given. In pellagrous encephalopathy 100 to 250 mg of niacinamide is given parenterally for a few days; this is followed by oral dosages. To this must be added oral thiamin and riboflavin in therapeutic quantities—five to ten times the recommended daily dietary allowances. As soon as the patient is able to feed himself, he should receive a well-balanced diet contributing 2800 to 4000 cal, which contains 2 g of protein per kilogram of body weight. Particular emphasis should be placed on inclusion of liver, eggs, milk, and meat.

Encephalopathy of Niacin Deficiency

Apart from the mental symptoms of pellagra, there exists a specific, clinically fairly defined encephalopathic syndrome which is due to niacin deficiency. Pellagrous signs are not present, but associated signs of malnutrition such as follicular keratinization or stomatitis may be present and are indicative of other concurrent deficiencies. The syndrome is characterized by a clouding of consciousness, cogwheel rigidity of the extremities, uncontrollable grasping and sucking reflexes, and at times coma. Many of the patients are old, debilitated, and malnourished. The syndrome is most frequent postoperatively (or after periods of high fever or delirium), following extensive parenteral infusions which are unaccompanied by vitamin supplementation.

The disorder responds specifically to administration of niacinamide in massive doses. From 300 to 500 mg of niacinamide should be given daily, in divided doses, together with generous, balanced supplementation with other vitamins (see previous section). Tube feeding may be necessary at first, followed by the dietary regimen outlined above for the treatment of pellagrous encephalopathy.

Wernicke's Encephalopathy

Wernicke's encephalopathy is a syndrome related to thiamin deficiency characterized by anorexia, nystagmus, double vision, ophthalmoplegia, ataxia, loss of memory, confusion, confabulations, and hallucinations, which may progress to stupor and coma. Thiamin deficiency is largely responsible for the condition, though associated insufficiencies of other water-soluble vitamins may also be involved. Parenteral and oral thiamin therapy (15 to 20 mg subcutaneously or 30 to 60 mg by mouth in divided doses) is specific and should be coupled with polyvalent vitamin supplementation, including ascorbic acid in large amounts. This is followed with a well-balanced, protein-rich diet.

In most cases of encephalopathy due to dietary insufficiency it is safe to assume that hepatic function is marginal, to say the least, if not insufficient. Thus in such cases, except for indications of massive necrosis of the liver and impending hepatic coma, a high-calorie, high-protein, moderate-fat, and high-carbohydrate diet should be given and continued until improvement of hepatic function and nutritional status are achieved. At this point the caloric intake should be adjusted to maintain the patient at his ideal weight.

Polyneuritis of Thiamin Deficiency

In thiamin deficiency, peripheral neurologic changes usually appear after the patient has exhibited symptoms of neurasthenia (see section on pellagrous encephalopathy). The peripheral polyneuritis of thiamin deficiency is bilateral and usually symmetrical. The lower extremities are primarily involved. The onset is usually manifested by numbness, tingling, or burning of the toes and feet and muscle cramps; this progresses gradually to sensory and motor loss in the feet and ankles and eventually involves the entire leg. It has been suggested that the polyneuritis of pregnancy, the neuritis of colitis, and the neural damage seen in many cachectic states are related to thiamin deficiency which may be associated with multiple deficiencies of the B complex vitamins.

The treatment of the polyneuritis of thiamin deficiency is that outlined above for Wernicke's syndrome. Acute, recent deficiencies respond better than lesions due to malnutrition of long standing where irreversible neural damage may be a factor. Because of the usual multiple deficiencies associated with such conditions and to prevent relapses, it is essential that the patient receive henceforth a diet which is based on a high intake of the protective foods.

In the long run, therapy of any of the neurologic manifestations of nutritional deficiencies and prevention of relapses should depend on the establishment of an improved dietary regimen for life. Reliance should be placed on a balanced diet which supplies liberal amounts of eggs, muscle and organ meats, milk and milk products, citrus fruits, tomatoes, green and yellow vegetables, and enriched cereals and cereal products.

Unfortunately, this is more easily said than done, since many patients with nutritional deficiencies come from a social and psychologic milieu which is not compatible with an adequate diet. A large proportion are chronic alcoholics in whom a major change in dietary habits is contingent on reduced alcohol consumption—a goal which is notoriously difficult to achieve. Others may be elderly individuals in the early stages of personality deterioration, or individuals with marginal mental status or social adaptability. In many cases, poverty and ignorance complicate the picture further. In the less developed areas of the world, abject poverty is a powerful and indisputable factor, which is frequently associated with ignorance and prejudice to block the establishment of what is considered a nutritionally adequate dietary.

Combined System Disease

Subacute degeneration of the posterior and lateral columns of the spinal cord is common in patients with pernicious anemia. The condition is characterized by myelin degeneration of the posterior and pyramidal tracts followed by sclerosis of the demyelinized axons. The peripheral nerves, subcortical areas in the motor region of the brain, and nerve plexuses of the gastrointestinal tract may also become involved. Paresthesias of the fingers and toes, loss of vibratory and position sense, loss of normal reflexes, weakness of the extremities, and mental deterioration follow. Early treatment with vitamin B_{12} (Chap. 33) arrests the progress of the neurologic involvement and restores functional integrity. Structural damage of long duration is irreversible.

Convulsive Disorders

In the past, idiopathic epilepsy has been treated with various dietary restrictions such as abstinence from meat, purines, or chlorides. Experience has shown that none of these regimens had any demonstrable effect. Later, ketogenic and dehydrating diets were in vogue.

The essential feature of the ketogenic diet is a food intake that prevents complete combustion of fat and results in formation of the ketone bodies acetone, acetoacetic acid, and β-hydroxybutyric acid (Chaps. 9 and 24). To achieve this the diet must be high in fat and contain negligible amounts of carbohydrate; about 1 g of protein per kilogram body weight is allowed. The usefulness of the diet was thought to be due to accumulation of ketone bodies, but it appears more likely to be the result of the attendant progressive dehydration.

The ketogenic diet is difficult to arrange, is unpalatable, lacks nutritional balance, and produces little benefit in patients over the age of 15. It is seldom used today and has been largely replaced by more effective drug therapy. A trial diet is justified, however, in children who fail to respond to currently available drugs. A more palatable diet containing the triglycerides of octanoic and decanoic acids (medium-chain triglycerides, MCT) has been introduced more recently. It contains 60 percent of the total daily calories in the form of MCT oil.

Severe pyridoxine deficiency may lead to epileptiform convulsions with abnormal electroencephalographic findings in infants (Chaps. 11 and 13).

Pyridoxine occurs in many different foods, and except under very unusual circumstances or experimental conditions, signs of pyridoxine deficiency are not found. To date, such instances of convulsive seizures have been reported only in infants fed synthetic formulas lacking pyridoxine or fed an ill-processed proprietary formula in which the vitamin was destroyed. The parenteral administration of 10 to 20 mg of pyridoxine followed by 3 mg per day by mouth results in prompt recovery.

Food and Nutrition in Psychiatric Disorders

The tie between man's food and his psyche is a strong one; it dates back to early infancy and is conditioned by a wealth of emotional experiences thereafter. For the infant each feeding experience and each food is fraught with reactions of pleasure or pain, satisfaction or frustration, acceptance or rejection. The nursing or feeding process is more than an alimentary function; it turns into a social and emotional experience under the impact of all associated stimuli on the infant's nervous system, especially if the same experience occurs repeatedly. Food may thus become identified with unconscious meanings which are far removed from the original concept. It may become a physical equivalent of love and acceptance, and an emotionally deprived individual may express his frustration in unconscious, stubborn self-starvation, as is the case in psychogenic marasmus in children or in anorexia nervosa in adults. Conversely, substitution symbolism may permit the frustrated individual to compensate for his feelings of rejection with psychogenic hyperphagia which leads to obesity. Anorexia or voraciousness may thus represent repudiation or indulgence of love or hate, sexual cravings, or social relationships. Compulsive food faddism, bizarre eating habits, periodic fasting, and self-imposed starvation may be symbolic expressions of defense against nonadmitted aggressive or sexual drives; they are not uncommon components in psychoneurotic disorders and hysterical states. In such conditions food has acquired substitute meanings which can frequently be discovered only by psychoanalytic means before the individual can be liberated from their deleterious effect on his nutritional status.

Most psychiatric disorders are the result of long-standing anxiety and tension, and the possibility of prolonged malnutrition is ever present. The longer the duration of the illness and the more tense the patient, the greater is the chance that malnutrition has undermined his physical health. In psychiatric cases with acute or chronic malnutrition, the assumption should always be made that the nutritional deficiency is multiple and drug and diet therapy should be formulated accordingly.

Much of the success of the most carefully formulated diet therapy depends on the patient's emotional reaction to the nutritionist, and the latter must at all times be aware of the importance of the personal relationship with the patient. In the patient's mind, the nutritionist who gives, withholds, or formulates foods is likely to be associated with the persons on whom he was dependent in childhood, and the intake and even assimilation of the diet may depend on whether the nutritionist can avoid creating unpleasant associations. A hurried, disinterested, or authoritarian attitude will induce distrust and rebellion in the patient, while permissiveness and friendly encouragement will tend to bring forth his cooperation. A negative reaction to the diet and the nutritionist can frequently be avoided by a show of genuine personal interest when the nutrition history is taken, by visiting the patient at mealtimes, and through careful administration of the diet food service to have attractively served meals and—what is even more important—friendly service of the food by the attendants.

Anorexia Nervosa

Subnormal food intake and inanition are frequent occurrences in psychoneuroses, psychoses, and addictions. Hypoalimentation to the point where it is the predominant symptom and endangers life is characteristic of the psychoneurotic disease entity anorexia nervosa. The disorder is found predominantly in younger women who are usually unmarried. The condition is characterized by an aversion to food which overrides all other considerations. The unconsciously self-imposed starvation is an attempt to serve as a solution to unconscious emotional conflicts. Whereas some workers consider the syndrome to be a hysterical manifestation, others believe that it arises against a schizoid background. Most cases develop between puberty and the thirties, and at times marriage may be the precipitating factor. The underlying basis for the conflict appears to be the patient's inability to accept a normal adult sex role; unconscious fear of oral impregnation and similar symbolic fantasies seem to play an important role.

Salient features are aversion to food, disavowal of hunger, severe and progressive inanition with consequent amenorrhea, and a lowered basal metabolic rate which reflects the depressant effects of the starvation. Despite the patient's utter frailty (a weight of 70 pounds is not uncommon), she will frequently continue her accustomed occupation and disclaim any disabling effect of her self-imposed starvation. There is no aversion to handling foods as such as long as they are intended for consumption by others. Progression to chronic mental illness occurs in some patients, while others, if untreated, may eventually succumb to the effects of their cachexia, particularly through the medium of an intercurrent infection to which they are able to offer only scant resistance.

Dietary Regimen

Treatment consists chiefly of psychotherapy and dietary regulation. Psychiatric treatment is essential for any permanent alleviation of the condition since the patient must gain insight into the cause of her disorder in order to avoid future relapses.

Severe cases are so badly debilitated that they can tolerate only small quantities of food, and feeding by polyethylene nasal catheter is necessary in these instances. Such patients receive hourly feedings of 50 to 100 ml of skim milk to which multivitamins, minerals, pepsin, pancreatic enzymes, and bile salts have been added to aid digestion and assimilation. If there is no complaint of gastric distention, glucose, egg yolks, soybean or corn oil, wetting agents (polysorbate 80), and additional skim milk powder may be added, and the mixture is thoroughly emulsified in a blender before administration. Aspiration of any remaining stomach contents before each feeding should be done routinely to prevent gastric distention.

If the patient is capable of self-feeding, she is first given a high-protein, high-vitamin diet in small quantities, which contributes no more than the caloric intake to which she was accustomed. At intervals of 5 or 6 days the caloric allotment is increased by 250 to 350 cal, until a daily intake of 3200 to 4000 cal is attained. There may be some gastric distress after each upgrading of the diet, but the contracted stomach adjusts relatively rapidly to the physical burden of a normal food intake. Occasionally, the patient's nutritive state improves to a point where she begins to eat spontaneously, without being urged. However, in most cases, many months on such a regimen may elapse before a satisfactory state of nutrition is attained and ovarian function, menstrual activity, and the basal metabolic rate return to normal. Continued psychiatric help may be needed to prevent recurrences.

Anorexia in Other Emotional Disorders

Hypoalimentation frequently accompanies a host of other psychiatric illnesses and neurotic states and serves to complicate the disease picture since the attendant chronic malnutrition adds physiobiologic stress to the primary emotional disturbance. Anorexia and self-imposed fasting are frequently seen in depressive states, in obsessional neuroses, in senile arteriosclerotic psychoses, in some schizophrenic states, and secondary to alcoholism and drug addictions. In most cases psychotherapy is needed before the patient's cooperation in following a corrective dietary regimen can be obtained.

Dietary Regimen

The nutritional rehabilitation of such patients must proceed on an individual basis, and no overall generalization can be made. If malnutrition is advanced, as is frequently the case in patients who have been institutionalized for long periods without adequate individualized dietary supervision, a dietary program should be followed as outlined above for the treatment of severe advanced anorexia nervosa. In the case of noninstitutionalized, ambulatory psychoneurotic individuals, the dietary rehabilitation takes the form of an adaptable tailor-made program. Emphasis must be placed on the protective foods and the meal plans outlined in Chap. 15, but a liberal attitude and permissiveness must be shown by a multiplicity of choices and a wide range of menus from which the patient may choose. Many psychoneurotic or neurotic persons are potential food faddists, and it is best not to encourage a neurotic preoccupation with foods by an emphasis on special food items or restrictive diets, or to turn the dinner table into the arena in which a neurotic struggle with authority is fought.

In the case of the working patient, it is particularly important to stress a generous breakfast which supplies one-third of the daily caloric intake and which includes eggs, milk, enriched cereal or bread, citrus fruits or citrus or tomato juice, in addition to less essential items, and if desired, another beverage of choice. Because of the previous nutritional neglect and inanition, the daily protein intake should amount to at least 2 g/kg body weight, and multivitamin supplementation is needed initially.

The patient should be encouraged to have at least one thick milk shake or eggnog each day, which is easily prepared in a blender and may compensate for any disorganized eating and snacking throughout the day when he is away from home. A nourishing cocktail is readily prepared by blending milk, skim milk powder, frozen orange juice concentrate, and raw egg yolks (it is preferable not to use raw egg whites too consistently because of the biotin-destroying potential of the avidin which they contain); to this, sugar and flavoring (vanilla, chocolate, etc.) is added and, unless there is a strenuous gustatory objection on the part of the patient, dried brewers' yeast. It is really not important to insist on specific measurements for each ingredient, since it is best not to surround the preparation of the daily food cocktail with an aura of compounding a prescription. It suffices to indicate a minimum of 1 cup of milk or skim milk, $1/4$ cup of skim milk powder, 2 egg yolks, and 2 tablespoons of orange juice concentrate. The patient can add to this liquids and flavoring and sweetening agents to his heart's content. The resulting food cocktail will compensate for a multitude of sins of nutritional omission committed through forgetfulness or passive neglect throughout the day. It is important to emphasize to the patient that this snack should not replace any regularly scheduled meals.

Dietary Considerations in Alcoholism

Approximately 10 percent of first admissions to psychiatric wards or mental hospitals in the United States belong to the alcoholic group. Chronic alcoholics usually do not consume an adequate diet, and while the characteristic liver damage is thought to be primarily the result of a direct toxicity of the consumed alcohol (Chap. 36), the frequently observed deficiency in the B complex vitamins is probably due mainly to inadequate nutrition rather than to any specific disturbance of intermediate metabolism. Thiamin deficiency is considered responsible for the peripheral nerve degeneration and central nervous system changes found in long-standing cases of chronic alcoholism (peripheral polyneuritis with paresthesias, sensory loss, motor weakness and tremors, cord lesions with sphincter dysfunction, leptomeningitis, and central nervous system changes with personality changes, hallucinosis, and amnesia). The impairment of nutrition may be furthered by the chronic gastritis which is not uncommon among alcoholics.

The therapy of alcoholism has two major aims: (1) cessation or reduction of alcohol intake, a notoriously difficult problem akin to the breaking of other addictive habits, be they compulsive overeating or reliance on drugs, and (2) nutritional rehabilitation, correction of deficiency states, and, if possible, repair of the hepatic and neural damage caused by inadequate nutrition.

The patient with delirium tremens may be treated by the intravenous administration of 100 ml of 25 percent glucose solution which contains 10 to 25 mg of thiamin in order to abort the acute attack. Preliminary sedation with paraldehyde is usually necessary. This is followed by intravenous feeding with electrolytes, glucose, amino acids, and polyvalent water-soluble vitamins (particularly thiamin, 10 to 20 mg, niacinamide, 50 to 100 mg, and riboflavin, pyridoxine, and pantothenic acid) until gastrointestinal function is restored. Thereafter a daily fluid intake of 3,000 ml is instituted, and the patient is given 15 to 30 mg of thiamin by mouth and small quantities of milk, as tolerated. This is followed with any quantity of the food cocktail, described in the previous section, which the patient can retain. If the patient tolerates food but is too incapacitated or uncooperative, he may have to be fed by tube, initially.

Once the patient has weathered the acute episode, he is given a balanced diet rich in protein and the B vitamins—pork, liver, kidney, beef, cheese, milk, legumes, and enriched cereals. (This may be supplemented with one Decavitamin Tablet, U.S.P., per meal.) The protective food cocktail (see above) should also be urged on the patient as an additional snack, particularly since it serves as a painless vehicle for relatively large amounts of high-quality proteins which are essential for partial rehabilitation of the commonly gravely damaged liver.

Chapter 35

Nutrition in Diseases of the Skin

The role of diet and nutrition in the causation and treatment of diseases of the skin has never been quite clearly defined, and even today there is little unanimity on the subject. Dermatologists have used a variety of special diets and nutritional factors in various combinations and at all conceivable dosage levels in the management of skin disorders, especially those of elusive etiology. As a result the literature is filled with a tremendous array of reports which range from enthusiastic announcements concerning the therapeutic value of vitamins to complete negation of their usefulness in treatment of skin disorders. The temptation is great to look upon a borderline dermatosis of unknown etiology, especially in the older patient, in terms of a nutritional deficiency, preferably a vitamin deficiency. On the other hand, in many cases specific therapy is directed toward a dermatologic lesion without attention to the nutritional status of the patient as a whole, which, though not specifically responsible for the disorder, may have a definite bearing on the appearance of frank clinical symptomatology. In the treatment of cutaneous diseases, dietary therapy or regulation may be effective in a number of ways: (1) It may eliminate causative factors, as in the withholding of offending allergens from the diet in allergic cutaneous manifestations. (2) It may clear up the cutaneous symptoms by its specific effect on the basic underlying disease picture, as in the case of diabetic vulvovaginitis. (3) It may improve the patient's general nutritional status or correct a specific deficiency, either one of which may have been responsible for the cutaneous condition, such as in nonspecific intertrigo of the obese or the pellagrous "wine sores" of the skid-row alcoholic.

Experimental observations in man and animals have shown that many nutritional deficiencies lead to conspicuous cutaneous disorders. However, in clinical practice, at least in the United States, it is rare to find distinctive cutaneous manifestations which would justify the diagnosis of a deficiency in one specific nutritional factor. Multiple deficiencies are found more commonly and exhibit a variety of cutaneous symptoms, including dryness, loss of elasticity, pallor, melanosis, scaling, nonspecific eruptions, and changes in the nails and hair.

Dermatologic Aspects of Specific Nutritional Factors

Protein Protein or amino acid deficiencies may cause the following cutaneous symptomatology in man: (1) the pellagra syndrome based on deficient tryptophan-niacin supply (Chap. 22), (2) the dermatosis and hypopigmentation of kwashiorkor (Chap. 22), and (3) deficient melanin formation and eczematoid eruptions in phenylketonuria (Chap. 32). Inadequate protein nutrition is reflected in the skin chiefly by nutritional edema and decreased resistance to infection.

Vitamin A In man, vitamin A is essential for maintenance of normal cell structure in epithelial surfaces, and conversely, hypovitaminosis A is responsible for follicular hyperkeratosis and keratinizing squamous metaplasia of mucosal surfaces. In extreme vitamin A deficiency, characteristic keratotic papules may appear at the site of the hair follicles on the extensor surfaces of the extremities and on the shoulders and lower abdomen. Dermatoses of milder degree are not infrequent in the United States, exhibiting a dry, scaly skin and occasional keratotic plugs at the site of hair follicles. Proper diet results in a gradual improvement. Skin disorders which are benefited by vitamin A therapy include Darier's disease (keratosis follicularis), pityriasis rubra pilaris, ichthyosis, keratosis pilaris, and at times chronic lichen simplex.

Excessive administration of vitamin A may result in hypervitaminosis A, a syndrome characterized by a scaly, rough, itchy skin, loss of hair, painful periostitis and other skeletal disturbances, and anorexia (see also Chap. 10).

A yellowish discoloration of the skin may be caused by an excessive intake of the precursor of vitamin A, carotene (from carrots, squash, and the like). This condition has only a temporary cosmetic significance; it is cured by elimination of the source of excessive carotene from the diet. Differential diagnosis from a true icteric condition is made by noting the absence of yellow color from the sclerae.

The B Complex Vitamins Members of the vitamin B complex are generally found associated together in foods, and for this reason deficiencies in a single vitamin are rarely found in clinical practice. Even though the stigmata of what appears to be a single deficiency may predominate, undernutrition with regard to several members of the group should always be suspected, and therapy should be directed toward supplying all the factors which may be missing and a totally adequate diet.

Thiamin Skin diseases resulting from a vitamin B$_1$ deficiency have not been reported. Severe thiamin deficiency, in the form of beriberi, is reflected in the skin only by the manifestation of edema.

Riboflavin The skin lesions characteristic of ariboflavinosis are believed to be perlèche, or cheilosis, fissuring of the skin in the angles of the mouth; seborrheic dermatitis about the nose, forehead, and scrotum; and a magenta tongue. In practice, such findings may often be caused by other factors and misinterpretation is not uncommon. For instance, in the toothless older person malocclusion predisposes to maceration of the tissues in the corners of the mouth; this may be followed by a chronic infection with a resulting angular stomatitis.

Niacin Pellagra, including its cutaneous manifestations, is discussed in detail in Chap. 22.

Pyridoxine Experimentally induced vitamin B$_6$ deficiency in man may produce seborrhealike lesions about the mouth, nose, eyes, and ears and general intertriginous eruptions in skin folds and moist areas. Pyridoxine therapy is specific for this condition. However, it is open to question whether patients presenting themselves with such symptomatology will necessarily benefit by pyridoxine therapy since the underlying cause may be much less specific.

Vitamin C The classic manifestation of ascorbic acid deficiency is scurvy. In the skin, scurvy may show secondary changes due to capillary fragility such as petechiae, ecchymoses, and purpura, as well as some melanosis and follicular hyperkeratosis. Vitamin C is essential for connective tissue formation and normal wound healing and should be supplied generously in case of extensive burns and skin injuries.

Vitamin D Vitamin D was used at one time as an adjunct in the treatment of cutaneous tuberculosis, but its use has been made obsolete by the advent of modern antibiotics and chemotherapy for this disease.

Vitamin K Vitamin K deficiency interferes with normal prothrombin synthesis in the liver and may thus be the cause of cutaneous purpura due to impaired blood clotting. This deficiency is encountered primarily in obstructive jaundice—where supportive vitamin K therapy and corrective surgery are indicated—and in hemorrhagic disease of the newborn.

Apparently, no other single vitamin plays a current, definite role in dermatology as replacement therapy. It must be emphasized, however, that a generalized improvement of the nutritional status may be valuable in the clearing up of skin disorders of dubious etiology when there is a reasonable prospect that malnutrition may be involved.

Unsaturated Fatty Acids Experimental work with infants indicates that the polyunsaturated acids, specifically linoleic and arachidonic acids, are essential for normal skin maintenance. Deficiency in these essential fatty acids may lead to eczematous dermatitis, and replacement therapy is specific. This should be kept in mind, particularly in cases of infantile eczema where the patient has been maintained for prolonged periods on a very restricted diet devoid of whole milk or vegetable oils (as is the case in elimination diets for multiple allergies).

The Dermatologic Aspects of Obesity

In the United States today, overeating and consequent obesity is probably the most frequent cause of skin disorders or of secondary complications of existing dermatoses. Dissipation of body heat by radiation and conduction is impaired by exaggerated subcutaneous fat deposits; consequently, obese persons overheat easily and sweat excessively. This profuse perspiration has an adverse effect on normal or inflamed skin, and excessive sweat retention underlies miliaria rubra (prickly heat). Because of the accumulation of heat and moisture between fatty skin folds and other intertriginous areas, the skin becomes macerated and the growth of potentially pathogenic fungi and bacteria is encouraged. Mechanical irritation in the form of chafing further favors intertriginous dermatoses in the obese. Much of the nonspecific intertrigo, pyoderma, superficial moniliasis, seborrhea, and eczematous dermatitis seen today may be laid at the doorstep of obesity. Also not to be discounted is the provocative influence of obesity on the emergence of latent diabetes, with its cutaneous complications, as well as the not infrequent aggravating influence of obesity on the course of psoriasis.

Special Diets

The staphylococcic pyodermas (furunculosis, hidradenitis) are particularly hard to manage because of the ready emergence of antibiotic-resistant strains, the survival of the pathogens in foci isolated by scarring, and the undesirability of long-continued antibiotic therapy. An empirical sharp restriction of carbohydrates in the diet seems to have a salutary effect on the course of these skin conditions. It is possible that a lowering of the glucose content of the skin occurs, which makes it a less favorable substrate for the responsible microorganism.

Diets very low in fats and carbohydrates have been recommended in the treatment of acne vulgaris. Presumably, a high fat and carbohydrate intake is reflected in increased sebaceous gland activity, which is a constant factor in this skin condition. The beneficial effect of such a dietary treatment appears open to question, and self-treatment by rigid dietary restriction on the part of the self-conscious teen-ager with acne should not be encouraged.

The dietary treatment of allergic skin manifestations is discussed in detail in Chap. 39.

Chapter 36

Nutrition and Alcohol

Alcoholism is a metabolic disease associated with a configuration of social, psychologic, and physiologic factors of varying proportions. An estimated 6 million obligate alcoholics live in the United States today. Firm incidence figures are not available because many alcoholics, particularly women, are not identified. The incidence tends to be high among the less advantaged social and economic population strata. Persons with a history of alcoholism have an overall death rate $2^1/_2$ to 3 times as high as average, standard risks. Chronic intake of large amounts of alcohol is associated with the development of a fatty liver and, ultimately, irreversible cirrhosis of the liver. Hepatic cirrhosis ranks eleventh among leading causes of death in the United States, accounting for approximately 28,000 annual deaths. (In addition, an estimated one-half of the annual 55,000 deaths due to automobile accidents is attributed to drunk driving.) Alcohol is the causative factor in the overwhelming majority of cases of fatal liver cirrhosis in the United States.

A generation of medical students, nutritionists, and physicians has been taught that the chronic, progressive malnutrition commonly associated with frank alcoholism is responsible for the characteristic alcoholic cirrhosis of the liver seen in the countries (primarily occidental and industrialized) where alcoholism is endemic, just as grossly inadequate and imbalanced diets in the poorer areas of the world are responsible for the liver damage seen there. The doctrine of nutritional damage to the liver has always been accepted in the past despite the fact that evidence for a primary causative role of nutritional deficiencies in the development of liver damage in *adult man* (rather than in children or laboratory animals) is scanty. It is plausible that the abundant evidence for nutritionally induced fatty metamorphosis of the liver, hepatic necrosis, and eventual cirrhosis in nonprimate *experimental animals* (particularly in rodents), in the past has led to the conclusion that similar mechanisms are operative in man. This hypothesis is no longer tenable in the light of experimental evidence obtained in primates and man during the recent decade, which indicates that liver damage associated with alcoholism is the result, at least in the major part, of a *direct* toxic effect of ethanol. Intercurrent malnutrition, however, may be a permissive factor in some cases; it may render a person more susceptible to viral or toxic agents, or it may potentiate alcohol-induced hepatic steatosis.

Metabolic Role and Physiology

Alcohol, as a food, contributes 7 cal/g ethanol oxidized, compared with carbohydrates and proteins (4 cal/g) or fats (9 cal/g). It has been estimated that alcohol contributes 5 to 10 percent of the total caloric intake in American diets. Of alcoholic drinks most frequently consumed, beer and hard cider contribute 3 to 6 percent, wines 9 to 21 percent, distilled spirits 30 to 50 percent, and some liqueurs up to 60 percent of alcohol by volume. Some alcoholic beverages do not necessarily contribute only nutritionally empty calories to the diet; beer and other fermented (but not *distilled*) drinks are a possible source of pantothenic acid, folic acid, other B complex vitamins, and phosphorus.

Alcohol is absorbed, primarily in the stomach, by simple diffusive transport without need for prior digestion. Alcohol in carbonated drinks (whiskey and soda, champagne) is more rapidly absorbed than when taken in the absence of carbon dioxide. Absorption of alcohol is most rapid from solutions containing 10 to 20 percent on an empty stomach; alcohol in the presence of large quantities of food, or in high concentrations, is absorbed less rapidly. The absorbed alcohol diffuses rapidly and uniformly throughout the fluid compartments of the body and is found in different tissues in proportion to their water content. In the central nervous system ethanol acts as a *depressant,* first in the phylogenetically more recent regions of the brain (affecting at first such parameters as acquired, learned inhibitions, judgment, personal behavior, and memory) and, after more prolonged exposure, in the more primitive regions, where progressively physical coordination and proprioception, and eventually the more fundamental functions like vision and respiration, are affected. The progressive effects of alcohol roughly parallel its concentration in the blood; in most localities in the United States a blood concentration of 100 to 150 mg per 100 ml is considered the upper limit for safe driving.

Ethanol has a number of effects on intestinal mucosal and cellular transport processes. It inhibits active cellular transport of sodium and potassium, amino acids, and glucose. At a 2 percent concentration in the lumen of the small intestine (a concentration that can be present in moderate drinkers) the absorption of a number of essential amino acids is inhibited. Alcohol ingestion may lead also to decreased absorption of fat and vitamin B_{12}. At the same time, ethanol stimulates triglyceride synthesis by the intestine with subsequent increased lymph triglyceride content. It has been suggested that this may contribute to alcoholic hyperlipemia and genesis of the alcohol-induced fatty liver.

Relation to Nutrition

There is no one set dietary pattern for persons who consume alcohol regularly, just as there is no one set pattern of the alcoholic intake of all such individuals. These vary from the extreme of the drinker who may drink only on certain occasions, through several types of moderate or "social" or "executive" drinkers, to the other extreme of the socially deviant, self-destructive alcoholic. A significant proportion of this population consumes a normal or near-normal diet. For instance, studies have shown that as a group, executive drinkers or social drinkers whose daily ethanol intake may be considerable, contrary to the popular assumption, have an adequate protein intake and seem to meet most of the recommended daily allowances for other essential nutrients even when obtaining 10 to 15 percent of their daily caloric intake from alcohol. A majority of moderate drinkers studied appears to add alcohol calories on top of a fairly unvarying and adequate daily food intake. This is not the case in those advanced alcoholics who have a drinking pattern characterized by several days of fairly uninterrupted heavy alcohol consumption (the "lost weekend" binge type) followed by a state of moderate to severe intoxication and gradual recovery. In these individuals, food intake is scanty at the height of their drinking bout and immediately thereafter, and their general nutritional status is usually precarious or poor. This type of advanced alcoholic individual substitutes ethanol for much of his normal food intake, and as a consequence his intake of proteins, essential minerals, and vitamins may be grossly deficient. It is in such individuals that the central and peripheral nervous system lesions due to vitamin deficiencies, described in Chap. 34, are found. To what extent malnutrition *contributes* to the production of liver disease in alcoholism is presently uncertain; recent studies, however, have demonstrated that the prime factors which determine the development of alcoholic liver injury are the *amount* and *duration* of alcohol intake rather than malnutrition.

Hepatic Effects of Ethanol

Administration of alcohol by mouth or intravenous infusion induces a rise in serum triglycerides concomitant with a fall in plasma-free fatty acids. It has been suggested that ethanol induces increased hepatic synthesis and release of triglycerides. Simultaneously, an accumulation of some of the newly synthesized triglycerides takes place in the liver cells, which does *not* become dissipated if additional alcohol is consumed soon again. It has now been demonstrated in man and experimental animals that the extent of liver fat accumulation depends on both the dose and duration of alcohol intake and hepatic morphology can be restored, in the beginning at least, by withdrawal of alcohol. Such hepatic fat accumulation is associated with striking ultrastructural changes within the liver cells, characterized by enlarged mitochondria and disturbed architecture of the endoplasmic reticulum. These alcohol-induced changes take place even in the presence of well-balanced diets and special diets high in protein and low in fat. These effects take place not only among individuals who habitually consume moderate to large amounts of alcohol; in nondrinkers *brief* experimental alcohol consumption (resulting in blood alcohol levels well *below* accepted legal limits for intoxication) display similar hepatotoxic effects. These are reversible at first, but they tend to become established with continued exposure to alcohol.

Dietary Consideration in Alcoholism

Even though it is no longer accepted that the development of a fatty liver and alcoholic cirrhosis (or the specific toxic effect of alcohol on the heart musculature) is the result of inadequate nutrition, the prophylactic role of a well-balanced diet, high in protein and providing adequate quantities of the water-soluble vitamins, is still as important as ever for the well-being of the alcohol-consuming individual. Such a diet will go far in preserving his general well-being; specifically, it will obviate the frequently observed manifestations of specific vitamin deficiencies in long-standing cases of chronic alcoholism which tend to disable the advanced alcoholic: pellagrous "wine sores," peripheral nerve degeneration with paresthesias ("burning feet"), sensory loss, and motor weakness (stumbling or shuffling gait), sphincter dysfunctions, and central nervous system deterioration with personality changes, amnesia, and hallucinations. A more detailed presentation of the vitamin deficiencies and peripheral and central nervous system damage of chronic, advanced alcoholism and their therapy and prevention is found in Chap. 34.

Chapter 37

Principles of
Parenteral Nutrition

Fluid Therapy

In the last three decades, parenteral fluid therapy has developed into a specialized body of knowledge without which modern surgery and medicine would be unfeasible. The proper application of parenteral fluid therapy and the consequent salvage of human lives is one of the major medical advances in our times. Fluid therapy has a variety of uses, the most important of which may be characterized as follows:

1 Prevention and treatment of shock by infusion of fluids which exert colloidal osmotic pressure. These fluids compensate for the blood volume lost through hemorrhage and replace the fluid which has left the circulatory compartment through increased capillary permeability; they tend to maintain the circulating blood volume and to reverse the trend of migration of fluid from the plasma to the interstitial spaces. Fluids used for this purpose include whole blood, blood plasma, human serum, albumin, and dextran.

2 Maintenance of normal fluid balance and replacement of abnormal losses of water through such routes as vomiting, diarrhea, tubal drainage, as well as profuse sweating in pyrexia. Such fluid therapy is also imperative for its "pump-priming" action in renal depression or renal shutdown after excessive losses of extracellular fluid (as in the dehydration of infantile diarrhea or cholera and shock).

3 Maintenance or restoration of electrolytes—sodium, potassium, magnesium, chloride, phosphate, calcium—to cover normal loss and particularly abnormal expenditure through the routes mentioned above and through renal dysfunction.

4 Specific therapy to compensate for imbalanced metabolic states such as those found in diabetic acidosis or coma, metabolic alkalosis, renal failure, and adrenal insufficiency.

5 Maintenance of nutrition, where the gastrointestinal route is contraindicated, unfeasible, or ineffective and where the need exists for immediate, effective provision of the required nutrients to the body tissues, as in critical states or before and after surgery.

This chapter deals primarily with the nutritional balance aspects of fluid therapy. A detailed discussion of the physiologic and therapeutic ramifications of electrolyte and fluid imbalance (such as the interrelationship between specific electrolytes and neuromuscular irritability or the effects of hyper- or hypopotassemia on cardiac function) is largely beyond the scope of this book.

Routes of Administration

Fluids may be administered by the intramuscular, subcutaneous, or intravenous routes. The subcutaneous route is used in hypodermoclysis, where large volumes of fluid may be readily injected into the lateral aspects of the thighs, flanks, and chest. The addition of hyaluronidase facilitates more rapid absorption of the fluid by the tissues and combats local distention. Only isotonic or nearly isotonic solutions should be administered by hypodermoclysis, and this route is inadvisable and commonly unsuccessful in individuals with cardiac decompensation and tissue edema, or with low serum protein levels; and in case of shock.

The intravenous route is indicated when rapid absorption is desirable, when the required volume is too great to be absorbed efficiently from the subcutaneous tissues, or when the solution is known to cause tissue irritation. Reactions to intravenous infusion may be rapid and dangerous, and for this reason only standard preparations of known performance should be used. Intravenous infusion may place an excessive burden on a decompensated heart, and thus in cardiovascular disease fluids must be given very slowly, in small quantities, and with frequent observation of the patient.

In cases of long-term intravenous feeding, solutions should be run into veins through fine plastic catheters. This reduces the danger of reactive thrombophlebitis and delays the day when the intern or nurse "runs out of veins" in which to start infusion.

The intramuscular route places a certain limit on the amount of fluid that may be injected, though the inclusion of hyaluronidase in the solution greatly enhances the volume absorbed by the tissues. The intramuscular route is frequently used for the provision of concentrated vitamin preparations.

Replacement of Fluid

If needed, parenteral water is best given by the intravenous infusion of 5 percent glucose (isotonic glucose) or 10 percent glucose solution. Five percent glucose in physiologic saline and 10 percent glucose solution are hypertonic and may lead to increased thrombophlebitic reactions; 10 percent is the highest percentage of glucose which will be moderately well tolerated by veins.

The rate of intravenous injection should not exceed the body's ability to handle the infused fluid. As a basic rule, a patient who depends on a parenteral water intake should receive 2,000 to 3,000 ml of fluid per day, provided kidney action is normal and there are no abnormal losses of fluids and electrolytes through vomiting, diarrhea, tubal drainage, and excessive sweating. The exact amount is regulated by experience, on the basis of the patient's urinary output; a daily production of about 1,000 ml of urine is the desirable aim. The slow injection of 5 or even 10 percent glucose solution in amounts sufficient to cover normal water expenditure does not supply more glucose than the patient can metabolize and simultaneously affords protection against ketosis and results in protein sparing. Glucose infusions, if given over a period exceeding 1 or 2 days, should be accompanied by parenteral vitamins (see section on vitamins, below).

Isotonic saline should not be used to supply the entire 24-hour fluid requirement, since this would provide an excess of sodium. Except during the first day of treatment, when specific replacement therapy may be indicated, the total fluid mixture given per 24-hour period should not contain more than 600 to 1,000 ml (or one-third of the total volume) of physiologic saline solution. Ordinarily 5 to 10 percent glucose and isotonic saline are used in a 2:1 ratio to meet fluid requirements.

The initial infusion of a mixture of 2 parts of 5 percent glucose and 1 part of isotonic saline (with or without 5 percent glucose) serves as a pump-priming solution to restore kidney function and urinary flow. If urine excretion does not follow such an infusion, severe renal impairment is indicated and demands careful, specific clinical management.

Replacement of Electrolytes

Replacement of part of the glucose solution with isotonic (physiologic) saline in the amounts suggested above supplies the basic requirement for the principal ions of extracellular fluids. If the patient is dependent on intravenous feeding for a number of days, 500 ml of an infusion containing about 4.25 percent sodium chloride and 3.12 percent potassium chloride should be introduced to the daily quota of glucose infusion, instead of the isotonic saline mentioned above, to provide an optimal supply of potassium. Balanced solutions of this type, or better yet, of the Butler-Talbot-Lowe type (with other added electrolytes and glucose), are commercially available. They contain sodium, potassium, magnesium, chloride, phosphate, and lactate in a ratio resembling the proportions of these cations and anions in normal plasma; glucose is usually added at a rate of 5 to 10 percent, and these balanced solutions may thus be used as basic maintenance solutions. Potassium-containing solutions should always be administered very slowly and should not be administered intravenously to a patient with renal depression or shutdown since potassium will be retained and will eventually reach cardiotoxic levels.

In correcting abnormal fluid and electrolyte losses due to concurrent vomiting or tubal drainage, volume-for-volume replacement is made with a solution which resembles the body fluid lost. A number of type-specific, ready-made solutions are available for such purposes. Lactated Ringer's solution (Hartman's solution) with or without added glucose may be employed as a general-purpose replacement solution. Excessive perspiration or diarrhea fluid may be replaced with the balanced solutions mentioned in the previous paragraph since their compositions are similar. Patients with abnormal body fluid losses receive the appropriate replacement solutions in addition to their basic quota of balanced fluids which are meant for daily maintenance of fluid and electrolytes.

Short-Term Intravenous Feeding

The daily requirement for protein may be met by the infusion of protein hydrolyzates and specially compounded amino acid mixtures; the equivalent, in the form of a 5 percent amino acid solution, of 1 g of protein per kilogram of body weight in adults and 2.5 g for infants can be met without too much difficulty by a 24-hour infusion schedule. The inclusion of a maximal quantity of glucose in the program serves to spare the infused amino acids so that they will be used for needed tissue protein synthesis and not for energy purposes.

Ten percent invert sugar (an equal mixture of fructose and glucose) and 10 percent fructose solution are also available to meet caloric needs. The fructose has been advocated for use in diabetics since it presumably need not be balanced simultaneously with insulin in order to be metabolized.

Human plasma and whole blood should not be used for the intravenous feeding of patients with depleted tissue proteins. These fluids are not particularly rich sources of assimilable protein; they contain excessive amounts of sodium in the quantities in which they would be useful, they are extremely expensive, and except for the latest specially processed preparations, they carry the danger of infection with the virus of homologous serum hepatitis (Chap. 27).

Total Intravenous Feeding (Hyperalimentation)

Until recently it has been difficult to provide a complete intravenous diet, primarily because it has been impossible to supply a full daily caloric complement by vein without compromising the patient in some respect. First, the fat infusions of the past fell short of the ideal in that they still induced undesirable side effects in a significant number of patients if used over prolonged periods. Second, supplying the patient's daily caloric requirement with the aid of intravenous glucose (instead of fat) created other problems: the amount of water which a sick adult can ordinarily handle safely is limited to approximately 35 to 50 ml/kg body weight, or about 3 to $3^{1}/_{2}$ liters per day. The caloric density of macronutrients other than fat is relatively low, and thus the solute concentration of a calorie-adequate infusion had to be high. Unfortunately, the concentration of solute which can be administered into a peripheral vein without causing thrombosis or phlebitis (with eventual sclerosis of the vessel) is limited to about twice isotonicity (the equivalent of a 10 percent dextrose solution).

Eventually two new parenteral infusion techniques were evolved for prolonged infusion of hypertonic solution. The first involved insertion of a catheter into the superior vena cava via the subclavian vein or via the external or internal jugular vein; sterile, nonpyrogenic solutions containing approximately 5 percent fibrin hydrolyzate (to supply the nitrogen requirement), 20 to 25 percent dextrose (calories) and 5 percent additional solute consisting of all required vitamins, minerals, and trace elements can then be infused slowly and continuously by pump into the relatively large and rapidly exchanging bloodstream in this site without damage to the blood vessel walls. The second method, preferably used for patients in whom prolonged hyperalimentation is anticipated, utilizes a permanently implanted plastic, external arteriovenous shunt of the type constructed in patients who require dialysis treatment with artificial kidneys. The solution is simply infused into the plastic shunt and mixes rapidly with blood streaming within the shunt, without compromising the neighboring peripheral vessels.

The lifesaving effects of total parenteral feeding have been proved in hundreds of patients who could no longer be nourished by way of the gastrointestinal tract, prior to contemplated surgery, because of malignant or other severe lesions. In other cases, after massive intestinal resections (which left the patient with an inadequate gut) or in overwhelming cases of regional enteritis or ulcerative colitis, recourse to successful long-term hyperalimentation has permitted a gradual reassumption of function by the surgically shortened intestinal remnant, or has ushered in a state of remission in the now resting gut, or resolution of inflammatory masses or fistulas. Even where subsequent surgery was still needed, the very marked restoration of the previously completely debilitated, malnourished, and cachectic patients prior to surgery usually made the difference between a very poor prognosis and a successful operation. Total hyperalimentation has been particularly successful in infants with congenital anomalies of the gastrointestinal tract which made normal nutrition (and thus continued survival) impossible. Such infants are now being fed parenterally for months (and grow and develop normally) until they are in an optimal state, and somewhat larger, for elective surgical repair of the defect.

Total hyperalimentation is not without risk. Infections of the catheters with suppurative phlebitis or even overwhelming septicemia are encountered when improper techniques are used. The recent development of parenteral fat emulsions which are free of reactions and can supply adequate amounts of calories via peripheral veins now make it possible to supply highly catabolic patients (those with peritonitis, severe burns, or massive fractures) with the calories they need despite poor alimentation, and thus to avert an otherwise inevitable and undesirable severe tissue breakdown with loss of lean body mass and nitrogen.

Vitamins

In instances where parenteral feeding is used for periods of 1 or 2 days only (and provided there is no evidence of previous nutritional depletion in the patient), there is no need for special vitamin supplementation. However, more prolonged intravenous feeding must be accompanied by parenteral administration of all vitamins in prophylactic quantities. Wherever there is evidence of long-continued previous depletion, the dosage should be from three to five times the recommended daily allowances (Table 22), or in case of vitamins not tabulated, three to five times the prophylactic daily requirement.

Vitamin supplementation is essential for two reasons: (1) patients who are sick enough to require parenteral maintenance are likely to require vitamin supplementation to compensate for existing or currently developing deficiencies; and (2) the need for vitamins to metabolize nutrients does not cease because of the peculiar route of administration of the major food elements. This is particularly important in the case of thiamin since the glucose, which is being furnished intravenously, requires thiamin for proper utilization. Profuse glucose infusion which is not accompanied by parenteral thiamin may produce central nervous system manifestations of athiaminosis in previously depleted individuals (Chaps. 22 and 34).

Additional aspects of parenteral feeding, including parenteral vitamin K and ascorbic acid supplementation, are discussed in Chap 38, Nutrition and Diet in Surgery and Surgical Conditions.

Chapter 38

Nutrition and Diet in Surgery and Surgical Conditions

Preoperative Nutrition and Surgical Risk

The state of nutrition of the surgical patient before and after an operation has an important bearing on the response during surgery and the rate of recovery. Deficiencies in protein, ascorbic acid, and vitamin K are particularly disadvantageous, if not hazardous. Hypoproteinemia, not uncommon if prolonged illness has preceded the operation, predisposes to anemia and poor tissue repair, delays the healing of fractures, reduces resistance to infection, and embarrasses cardiac and pulmonary function. Prolonged malnutrition may be compounded by liver impairment, which makes for further protein deficiency and intolerance to anesthesia. Ascorbic acid deficiency predisposes to poor wound healing and dehiscence of surgical incisions, and vitamin K deficiency makes for hypoprothrombinemia with an attendant impairment of blood clotting; such a bleeding tendency results in an undesirable bloody surgical field. In an effort to reduce surgical morbidity and mortality, the surgeon must evaluate the patient's nutritional state prior to surgery and correct preoperatively any suspected or existing nutritional deficiencies. Whenever immediate surgery is indicated, the risk of operating on a malnourished individual with doubtful powers of recovery should be weighed carefully against a temporary postponement which would permit the building up of the patient's nutritional status.

Replenishing the surgical patient's nutritional reserves is particularly important since the circumstances which lead to operations commonly predispose to nutritional depletion. Thus prior to the scheduled surgery the patient may have been acutely ill with sufficient anorexia or pain to interfere with dietary intake for days and weeks; vomiting, diarrhea, and occult or overt bleeding frequently contribute further to the patient's depletion. In the presence of trauma, fractures, or infection, or after immobilization of the body (when a patient is bedridden for days prior to an operation), a rapid tissue protein breakdown takes place, as evidenced by an increased excretion of nitrogen in the urine. In the case of burns there is very considerable external protein loss due to serum seepage, in addition to increased catabolism of tissue proteins.

In severe illness or injury when extensive amounts of nitrogen are lost in the urine, there is usually an associated large-scale excretion of potassium. Sodium and chloride losses due to vomiting and diarrhea may be quite marked, and iron-deficiency anemia looms whenever the patient has had a significant blood loss. Calcium reserves, essential for prompt healing of fractures, may be depleted in elderly patients, if they have been bedridden for a long time before surgical (open) reduction of fractures of the hip are attempted, because prolonged immobilization favors disuse demineralization of the skeletal system.

Extreme overnutrition is also detrimental for the preoperative patient. Obesity interferes with surgical exposure, weakens the healing surgical incision, predisposes to future disruptions and abdominal herniations, and delays postoperative ambulation, thus increasing the risk of ileus and pneumonia. Therefore correction of extreme obesity is most desirable before elective surgery is scheduled.

Evaluation of Nutritional Status

Measurement of the patient's weight and observation of any weight changes are the most practical way of evaluating protein deficiency. In most patients, weight loss or underweight per se may be considered indicative of protein loss or depletion. In such appraisals, the physician must guard against misleading weight changes which are caused by abnormal retention or excretion of fluids. In the hospitalized patient, fluid input and output data permit the appraisal of true body weight changes.

Total blood volume is another criterion of body weight status and, indirectly, protein loss; the volume of whole blood falls 50 to 100 ml for each pound of true body weight which is lost.

Clinically recognizable signs and symptoms of vitamin deficiency should be looked for but will seldom be found. Indications of subclinical deficiencies may be obtained however, by taking a careful and detailed dietary history. Prothrombin time determinations should be done routinely to detect hypopro- thrombinemia, which may be the result of vitamin K deficiency or defective liver function.

Blood chloride determinations are necessary to detect chloride depletion in patients with kidney damage and those with a history of extensive vomiting or diarrhea. Potassium deficiency may be expected in patients who did not have oral or tube feedings for 4 to 7 days prior to surgery and did not receive corrective parenteral potassium replacement.

Iron-deficiency anemia must be expected in patients with long-standing peptic ulcers, metromenorrhagia, hemorrhoids, or gastrointestinal malignan- cies; a history of biliary obstruction should alert the surgeon to the possibility of deficiency in the fat-soluble vitamins, particularly vitamin K.

Preoperative Correction of Deficiencies

Whenever possible, the undernourished preoperative patient should receive a high-protein, high-calorie diet, supplemented by multivitamin preparations of therapeutic strength. Oral intake should be encouraged but not forced. Weight should be taken every day, and actual food intake and fluid intake and output should be recorded in an effort to distinguish between a true weight gain and fluid retention. When necessary, tube feedings using small polyethylene or polyvinyl tubes should be given, with emphasis on a high protein intake (Chap. 23).

Small doses of testosterone may be administered to encourage a positive nitrogen balance, and if fat absorption is limited by pancreatic or liver disease, pancreatin or wetting agents like polysorbate 80 are useful.

When circumstances such as complete obstruction, inability to retain food, or severe injury or burn make intravenous feeding necessary, a supreme effort must be made to supply a maximum of amino acids and of glucose. Mixtures containing 50 g of protein-equivalent and 200 g of glucose per 1,300 ml of fluid may be prepared by adding 300 ml of 50 percent glucose solution to 1,000 ml of a 5 percent protein hydrolyzate solution which also contains 5 percent glucose. Up to 3,900 ml of such a mixture may be infused continuously over a 24-hour period, thus supplying 150 g of protein and 3000 cal per day. Serum electrolyte determinations will indicate the extent to which sodium chloride and potassium must be furnished. Parenteral vitamin supplementation in therapeutic dosages may be advisable, with particular emphasis on vitamin K and ascorbic acid. (See Chap. 37 for the quantitative aspects of parenteral feeding.)

Preoperative Dietary Routine

Ordinarily, food is forbidden after 6 P.M. on the evening preceding the scheduled surgery, and oral fluids are not given after midnight if the patient is to have general anesthesia or major surgery with spinal anesthesia. This is done to assure an empty stomach and to forestall the dangerous possibility of vomiting and aspiration of the vomitus either under anesthesia during surgery or during recovery from anesthesia. Food in the gastrointestinal tract also increases the likelihood of retention and distention during postoperative ileus.

When surgery of the intestinal tract is involved, the preoperative fast is usually begun at noon of the preceding day in an effort to obtain an empty upper bowel, and a preoperative cleansing enema serves to empty the colon. In case of intestinal obstruction, all proximal intestinal contents are removed by suction tube.

To forestall a last-minute depletion before surgery, patients subject to a prolonged preoperative fast should receive parenteral feedings for as long as practical. This is particularly important to avoid fluid deficits; any possible acidosis or alkalosis must also be corrected at this point by appropriate fluid therapy.

A more leisurely preparation of the patient awaiting gastrointestinal surgery has become possible with the advent of the "elemental" chemical formula described in Chap. 25. It provides all known nutritional requirements in soluble form, is fully absorbed in the small intestine, and results in practically no fecal residue.

Postoperative Feeding

Blood loss during the operation and postoperative blood pressure are the criteria for any blood or plasma requirements. Patients in a poor nutritional state and those with extensive burns or traumatic wounds, intestinal obstruction, or suspected intermittent internal blood loss may require significant quantities of whole blood or plasma postoperatively.

Five percent glucose solution is ordinarily infused intravenously during and after major surgery. Two to three liters should be given during the first 24 hours, provided there is no cardiac decompensation which contraindicates this volume of fluid. Following major trauma or surgery there is usually a depression in urinary output; for this reason the patient should not receive intravenous saline for the first 48 hours after surgery since it may lead to sodium retention with a consequent increase in tissue fluid. A reduced urinary output of 500 to 750 ml is to be expected during the first 48 hours; thereafter, enough intravenous or oral (where surgery did not involve the gastrointestinal tract) fluids should be administered to obtain a daily urinary output of about 1,000 ml.

Patients who have postoperative fluid loss through drainage tubes, suction, or diarrhea should receive specific replacements as outlined in Chap. 37. Particular attention must be paid to restoration of potassium losses by intravenous infusion. Blood potassium determinations will indicate the need for supplementation. The potassium may be furnished as part of the balanced replacement infusion, or if the potassium deficit is significant and the serum level drops below 12 mg per 100 ml, potassium chloride may be administered by a slow infusion of a 0.2 to 0.25 percent solution. Potassium should not be infused when urinary output is subnormal since cardiotoxic blood levels may be reached. In case of doubt, electrocardiographic readings should be used to rule out the danger of hyperkalemia.

If the timetable for provision of food in the postoperative period were based on the strength and healing of gastrointestinal surgical wounds, the oral intake of nutrients would have to be delayed until well into convalescence, to about the ninth to twelfth day. As it is, in most cases resumption of oral feedings is based on the return of gastrointestinal function. For the first 24 to 48 hours after abdominal surgery, gastrointestinal motility and secretion are usually inhibited. Afterward there is a gradual return of motility and normal gastrointestinal secretory activity. The gastrointestinal tract is ready to accept food again when the renewed gastrointestinal activity manifests itself by audible peristalsis, when the abdomen is soft and flat, and when there is free passage of fecal matter, mucus, or gas from the rectum. At this point about 1 ounce of water may be given every hour by mouth; this amount is gradually increased, as tolerated, until 6- to 8-ounce quantities are retained. Semiconscious or stuporous patients should not receive anything by mouth until the danger of aspiration of vomitus has passed.

Once the patient retains fluids, a clear liquid diet may be given (Chap. 23). Though this diet is inadequate in practically all essential nutrients, it fulfills the fluid requirements and contributes some calories, sodium, and potassium. A more desirable substitute, recently available, is represented by the chemically defined, nutritionally complete, soluble and predigested, clear fluid formula of the "elemental" type described in Chap. 25.

This is followed by a full liquid diet.(Chap. 23). The nature of the operation and clinical judgment of the attending physician will determine the time at which this diet is instituted; the sooner this is done, the greater is the chance of reversing the negative nitrogen balance which almost invariably follows surgery. Patients who have adequate reserves are not harmed by 1 or 2 days of postoperative abstinence from adequate food intake; however, fasting a traumatized patient who may have been depleted before his operation is hardly beneficial. A full liquid diet, high in proteins and calories, is instrumental in reversing tissue protein catabolism and serves to prevent ketosis, which is inimical to prompt wound healing. If postoperative abstinence from oral foods is enforced for prolonged periods (as may be the case after peritonitis and major intestinal surgery), the patient, after first experiencing a strong appetite and later intense hunger sensations, may eventually develop an indifference and even repugnance to foods. Later, once oral foods are permitted, it may require days until the subject overcomes the feeling of weakness and depression which result from his enforced starvation and recovers a normal appetite.

If the patient tolerates the full liquid diet and improvement is noted, a soft diet is introduced (Chap. 23), which is followed in time by a full general diet. Tissue repair and attainment of physiologic equilibrium will be aided by a balanced diet which provides a generous supply of protein and liberal intake of calories. To that end it is important that the patient be urged to consume all the food ordered for him and that a record of actual intake be kept; if he displays a desultory appetite and much of the food remains on his tray, the food cocktails mentioned in Chaps. 23 and 34 should be given between meals and at bedtime.

Dietary Regimen after Gastric Surgery

Full intravenous feeding must be used for the first day or two if suction drainage is maintained. Once the adynamic ileus has passed and intestinal function is manifested by physical signs, 2-ounce portions of water, and later clear liquids, may be given through the stomach tube which is already in place. If there is no ill effect or distention, this is gradually followed by multiple small portions of a tubal liquid diet given at 2-hour intervals. Any remaining residue must be aspirated and feedings spaced further apart; small oral feedings of a full liquid diet are next. By the end of 4 days most patients have taken a full liquid diet by mouth in small multiple feedings and are ready for six feedings per day of a soft, bland diet (Chaps. 23 and 25). The size of the feedings is adjusted to the patient's tolerance and is increased gradually. Multiple vitamin supplementation should be routine during the period of convalescence.

The surgeon's clinical judgment will determine when the patient is ready for regular feedings of a bland diet; the surgeon will also decide how long this diet is to be followed after dismissal from the hospital.

Dietary Management of Postgastrectomy Malnutrition and the Dumping Syndrome (Jejunal Hyperosmolic Syndrome)

Postoperative nutritional problems are frequent in patients after subtotal gastrectomy and occur in almost all patients subjected to total or near-total gastrectomy. The main cause of undernutrition after gastric surgery is failure of patients to eat adequately. This, in turn, is related in most instances to the so-called "dumping syndrome," which becomes established in many patients following gastrectomy. The dumping syndrome consists of attacks of epigastric discomfort, pallor, weakness, sweating, quickening pulse, nausea, and malaise, usually 10 to 20 minutes after a meal; the patient is usually forced to seek relief by lying down for a while. After the patient once has this experience, he becomes increasingly wary of eating, and his food intake may fall below the desired level.

In the postgastrectomy patient, the resected stomach no longer serves as an effective storage-and-dispensing organ to meter out small, measured quantities of food into the small intestine at regular intervals. It is commonly believed that the postgastrectomy dumping syndrome, which may persist for years after surgery, is due to a sudden reduction in blood plasma volume in the peripheral circulation, secondary to the drawing of large quantities of fluid from the bloodstream into the intestine following the rapid introduction of large quantities of hypertonic foods into the jejunum. The hypovolemic shocklike symptoms, coupled with the effects of the gross distention of the jejunum which occurs when the osmotic action of the indwelling food attracts large amounts of fluid, are apparently responsible for the clinical picture of the dumping syndrome.

Nutrients differ in their ability to cause the dumping syndrome. Large quantities of hypertonic solutions will invariably precipitate it. Proteins, particularly in the form of meat, rarely cause symptoms. In the usual diet, carbohydrate is the chief offender, and finely emulsified fat next, with fat in normal form and protein causing the least distress. Solid foods are tolerated better than liquids.

Dietary management represents the best approach to alleviation of the dumping syndrome, and a strict dietary regimen almost invariably relieves the condition. The patient must avoid large meals; food should be given in small amounts at frequent intervals. The ideal regimen consists of six to eight small daily feedings, high in protein, low in carbohydrate, and containing moderate amounts of fat. Sugars, which have a strong osmolar effect, must be avoided; artificial sweeteners may be substituted. Milk and dishes containing milk (custards, milk shakes, eggnogs) frequently precipitate symptoms and should be omitted. Fluids should be withheld during meals and for an hour after eating. It is important that fluids taken between meals contain little or no sugar; soft drinks and fruit juices are notorious offenders. Once this regimen has achieved its purpose and suppressed dumping syndrome distress for a prolonged period, judicious attempts may be made to liberalize the dietary pattern.

Aside from the dumping syndrome, the patient after gastrectomy can expect some degree of aberration of absorptive function, including steatorrhea. These anomalies may be attributed to the changed, postoperative chemistry of the intestinal tract (such as deficiency or absence of gastric hydrochloric acid and its sequellae) or to the altered anatomic and physiologic relationships. Here, too, even in the absence of the overt dumping syndrome, dietary precautions must be taken to avoid eventual undernutrition. The diet should deemphasize carbohydrates, and it should be high in protein since it is least apt to stimulate the dumping syndrome and its absorption is somewhat impaired. When absorptive defects do exist, they are proportionate to the amount of fat or protein ingested, so that an increased intake results in adequate absorption of the nutrient. Nutritional improvement can be expected in most gastrectomized patients when they are fed a diet high in fat and protein, limited in carbohydrate content and the food is given in small amounts at frequent intervals.

Last but not least, after gastrectomy the physician must be on the lookout for the subsequent development of anemias in the patient since in the absence of adequate gastric hydrochloric acid secretion or elaboration of intrinsic factor, the absorption of iron and of vitamin B_{12}, respectively, may be impaired or completely interrupted. Patients who have had a Billroth II gastrectomy are particularly prone to exhibit abnormalities in hemoglobin levels, serum vitamin B_{12} levels, and serum iron. Atrophic gastritis is likely to develop in postgastrectomy patients (possibly owing to intestinal reflux) and contributes significantly to late nutritional deficiencies.

Dietary Regimen after Colostomy, Ileostomy, or Intestinal Resection

Full intravenous feeding is usually essential for the first 4 to 7 days, during which it is desirable to permit undisturbed healing of the anastomoses. Suction is maintained to avoid any distention during this period. Once intestinal function is restored, 2-ounce portions of water are given by tube, 2 hours apart. This is followed by a clear liquid diet, given for 1 day. It is essential to avoid any traumatization of the intestine with solid food residues; consequently, the patient receives a minimal-residue diet for the next 3 days of his convalescence. During the next 4 days this diet is modified to a low-residue diet (Chap. 25), and eventually, and very cautiously, to a bland diet. Multiple vitamin supplementation is routine during convalescence. The attending surgeon will determine the nature of the patient's diet during his last days in the hospital and the desirable diet after dismissal. The detailed meal planning, in accordance with the prescribed diet, should be worked out with the hospital dietitian.

Dietary Regimen in Surgery of the Lower Intestine

In order to minimize intestinal contents before surgery and to avoid stools during the first postoperative days, the patient is placed on a minimum-residue diet for several days before the operation and during his convalescence thereafter. Intravenous feeding is not customary after elective rectal or anal surgery. Immediately after the operation, the minimum-residue diet is quantitatively restricted to half portions for a period of 4 days, to reduce fecal accumulations. Passage of stools is also prevented by suitable medication with opium derivatives which immobilize the intestine. Additional aspects of nutrition related to surgical conditions are discussed in Chap. 37, Principles of Parenteral Nutrition.

The Minimum-Residue Diet

The principles of minimum- and low-residue diets are discussed in Chap. 25. The following is an elaboration with emphasis on minimal residues.

Permissible foods	*Foods excluded*
Decaffeinated coffee, soft drinks	Milk, milk drinks
Precooked infant cereals, cooked refined cereals free of all bran	Any other cereals
Toasted, enriched white bread, soda crackers	Breads, crackers, or rolls made with whole-grain flour or bran
Well-trimmed tender meat, fish, and fowl, broiled, baked, or boiled; hard-cooked eggs, cottage cheese	All other meats, eggs, or cheese
Vegetable oils, margarine (in moderation only)	All other fats
Boiled noodles, spaghetti, macaroni, white rice	Potatoes in any form
Clear or strained fruit juices	All fruits
	All vegetables
Consommé, clear skimmed broths	All other soups
Light cakes, cookies, jello, sherbets, all without nuts or fruit	Rich pastries, pie, whipped cream, ice cream, custard
Sugar, jelly, honey, syrups, sugar candy	All candy containing nuts or fruit; marmalade, jam

Sample Menu

(Contains approximately 85 g protein, 55 g fat, 240 g carbohydrate, and 1800 kcal. Serve only the listed fluids with each meal. Additional fluids are permissible between meals.)

BREAKFAST
Precooked, enriched infant rice cereal, with syrup (¹/₂ cup)
2 hard-cooked eggs
1 slice white toast, jelly
1 pat margarine
Decaffeinated coffee, sugar

MIDMORNING
Strained orange juice (¹/₂ cup)

LUNCH
Broiled fish fillet, lemon (4 oz)
Boiled rice (¹/₂ cup)
1 pat margarine
1 slice white toast, jelly
Fruit-flavored jello (¹/₂ cup)
Decaffeinated coffee, sugar

MIDAFTERNOON
Sweet apple cider (¹/₂ cup)

DINNER
Broiled liver (4 oz)
Noodles ($^1/_2$ cup)
1 pat margarine
1 slice white toast, jelly
Cottage cheese (3 oz)
Sherbet ($^1/_3$ cup)
Tea, sugar

BEDTIME SNACK
Grape juice
Vanilla wafers

Nutrition and Wound Healing in Trauma

After extensive traumatic damage to any region of the body (through accident or by surgery), there occurs in the otherwise well-nourished and healthy person a marked loss of protein coupled with a rise in urinary potassium, sulfur, phosphorus, and protein breakdown products. This abnormal tissue catabolism reaches its peak 5 to 8 days after injury. Following less severe trauma, a more moderate protein loss takes place which may generally be attributed to a low caloric intake (or misguided caloric restriction) and which, usually, can be reversed by adequate oral or parenteral feeding. In the case of more serious trauma, an adequate parenteral supply of calories and amino acids can greatly diminish the undesirable loss of tissue nitrogen; in the presence of infection, this additional complication tends to counteract achievement of nitrogen equilibrium and a significant negative nitrogen balance may result. In any event strong efforts should be made within the framework of the injury to supply optimal quantities of calories, nitrogen, and electrolytes.

In the case of major trauma, attendant shock or near-shock will be accompanied by renal suppression; this may result in increased nitrogen and potassium blood levels until urinary excretion becomes normal. Blood or plasma transfusions are necessary to abate the state of shock and counteract any tissue edema which is inimical to optimal wound healing.

Tissue repair is a complex process which involves intense histologic and biochemical activity. Under ideal conditions (as in the case of surgical incisions), the wound is clean, is relatively free of pathogenic organisms, and contains little traumatized or dead tissue. The wound surfaces are separated by a fibrin clot interspersed with red blood cells. Wandering mesenchymal connective tissue cells migrate toward the fibrin strands which organize in the blood clot and an intercellular ground matrix of mucopolysaccharides and collagen is laid down. As the fibroblasts mature, capillaries invade the area and solidifying collagen strands strengthen the new tissue. Vascularity is essential for an adequate supply of nutrients and humoral anti-infective action and promotes rapid healing.

Nutritional considerations in wound healing are primarily the patient's blood protein levels and his supply of calories, ascorbic acid, and vitamin K. Hypoproteinemia is detrimental to wound healing for two reasons: (1) it results in edema, which tends to separate the wound edges and delays fibroplasia; and (2) it results in a relative local lack of amino acids. A high-protein diet is indicated during the recovery from traumatic injury, and elective surgery—a foreseeable injury—should be preceded by a prophylactic high-protein regimen. An adequate supply of calories is essential to prevent the tissue breakdown attendant on the body's attempts to utilize proteins for energy purposes in less than optimally nourished individuals.

Vitamin C is essential for the laying down of intercellular matrix and maturation of collagen and encourages prompt fibroplasia and capillary invasion of the tissue defect; a deficiency in this vitamin has a serious inhibitory effect on wound healing. Prophylactic oral or parenteral administration of ascorbic acid before elective surgery and during recovery from traumatic injury is thus indicated to assure prompt and optimal healing and to prevent wound dehiscence. From 100 to 200 mg daily suffices in well-nourished individuals; where malnutrition is suspected, 500 mg or more daily will soon produce tissue saturation.

Vitamin K deficiency may lower the blood prothrombin level to the point where blood clotting is impaired. In such instances, blood which slowly extravasates from the capillaries surrounding the wound tends to separate the wound surfaces excessively and interferes with optimal healing. Ordinarily the possibility of vitamin K deficiency is slight; however, when jaundice is present or liver damage is suspected—circumstances which make for impaired intestinal vitamin K absorption and prothrombin formation—prophylactic, parenteral vitamin K administration is indicated.

Among other vitamins, pyridoxine and pantothenic acid seem to play specific roles in antibody formation and foreign-body response and thus indirectly to promote prompt healing through suppression of infection.

A positive calcium balance should be maintained during convalescence after fractures in order to make calcium readily available for callus formation and to avoid partial demineralization of existing skeletal structures for this purpose. Simultaneously, adequate vitamin D must ensure intestinal uptake of the dietary calcium. Likewise, dietary supplementation with inorganic phosphate salts (1,000 to 1,200 mg of phosphorus daily) appears to counteract the usual skeletal demineralization following trauma and therapeutic immobilization, to stimulate prompt and greater callus formation, and to shorten the time of clinical union of the fracture.

In summary, a well-balanced diet, rich in protein and calories and high in vitamin C, which supplies all essential nutrients, is a basic requirement for prompt recovery from traumatic injury; in selected cases multivitamin supplementation should be part of the regimen.

Nutrition after Burns and Radiation Injury

The first characteristic local manifestations of a burn are due to distention of capillaries and increased capillary permeability. Plasma fluid rapidly collects in the affected tissues and produces edema under the overlying epidermis. Where the burn was extensive enough to damage subcutaneous tissues, the epidermis sloughs off rapidly and large amounts of fluid are liberated from the tissues and ooze from the burned area. This fluid contains all the soluble constituents of blood plasma at a similar concentration as well as plasma proteins at a somewhat lower concentration (at about 60 percent of normal plasma levels).

The pain of the injury may result in neurogenic vascular shock and collapse, depending on the severity of the injury. Secondary shock due to loss of plasma proteins is bound to develop gradually in deep and extensive burns, as the fluid which exudes continuously from the burned area depletes the circulating serum proteins. Fluid which is no longer held in the circulatory compartment by the colloidal osmotic pressure of the serum proteins migrates into the tissues, the circulating blood volume becomes inadequate, and the erythrocyte/fluid ratio increases to the point where the blood flows less easily through the capillary bed.

When more than 10 to 15 percent of the body surface is involved in the burn, systemic therapy directed against shock and plasma protein loss becomes more important than local treatment of the wound proper, and parenteral support and replacement become crucial. Experience has shown that during the first 24 hours the patient should receive 1 ml of whole blood and/or plasma and 1 ml of replacement electrolyte solution per kilogram of body weight for every percent of body surface which was burned. Lactated Ringer's solution (Hartman's solution) is a suitable electrolyte replacement fluid; in its absence, isotonic saline may be used but is less efficacious. (According to recent studies the oral administration of saline is beneficial in combating burn shock. In view of this, the oral fluid mentioned in the next paragraph should preferably contain some isotonic saline or clear consommé.)

In addition to the parenteral support, the patient should receive 2,000 to 2,500 ml of oral fluid in the form of a clear liquid diet (Chap. 23) in order to prevent renal shutdown; if the patient cannot retain oral fluids, a similar quantity of 5 percent glucose solution is administered intravenously during the first 24 hours. In view of the primary parenteral support already mentioned, such an intravenous regimen may exceed the patient's ability to handle this amount of fluid and he must be watched carefully for clinical signs of circulatory overload.

During the second day the infusion of blood (or plasma) and electrolyte replacement solution is decreased to 50 percent of the first-day level. Again, 2 to 2½ liters of fluid is administered by tube or mouth in the form of juices, sugar water, or tea, and 500 to 1,000 mg of vitamin C is given orally in addition to complete multivitamin supplementation (with emphasis on the B complex) in therapeutic doses. A high-protein diet may be started by tube, in multiple small feedings (Chap. 23).

By the third day, the patient may tolerate a full liquid diet; emphasis must be put on a high protein intake (2 to 2½ g/kg body weight) to replace the extensive protein loss through the exudate at the site of the burn. Vitamin C supplementation must be continued to counteract the lowering of serum ascorbic acid values which usually accompanies major burns and to promote wound healing. The calorie requirement of the burn patient is particularly high because of the characteristic tissue catabolism, particularly if there is superimposed infection and fever. Thus an intake of 4000 to 7000 cal per day should be striven for in severe burn injuries. The principles discussed in the previous section which pertain to the healing of traumatic wounds also hold true in the case of burns and should guide the nutritional management of the patient throughout the rest of his convalescence.

To date no specific forms of nutritional management have been generally agreed upon as suitable in the case of acute radiation injury. A high-calorie diet and vitamin supplementation have been recommended on a more or less empirical basis. Some clinicians advocate the use of pyridoxine (100 mg daily, by mouth, in divided doses). If the patient is acutely ill, parenteral feeding is indicated and the management becomes that of a thermal burn.

Chapter 39

Food Allergy

Allergy

Allergy may be defined as an acquired, fixed alteration in the reaction of living tissues to exposure to specific substances which are innocuous to the majority of members of the same species under identical circumstances and in similar quantities. The offending substance, the allergen, must be capable of stimulating the production of specific antibodies in the body of the susceptible individual. Once such initial sensitization has taken place, subsequent exposures to the allergen will result in the interaction of the allergen with the specific antibodies present in the general circulation or in fixed tissues. This interaction produces the abnormal manifestations. It is believed that much of the allergic symptomatology may be explained on the basis of the release of histamine or a histaminelike substance by the sensitized cell and the reaction of the surrounding capillaries and tissues to this substance. Most allergens are protein in nature; however, nonprotein allergens also exist, and even physical agents like sunlight and cold are known to precipitate allergic reactions. The predisposition to allergic sensitization is familial; it is estimated that about 9 percent of the population carry an inherited predisposition to allergic sensitization. Many of these individuals become sensitized to one or more allergens in infancy or childhood; others become sensitized later in life, while some individuals with the inherited potential never acquire a frank clinical allergy.

Clinical manifestations of allergy include bronchial asthma, hay fever, perennial rhinitis, hives, angioneurotic edema, gastrointestinal symptoms, headaches, dermatitides, and others. The route of exposure varies, and the allergen may trigger a reaction after contact, ingestion, inhalation, or injection. The allergic response may be immediate or may be delayed for hours or even days. The response to a specific allergen need not be identical in different individuals. Whereas one allergic patient may react to the ingestion of certain fish proteins or inhalation of horse dandruff with a mild eczematoid dermatitis, another sensitized individual may react with violent paroxysms of vomiting or with a delayed migraine attack. However, the reaction of each individual to a given allergen is usually specific and characteristic.

Food Allergy

Food allergy connotes the ability to react to the ingestion of specific food antigens. Allergic reaction to specific foods may manifest itself in the form of allergic rhinitis, bronchial asthma, urticaria, angioneurotic edema, dermatitis, pruritis, headache, allergic labyrinthitis and conjunctivitis, nausea, vomiting, diarrhea, pylorospasm, colic, spastic constipation, occult gastrointestinal bleeding, mucous colitis, perianal eczema and pruritis, and rarely, in the form of generalized systemic reactions with circulatory collapse, shock and even death.

The incidence of food allergy depends to a great extent on age. In infants and young children, food allergy is not uncommon but a tendency toward gradual, spontaneous disappearance or amelioration of the condition is noticeable in many individuals after the sixth year. Nevertheless, there is a higher incidence of food allergy in adults than in children, though in many cases it is not as readily diagnosed.

Food allergens are predominantly protein in nature. Any major alteration in the molecular structure usually results in loss of allergenic potential. Thus digestion, with the attendant splitting of the molecules into peptides and amino acids, renders the protein nonallergenic, depending on the extent of hydrolytic degradation. Denaturation of many proteins also results in loss of their allergenic potential because of the attendant molecular rearrangement. Thus raw or pasteurized milk may give rise to allergic reactions in a person hypersensitive to the lactoglobulins or lactalbumins which it contains, while thoroughly boiled milk (or evaporated milk), its offending proteins denatured, may be consumed by the same individual without untoward reactions.

In very rare instances the original sensitization may have taken place in utero after some antigenic material managed to pass the placental barrier. It is assumed that ordinarily the offending allergen produces the original sensitization of the individual after it has been ingested and after small quantities of the nondigested material have passed intact through the mucosal barrier into the bloodstream. There is sufficient evidence to show that the gastrointestinal tract of the newborn is relatively permeable to small amounts of undigested, unaltered food components and remains so for the first 3 to 6 months.

Although many foods may be implicated in allergy, the most common offenders are wheat, milk, eggs, fish (or seafoods), chocolate, corn, nuts, strawberries, chicken, and pork. The complete list of food allergens is larger and includes, among others, oatmeal, rye, and other grains, cottonseed, the legumes, tomatoes, potatoes, beef, mustard, cucumbers, garlic, citrus fruits, and even human milk. Foods rarely if ever proved allergenic are rice, lamb, gelatin, peaches, pears, carrots, lettuce, artichokes, sesame oil, and apples.

Diagnosis

A diagnosis of food allergy may be established with the aid of a detailed food history, food diaries, elimination diets, or cutaneous tests. Intracutaneous injection and scratch or patch tests are not as useful in the detection of food allergies as they are in the diagnosis of allergies due to specific contactants or inhalants: frequently, an allergen which regularly triggers an allergic reaction on ingestion will not give a positive reaction by skin test. In such cases one may have encountered a specificity of target tissues, or equally plausibly, the extract used in the intracutaneous or scarification test has been rendered ineffective by the chemical or physical processes involved in its preparation or sterilization. (Irreversible denaturation may take place during heating or extracting with nonaqueous organic solvents.) Scratch and patch tests frequently reveal skin sensitivity to so many substances that the tests are of little help in selecting the specific food(s) or food constituent(s) responsible for the patient's symptoms. On the other hand, the finding of precipitin antibodies to bovine milk in the blood serum of infants (by immunoelectrophoresis) has proved a reliable diagnostic sign in allergy to cow's milk.

A careful diet history is often very helpful in establishing a tentative diagnosis and in pinpointing the offending food. Questions should be so designed as to elicit from the patient any effects of the ingestion of the food commonly implicated in his allergies and any observations made by the patient with respect to parallel periodicity pertaining to certain foods and untoward symptoms. Often the patient's food dislikes turn out to be protective devices arrived at by unconscious trial and error. Thus an intense aversion to cow's milk on the part of a young child with symptomatology which could be of allergic origin should alert the interviewer to the possibility of a specific hypersensitivity.

Food allergies often remain unrecognized unless a detailed food diary is kept by the patient. In it the subject lists all food items eaten at any time for several weeks (and the ingredients of mixed dishes consumed) and notes any undesirable reaction. This permits an eventual correlation of repeated symptoms with the repeated ingestion of suspect foods. Such foods are then excluded from the diet, and their allergenicity is subsequently proved or disproved by dietary "on-and-off" experimentation.

The most concrete diagnostic tools are elimination diets. These are best used after a careful history has been taken and after a preliminary food diary has yielded helpful background data.

Elimination Diets

Elimination diets are used when symptoms occur so frequently that allergy to a commonly eaten food may be justifiably suspected. The patient is given a sharply restricted list of foods consisting of a few items which are ordinarily not implicated in excitation of allergic reactions. He is limited to this narrow choice of foods for a period of 1 or 2 weeks and told to record any unusual symptomatology. If during this preliminary trial the patient's habitual symptoms (gastrointestinal disturbances, headaches, and the like) do not clear up or become intensified, it is assumed that the offending allergen is one of the foods in the basic diet list; at this point a new basic diet list is given which does not include most of the foods originally permitted. If, however, the patient is relieved of his symptoms after consuming the sharply restricted basic diet during the trial period, the assumption is made that the foods to which he reacts are not present in his diet. New foods are now added to the trial diet, one at a time, at 4-day intervals. If these do not precipitate untoward reactions, they are cleared of further suspicion. If symptoms return, the food most recently added to the diet falls under suspicion. It is therefore again excluded, and when subsequently the symptoms remit, this constitutes tentative evidence that the particular food is specifically involved in excitation of the allergic symptomatology. This tentative evidence is now confirmed or discarded by a repeated inclusion and exclusion of the suspected food at 3- to 4-day intervals. The diagnosis is confirmed if symptoms consistently develop after the particular food has been admitted to the permissible diet for one to three feedings and if they consistently remit after exclusion of the offending food substance from the diet.

Trial Diet in Suspected Food Allergy

This trial diet includes only foods known to be hypoallergenic. Foods or fluids not specified in the starting diet are not permitted. Since the exact composition of the diet must be known at all times, the consumption of meals prepared in restaurants or by persons not familiar with the patient's problem is contraindicated. If no allergic reactions occur after the patient has followed this diet for

15 days, other foods, as ordered by the physician, are added singly at intervals of 4 days. If symptoms persist, the diet may be restricted initially to 2,000 or 3,000 ml of whole milk per day. If the patient subsequently remains asymptomatic, the food items listed for the basic trial diet are introduced singly at 4-day intervals and the offending substance is eliminated once it has been pinpointed by resumption of symptoms. Thereafter, other foods are gradually added to the permissible list.

Permissible foods in the basic trial diet

Cooked rice and pure rice cereal and rice biscuits which do not contain other
    admixed cereals
Peaches or pears (only canned, cooked, or frozen at first; later the fresh fruit
    may be included)
Lamb (without the addition of other fats or flour for gravies)
Carrots
Gelatin desserts made from pure gelatin and the permissible fruits
Water, salt, sugar, and jams or jellies made from the permissible fruits

Such a diet will not meet the patient's vitamin requirements, and supplementation becomes desirable if this highly restricted regimen is continued for several weeks. Since allergy to one or more ingredients of the pharmaceutical vitamin preparations may exist, supplementation must be deferred until therapeutic response to the basic diet has been obtained. The subsequent addition of vitamins must be treated like the addition of any other new food items, and the patient should be on the lookout for any possible reactions.

Early additions to the basic diet include:

Lemons and lemonade	Prunes
Tea	Peas
Coffee	Asparagus
Lettuce	Rye (*Caution:* ordinary rye bread contains
Artichokes	wheat)
Olive oil	Chicken
Squash	Potatoes
Tapioca puddings	Tomatoes
Apples	Beef
Apricots	

Other additions are made gradually until a normal food choice is again possible, with exception of the specific few food items which excited an allergic response.

Simple Elimination Diets

If a carefully taken diet history and a dependable food diary have strongly pinpointed the offending allergens, the physician may wish to spare the patient the stringent dietary restriction which is entailed in the severe trial diet described in the previous section. In such cases the patient may be placed on a standard specific elimination diet, which is a general diet from which a specific food or food group notorious as an allergenic excitant has been excluded. For example, the patient will exclude from his diet during a 4-week period all wheat or wheat derivatives if a diet history and food diary appear to implicate wheat strongly as the allergenic offender. Other foods or food groups commonly eliminated are seafoods, milk, eggs, nuts, and chocolate.

Few patients find abstinence from such food items for a limited time objectionable. Patients on elimination diets must be warned against products which may contain a banned item in disguised form. Commercially processed or packaged food items often harbor a specific allergen when this is not expected, and the patient must acquire the habit of cautiously examining the list of ingredients on all labels and packages. Once the subject has become asymptomatic, the diet is continued and specific banned items, which may contain the basic allergen in semidenatured or otherwise altered and nonreactive form, are cautiously reintroduced at monthly intervals. In such a fashion it is possible to narrow down the list of prohibited food items considerably. For instance, the allergic individual may react to pasteurized milk or cream but may find that he can consume boiled or evaporated milk without dire consequences.

Permanent Treatment of Food Allergy

Exclusion of the offending allergen from the dietary is the only effective specific treatment. Parenteral desensitization does not usually warrant the effort because of the overwhelmingly frequent lack of success. Oral desensitization, through complete elimination of the excitant, followed by cautious reintroduction in gradually increasing quantities, has its advocates but is rarely effective. Abstinence from the allergen in its active forms is the most effective treatment, and the previously mentioned habit of reading food labels and anticipating offending ingredients in prepared foods must thus become second nature. Hypersensitivity to an allergen may decrease or even disappear spontaneously as the patient grows older, and therefore cautious trials at reinclusion should be made from time to time. This is particularly important in the case of infants and children, where food allergies frequently do not persist past the sixth year or past adolescence.

Nutrition in Infant Allergies

The nutritional state of infants with food allergies is likely to be poor for a variety of reasons. The offending foods may be rejected by the infant or young child since it appears to be aware of the consequences which usually ensue, or the implicated foods may have been excluded from the diet on the physician's advice. If the offending food contains essential nutrients which are traditionally supplied by it alone—for instance, calcium in the case of milk—then the food allergy may have a far-reaching deleterious effect on the patient's nutritional state, growth, and development. The interference with adequate nutrition may be less specific, though just as extensive, when the symptomatology is such as to limit the infant's general appetite, as is the case in recurrent allergic rhinitis with nasal obstruction. In other cases, gastrointestinal allergic reactions, such as edema of the intestinal mucosa or constant, recurrent diarrhea, may directly interfere with absorption of a variety of ingested nutrients, with subsequent multiple nutritional deficiencies.

The foods most frequently implicated in infant allergies are wheat, milk, egg, and citrus juices. Therefore potentially allergic infants should not receive mixed infant cereals (which contain wheat) when they are fed their first solids; rice is probably the most hypoallergenic of the commonly eaten cereals, and it is advisable to limit the infant initially to rice cereal. Oat and barley cereals may be introduced later, during the fourth or fifth month, but the consumption of wheat is best delayed until after the sixth month, and at that point the parent should be on the lookout for possible reactions.

For similar reasons, the consumption of egg white, which is a potent sensitizer, is usually deferred until the tenth month in all infants, not just those with a known allergic propensity. Egg yolk, on the other hand, is less allergenic, and heat denaturation renders egg yolks nonreactive. Thus prophylactic exclusion of egg yolks during the early months is not necessary if the egg yolk is hard-boiled prior to feeding or if it is commercially prepared strained egg yolk which is heat-sterilized in the normal course of processing.

Contrary to a widespread notion, the allergy associated with consumption of orange juice is apparently a specific hypersensitivity to the proteins contained in orange seeds. The pure juice sack "meat" of oranges does not arouse allergic reactions in infants or children known to react to orange juice. Orange-peel oil also causes undesirable gastrointestinal reactions and may precipitate a nonspecific dermatitis, but there is convincing evidence that the reactions to citrus-peel oil are not in the nature of a true allergic hypersensitivity based on an antigen-induced immune body response, and that a simple chemical contact irritation is involved. Improperly prepared orange juice may contain excessive amounts of peel oil or of seed proteins which have leached into the juice from broken seeds and may therefore cause reactions in susceptible children. Hypersensitive infants who react to orange juice should receive their daily vitamin C quota in other vitamin C–containing or enriched fruit juices, or through supplementation with pure ascorbic acid in the form of tablets, or as part of a multivitamin preparation.

From a nutritional standpoint, allergy to milk is the most serious of the commonly encountered food allergies since milk supplies the basic nutritional requirements in early infancy. Allergy to breast milk has been demonstrated but is very rare. Allergy to raw or pasteurized cow's milk is considerably more frequent; its incidence among infants has been variously reported as anywhere from 0.3 to 1.5 percent and more.

The major proteins in milk are casein, albumin(s), and globulin(s). The same casein is found in milk from different species of animals; lactalbumins and lactoglobulins, however, are largely species-specific. In most cases of cow's milk allergy, hypersensitivity to casein is not involved; the allergic reaction is due to the presence of lactoglobulins (which are potent sensitizers) and lactalbumins (which are next in allergenic potential). In many cases of cow's milk allergy it is thus possible to feed the infant evaporated milk (in which the offending lactoglobulins and lactalbumins have been largely heat-denatured) without untoward reactions. It is also profitable to try the substitution of goat's milk, since the latter contains lactoglobulins and lactalbumins with a different molecular composition from those of cow's milk, and consumption of goat's milk may thus prove to be innocuous. If evaporated milk and goat's milk produce allergic reactions, a milk substitute must be resorted to.

The study of milk sensitivity may be complicated by individual variations in degree of sensitivity, differing antibody responses, and pathophysiologic changes. Thus the ingestion of cow's milk in sensitized infants may cause the occult loss of significant quantities of blood into the gastrointestinal tract with

Table 40   Meat Base Infant Formula for Use in Milk Allergy—Formula I

This preparation simulates the composition of cow's milk except for vitamin A. It has a pleasant, somewhat sweet flavor and is fed by nursing bottle in the usual manner. Vitamins A and D are necessary in conjunction with the use of this preparation.

	For home preparation	For preparation where scales are available	
Strained beef heart*	1²/₃ jar (or 5¹/₂ fl oz)	165.0	g
Oil: sesame, olive	1 tbsp and ¹/₂ tsp	12.50	g
Granulated sugar	4¹/₄ tsp	14.85	g
Potato starch	2¹/₂ tsp	8.00	g
Calcium Lactate (Hydrous), U.S.P.	2 tsp	4.675	g
Dibasic Sodium Phosphate, U.S.P.	³/₄ tsp (¹/₂ and ¹/₄; both salts available at drugstores)	1.76	g
Hot water	10 fl oz	293.2	ml

Measure all ingredients and finish by adding the hot water. Stir thoroughly, breaking up all clumps. Heat the resulting mixture in the top part of a double boiler until it thickens, with intermittent thorough stirring to prevent lumping. Transfer the thickened hot contents into two standard nursing bottles. Cap with nursing nipple *through which six holes have been punched with a red-hot straightened paper clip.* Sterilize in the usual terminal sterilization manner.

*Substitute strained lamb in case of allergy to beef.

Table 41 Meat Base Infant Formulas for Use in Milk Allergy— Formula II

This preparation simulates the composition of human breast milk except for vitamin A. The formula has a pleasant, somewhat sweet flavor and is fed by nursing bottle in the usual manner. Vitamins A and D are necessary in conjunction with the use of this preparation.

	For home preparation	For preparation where scales are available
Strained beef heart*	5 tbsp	72.8 g
Oil: sesame, olive	1 tbsp and 1¹/₄ tsp	15.35 g
Karo syrup	2 tbsp and 1 tsp	39.24 g
Potato starch	2¹/₂ tsp	8.0 g
Calcium Lactate (Hydrous), U.S.P. (available at drugstores)	¹/₂ tsp	1.30 g
Hot water	12¹/₄ fl oz	363.3 ml

Alternate Formula IIa

This preparation requires no calcium lactate. It is low in thiamin and requires thiamin supplementation in addition to vitamins A and D.

Strained chicken (Heinz)†	2 tbsp and 1 tsp	33.25 g
Strained beef heart*	2 tbsp and 1³/₄ tsp	36.40 g
Oil: sesame, olive	1 tbsp and 1 tsp	14.10 g
Karo syrup	2 tbsp and 1 tsp	40.80 g
Potato starch	2¹/₂ tsp	8.00 g
Hot water	12¹/₂ fl oz	367.4 ml

Measure or weigh all ingredients and finish by adding the hot water. Stir thoroughly, breaking up all clumps. Heat the resulting mixture in the top part of a double boiler until it thickens, with intermittent thorough stirring to prevent lumping. Transfer the thickened hot contents into two standard nursing bottles. Cap with nursing nipple *through which six holes have been punched with a red-hot straightened paper clip.* Sterilize in the usual terminal sterilization manner.

*Substitute strained lamb in case of allergy to beef.
†Contains 680 mg calcium per 100 g.

resultant hypochromic, microcytic anemia. (A changeover to heat-processed cow's milk formula or to a soybean formula has resulted in cessation or greatly diminished bleeding in a group of such children with proved antibodies to cow's milk.)

Soybean preparations are commonly used as milk substitutes since soybean protein contains all the essential amino acids and soybeans contribute beneficial quantities of carbohydrates, fat, vitamins, and minerals. A number of soybean-based "milk" formulas are commercially available and extensively used. Nevertheless, caution is advisable before use of soybean substitutes for milk because they may be just as allergenic and there is evidence that in a general population of older children approximately 5 percent are sensitive to soybean derivatives. (This fairly high percentage may be partially due to the fact that a certain percentage of infants deemed allergic to milk is reared with the aid of soy formulas.) A child sensitized to soybeans may also show cross-sensitization to other legumes (peanuts, peas, green beans) and will be exposed to many "hidden" soy derivatives in his daily food since soy flour, rich in protein, is nowadays frequently found in bakery goods, sausages, soups, crackers, and candies.

Meat Base Formulas

Meat base formulas and protein hydrolyzate mixtures may also be used as substitutes in case of intolerance to cow's milk. Meat base formulas are especially useful in instances where infants allergic to cow's milk fail to respond to substitution with soybean milk. Strained meats have an essential amino acid pattern which readily fulfills the infant's growth requirements. Liquid meat base formulas may be compounded which have a chemical composition very similar to that of either breast milk or cow's milk. Their taste is pleasant; they are readily accepted by infants; and the stools they produce are very similar in appearance and frequency to stools formed in nonallergic infants who are fed cow's milk. In recent years, such meat base formulas have been used successfully in alleviation of infantile eczema and in treatment of gastrointestinal disturbances in early infancy due to hypersensitivity to cow's milk and soybean formulas. Detailed directions for the preparation of meat base formulas which simulate the composition of breast milk and cow's milk may be found in Tables 40 and 41.

Part Five

Additional Aspects
of Human Nutrition

Chapter 40

Nutrition in Emergencies

In the history of mankind, physical progress and the accomplishments of technology have somewhat decreased the frequency and reduced the severity of the impact of natural disasters. On the other hand, neither passage of time nor the attainments of civilization have effected a noticeable reduction in the incidence of wars. Major catastrophes, whether natural or man-made, are still part of the life cycle of twentieth-century man; and emergency feeding of individuals or large population groups under conditions of war and natural disasters or after famine or prolonged starvation remains a realistic topic which has a place in a comprehensive discussion of human nutrition.

Characteristics of Emergency Feeding

The goals of emergency feeding are similar in most types of natural or man-made catastrophes: to keep alive people who have been dislocated or deprived of access to food, to maintain their morale, and to supply them with enough sustenance to enable them to carry out their functions until a normal or near-normal pattern of life can be restored. Emergency feeding includes provision of meals not only to evacuees, but also to essential workers engaged in physical tasks like rescue work, fire fighting, clearing debris, etc., which frequently accompany major disasters. Feeding of especially vulnerable groups is almost always involved. Thus in any planning, special provisions must be made for the feeding of infants, pregnant and lactating women, and the sick and injured.

In emergency feeding emphasis is not on maintenance of nutritional standards and fulfillments of long-term nutritional requirements, but on two major objectives: the first is immediate provision of warm foods and beverages to relieve tension, assuage fears and anxiety, boost morale, and provide a physical lift for emergency workers engaged in strenuous activity; the second, a long-range objective, is the orderly provision of food to the population for as long as possible without precipitating impairment of individual function. Whereas the first is a short-range objective which can be attained with the efficient around-the-clock distribution of hot coffee, baked goods, and soups, the second objective calls for a certain amount of nutritional planning.

Individual Nutritional Allowances in Emergency Feeding

Under the conditions of most natural disasters, only a limited region is devastated and it is expected that a near-normal status will prevail in the balance of the country so that it is unlikely that emergency feeding in the true sense of the word will be required for much longer than 1 week.

A curtailment of intake for 1 to 3 weeks is usually well tolerated by healthy individuals over 4 years of age who are not subject to special needs by virtue of hard physical labor, injury, pregnancy, or lactation, provided basic caloric needs are fulfilled and that foods of nutritionally heterogeneous nature like bread, legumes, and milk are used as mainstays of the diet. However, if the emergency feeding must continue for periods of 4 weeks or more, fulfillment of caloric needs alone will not suffice, and attention must be paid to the supply of proteins and of the water-soluble vitamins, with particular emphasis on thiamin, which is the first to become depleted. By virtue of accumulated body reserves, the supply of fats, fat-soluble vitamins, and minerals usually does not become critical until the deprivation has persisted for several months. In general, nutritional allowances for brief disaster periods are less exacting, from the standpoint of quality and quantity, than allowances for prolonged periods.

For survival during the first few days, the provision of water is of primary importance, whereas that of solid food is secondary. If water is provided, man can survive even without any food for several days as long as he does not have to engage in physical exertion; he uses body tissues as sources of energy. (As time goes by, however, he will lose weight steadily and will become progressively weaker until death ensues.) If no water is provided, the average adult will lose about 1.5 liters of water daily through the kidney, lungs, skin, and bowel. He will die once these losses total about 9 liters—roughly 20 percent of his body water. Thus, within favorable limits of temperature and physical work, survival without water or food for up to 6 days is a possibility.

A number of factors govern the rate of loss of body water. High temperatures and physical work increase the loss of sweat from the skin. Loss of water by way of the kidney is controlled by the osmotic balance; there is an irreducible minimum of urine which the kidney must produce to excrete osmotically active substances, mainly urea from protein breakdown and sodium chloride from the blood. If the body is depleted of osmotically active substances, the kidney cannot conserve water efficiently, and there is accelerated loss. If the kidney is confronted with too much urea from degradation of protein foods, it is forced to use extra water to excrete this waste product. A high salt intake forces a similar increase in urine volume. Thus the ration must provide the proper amounts of protein and salt to permit conservation of body water. If the body produces osmotically active materials which the kidney must excrete, these also increase the rate of water loss. This is likely to occur during starvation when the body's fat depots are metabolized and tissue proteins are broken down to provide energy, resulting in ketosis and the excessive release of nitrogenous wastes. Ketosis will also be encouraged if the proportion of fat in the diet is excessive. The ration can and should prevent ketosis. Carbohydrates should provide the bulk of the calories furnished by the emergency ration; they exert both a protein-sparing and antiketogenic effect, and they have the ability to conserve water and electrolytes even when supplied in amounts as low as 100 g daily.

Under optimal conditions the minimum daily water requirement to prevent dehydration is 1 liter. Since ideal conditions are not likely to be met, a fluid intake of about 2 liters per person per day must be anticipated.

Ideally, the accompanying solid ration should provide about 2 g of salt per 1000 cal to replace daily losses and protect the water economy of the body. When the solid ration provides 5 to 10 percent of calories in the form of protein, loss of tissue protein is minimized and body water is protected. Larger proportions of protein give rise to undesirably large amounts of urea and thus increase the daily water requirement. The ration should provide less than 50 percent of calories from fat to avoid the production of ketonelike metabolites which raise the daily urinary water loss. Food products made from common cereal grains fit well into this profile of the ideal short-term survival ration.

The following recommendations for minimal nutritional allowances have been made by the Advisory Committee on Emergency Feeding to the New York City Office of Civil Defense for short-term disaster feeding.

Essential workers should receive 4 quarts of water daily and a meal every 4 hours, during working hours, which provides per feeding:

1400 kcal
25 g protein
0.875 mg thiamin[1]

Healthy, uninjured persons (excluding pregnant and lactating women) 4 years of age or over who are not engaged in essential emergency work should receive the following daily allowance:

1 qt water
1600 kcal
35 g protein
1 mg thiamin[1]

The minimal allowance for emergencies not exceeding 1 week, for infants up to 6 months, is:

110 kcal/kg
3.2 g protein/kg
0.4 mg thiamin/kg[1]

Similar allowances for children 6 months to 4 years old:

1200 kcal
35 g protein
0.6 mg thiamin[1]

Allowances for pregnant women:

2400 kcal
80 g protein
1.2 mg thiamin[1]

Allowances for lactating women:

3000 kcal
95 g protein
1.5 mg thiamin[1]

Because of their special needs, most of the available milk must be allocated to the last four groups. (Injured and burned patients will require the balance.) Milk should be allocated in accordance with the following order of descending priority: (1) infants, pregnant and lactating women, (2) children 6 months to 3 years of age, (3) children 4 years and over.

---

[1]In all probability foods supplying the indicated amount of protein will concomitantly supply enough thiamin to prevent clinical deficiency symptoms within the brief period for which this program is suggested.

Effective allowances for injured and burned patients cannot be formulated without attention to the individual case. The maintenance of fluid and electrolyte balance during the first day is crucial and a matter of clinical judgment; decisions concerning this and subsequent minimal nutritional maintenance must be left to the medical personnel in charge of these patients. It must be kept in mind, however, that the nutritional requirements of this group are decidedly higher and more exacting than those of uninjured individuals. It is also understood that during emergency conditions special diets will not be available for those affected with chronic ailments, so that diabetics will have to rely on insulin, and peptic ulcer patients on antacids, for maintenance of health.

The source of the enumerated minimal requirements will depend on whatever stockpiles of food are available. If facilities for baking are available or can be made to operate, bread made from standard enriched flour and 4 percent or more skim milk solids (this exceeds the milk solid content of most commercial breads) can well serve as the mainstay of the emergency diet. Butter or margarine, if available, may be used in conjunction with the bread to meet some of the higher caloric needs of those engaged in essential physical labor. When simple canteen-type facilities are available, mixed soups and stews are often the most satisfactory items of service. The major foods which constitute the backbone of emergency feeding are enumerated in the next section.

Foods for Stockpiling

Foods best adapted for stockpiling against future emergencies or for relief shipment into devastated areas must be stable against deterioration and should contain a maximum of nourishing solids and a minimum of unessential water. Enriched flour, polished enriched rice, dehydrated potatoes, sugar, fats, oils, and canned modified butter, margarine, or shortening are invaluable concentrated sources of needed calories. They do not, however, contribute high-quality proteins, vitamins, and minerals in generous quantities. Dried nonfat milk, powdered eggs, dried beans and peas, canned meats and fish, and dry hard cheese are examples of rich sources of the more essential nutrients without which any prolonged emergency feeding effort is hazardous.

Dried skim milk is probably the most valuable concentrated, stable emergency food from a nutritional and practical viewpoint. It can be used as an enriching ingredient for whatever emergency staple is used as the mainstay of the diet, be it bread, soup, or stews. More important yet, it may be reconstituted into an acceptable liquid product of varying strength to fill the needs of the groups which are particularly vulnerable or have special feeding requirements, like young infants, pregnant and lactating women, and the injured and burned. For all practical purposes dried skim milk retains the important nutritive values of the parent product, and technological advances in its processing yield an instantly wettable product which is easily reconstituted. Dry milk has repeatedly proved its merit in successful supplementation of the intake of undernourished people or rehabilitation of starving prisoners of war or inmates of concentration camps.

Dried powdered eggs lack the high calcium content which makes dried milk the ideal food to be stockpiled for the feeding of infants and pregnant or lactating women, but they are probably second to milk powder in the order of desirable, highly concentrated, nutritious staples for emergency feeding.

Canned foods lend themselves especially well to stockpiling because of their low perishability, safety, convenience, and the mechanical stability of the individual unit. The weight and bulkiness of canned foods need not be a disadvantage as long as selectivity is maintained in stockpiling. Canned fruits and vegetables containing anywhere from 75 to 95 percent water, depending on the variety, do not necessarily represent a good choice. (However, in times of emergency, potable water is often the greatest need, and canned fruits and vegetables, if available, will serve as a safe source of fluids.) Canned pressed meats constitute a very satisfactory source of proteins, fat, and essential micronutrients. Canned fish falls into the same category, particularly if the product is rich in calcium because of retained softened, edible bones (canned salmon) and contains added oil, which would represent a welcome source of calories (sardines, tuna). Canned modified butter or margarine and canned oil or shortening should be part of any planned emergency food reserve, as well as canned nonsweetened evaporated milk and staples like canned beans.

Radioactive Contamination

A discussion of emergency feeding would be incomplete without the mention of the special problem created by accidental or intentional nuclear explosion. Contamination with radioactive fallout makes foods or water dangerous and unfit for consumption. This hazard is negligible if the food is mechanically protected by its container from the admixture of radioactive dust. In this respect, substantial, airtight containers—cans or jars—are preferable to single-layer paper wrappers with seals which are not necessarily impervious or intact; cardboard boxes which have inner paper liners and are protected by outer shipping cartons are also considered safe. Published experimental evidence indicates that foods in unbroken sealed packages, cans, or jars are safe for consumption if the exterior of the container is thoroughly washed with a detergent solution to remove any radioactive substances and provided that extreme care is taken to avoid contamination of the contents when they are removed from the container (or when the "decontaminated" but still suspect wrapping material is removed from the contents). Foods which have a protective skin (most fruits, some vegetables) may be used if they are thoroughly washed with a detergent solution, rinsed, and then peeled under painstaking precautions to avoid contact of the possibly still contaminated skin with the interior edible portion. Cooperative studies conducted by the U.S.

Atomic Energy Commission and the National Canners Association have shown that induced radioactivity is not set up in canned foods which have been exposed to the intense radiation encountered near the center of nuclear blasts. Until the public water supply has been cleared of the suspicion of lingering radioactive contamination, packaged fluids such as bottled or canned fruit juices and soft drinks should be consumed.

All wash water, rinse water, rubber gloves, and rags used in decontaminating foods are best disposed of by burying them deep in ground so chosen that the likelihood of the leaching of radioactive wastes into public water supplies is small.

Nutritional Rehabilitation Following Starvation

The problem of refeeding starved populations or inmates of prisoner-of-war or concentration camps arises in times of war, famine, or major natural disaster. Previously starved individuals should not be permitted to eat ad libitum, since, depending on the length of the period of starvation, this may result in reflex overloading with distention, and nausea, vomiting, and diarrhea may occur. Moreover, severely starved individuals may be too weak to feed themselves and may therefore succumb within the sight of food if they are not aided by a planned effort at nutritional rehabilitation.

Severe cases of inanition may be so badly debilitated that they can tolerate only small quantities of food without distress. In extreme instances the use of the stomach tube may be advisable. Such patients receive frequent small feedings of skim milk (50 to 100 ml at hourly intervals). If this produces no untoward reactions, small quantities of skim milk powder, sugar, and egg yolks (or powdered egg) are added to the skim milk and the mixture is thoroughly homogenized. It is advisable to aspirate any remaining stomach contents through the indwelling catheter before new feedings are given. If such a regimen does not bring about rapid improvement, a trial at parenteral feeding may be made. (Large-scale initial parenteral feeding attempts without individual selection are not practical, nor have they proved very desirable or necessary from the standpoint of superior results.)

Persons in a very depleted state but able to feed themselves are given small quantities of easily digested food at frequent intervals. Reconstituted skim milk made from nonfat milk powder and water is a very practical first food. Its concentration may be increased and sugar and powdered egg admixed if the first feedings pass uneventfully. Easily digested solid foods (bread, soups) are given next in small amounts and at frequent intervals. Fats should be avoided at first because they are often poorly digested and tolerated by severely starved individuals. Because of the danger of producing gastric distress by overfeeding, individual reaction is the guide to the increase in the amount of food given at any one meal; eventually a normal pattern of three major meals is arrived at, with in-between-meal feedings as needed.

The primary need in refeeding starved persons is for an abundant provision of calories. The rate of recovery is roughly proportional to the calories supplied. An attempt is therefore made to upgrade the food allotment gradually from about 1500 cal until a daily intake of 3000 to 4000 cal is obtained. Intakes in excess of 5000 cal are unnecessary and do not speed recovery. A diet rich in high-quality protein should be given because of the need for essential amino acids for tissue rehabilitation. Special vitamin supplementation is not crucial in the first days of rehabilitation except where specific clinical deficiencies exist. Prophylactic multivitamin supplementation may be desirable and does no harm during the long period of recovery.

Before body weight is fully restored and full working capacity is attained, the subject may go through a phase during which the previously depressed metabolic rate increases beyond its level during the period of inanition and even beyond the normal prestarvation level. Similarly, the previously subnormal blood flow and pulse rate may accelerate beyond normal control values. Some clinicians like to interpret this as a rebound from the panhypopituitarism which is characteristic of prolonged and severe starvation. The unconscious habit of energy conservation acquired during long periods of deprivation is usually not abandoned hastily; therefore physical rehabilitation through exercise may have to be enforced. The recovering subjects may also become more difficult to manage as physical vigor returns because at this point the starvation-caused depression and lack of initiative may well be replaced by overt manifestations of previously repressed irritation and hostility.

Full recovery from long-term undernutrition is a slow process. In instances of severe, prolonged starvation in adults where the weight loss exceeds 25 percent, full functional rehabilitation may be delayed for as long as a year, even with the best of treatment; in the case of children, the recovery period may be considerably shorter (but may leave residual damage), whereas elderly subjects may require an even longer period in which to achieve complete or near-complete restoration.

Chapter 41

Food Poisoning and Food Toxicology

Food Poisoning

Food poisoning is a loosely used blanket term which may connote a multitude of widely divergent etiologies. From a statistical standpoint, food poisoning is not an important cause of severe illness or death. Nevertheless, the number of outbreaks which do occur each year, their dramatic nature, their epidemiologic peculiarities, the trauma and suffering, the occasional fatalities, and the resulting publicity suffice to endow the subject with an importance which cannot be ignored, even though it may be somewhat out of proportion to its actual public health significance. Foods which produce toxic reactions are either carriers of microbial infections and preformed microbial toxins or sources of poisons which are an inherent part of the composition of the particular plant, fungus, or animal.

Occasionally excessive residues of insecticides and fungicides applied in the form of sprays and dusts may be encountered on unwashed fruits or vegetables; such residues do not usually give rise to acute attacks of food poisoning, but they must be eliminated carefully to avoid any toxic cumulative effects. This chapter is limited to a discussion of toxic factors which may be found in foods and of the traditional concept of "food poisoning," and no attempt is made to discuss the vast spectrum of microbial infections which may be contracted by ingestion of contaminated foods and beverages (typhoid fever, amoebic dysentery, streptococcic septic sore throat, etc.).

Bacterial Infections

Many cases of food poisoning are the result of ingesting foods contaminated with pathogenic bacteria. The majority of such outbreaks are due to organisms of the *Salmonella* group, of which about 200 different serotypes have been recognized as pathogenic for man. The symptoms of food-borne infection with such organisms are basically alike. They are characterized by nausea and vomiting, abdominal cramps, diarrhea, headache and fever, and general prostration. There is usually an asymptomatic incubation period of from $1/2$ to $1^1/2$ days, followed by an abrupt onset. Attacks are of varying severity and usually last 1 to 2 days; they are rarely severe enough to be fatal.

Outbreaks of this type of acute gastroenteritis are usually characterized by an interesting epidemiology since in most cases large numbers of individuals who partook of the same contaminated food—at a restaurant, picnic, or wedding dinner—will be affected. Frequent sources of infection are human carriers who act as food handlers, insects which spread the pathogen from fecal sources to the food, and unsanitary contaminated ingredients or containers which were used in preparation of the food product or meal. Cases are known where poorly stored foods were contaminated with *Salmonella* organisms through the excreta of infected rodents.

Botulinus Poisoning

Botulism is a true poisoning in the sense that the pathologic syndrome is due to the ingestion of a toxic substance found preformed in the food. Botulism is caused by the ingestion of a potent toxin elaborated and secreted by different strains of *Clostridium botulinum*, an anaerobic, spore-forming organism which is widely distributed in soils. The bacterium grows readily under anaerobic conditions in improperly sterilized, preserved foods which have a near-neutral or slightly alkaline reaction. (The organism does not grow in a medium with a pH of 4.1 or lower.) Early outbreaks of botulism in Europe were caused by improperly preserved sausages. In the United States, since 1925, all commercially canned nonacid foods are heat-sterilized by retorting under pressure at temperatures far above the boiling point for prolonged periods to assure complete destruction of botulinus spores and consequent safety from botulism. At present, most instances of botulinus poisoning are caused by the ingestion of improperly sterilized, home-preserved nonacid foods, especially corn and string beans. In the canning process, boiling alone is not enough to assure complete sterilization of home-canned low-acid foods; a pressure cooker must be used to sterilize such foods at temperatures of 240°F or more for appropriate periods, which vary with the size of the container, the processing method, and the particular variety of food.

The toxin of *C. botulinum* is one of the most potent poisons known. The ingestion of even minute quantities will result in a severe syndrome which may be fatal within 2 to 10 days. Symptoms include headache, nausea, prostration, oculomotor abnormalities, blindness, progressive difficulty in swallowing and talking, ascending paralysis, and death. Treatment is primarily supportive, in addition to the administration of a polyvalent botulinus antitoxin (or of strain-specific antitoxins if the type of organism involved can be ascertained). The antitoxin is effective largely in instances where only small quantities of the toxin have been consumed and where prophylactic administration was started before onset of symptoms. The mortality in botulism is about 65 percent.

The toxin is heat-labile and may be inactivated by boiling for about 15 minutes. This fact may be responsible for the prevention of many instances of botulism because even though a particular jar or can of home-canned food may have supported growth of the organism, subsequent routine cooking by the unsuspecting homemaker may have inactivated the toxin.

Staphylococcus Enterotoxin Poisoning

The most common type of food poisoning is based on ingestion of a preformed toxin elaborated by organisms of the genus *Staphylococcus*. It is difficult to exclude staphylococci from foods since the organisms are ever-present on human skin and are constantly discharged from the human respiratory tract and suspended on droplets of moisture or dust particles. Food handlers with cutaneous infections are a major source of this specific contamination of foods. Staphylococci grow in cream fillings, custards, puddings, hollandaise sauce, and other starch-, egg-, and milk-containing mixtures (meats and meat combinations will also support their growth). Rapidly growing staphylococci may elaborate their specific enterotoxin within a few hours in fertile media like cream puffs and custard pies if growth is not deterred by proper refrigeration. Warm foods or foods permitted to stand for prolonged periods at room temperature in the summer months constitute an open invitation for this type of food poisoning.

As the name implies, the staphylococcus enterotoxin acts primarily on the gastrointestinal tract. Since a preformed poisonous substance is involved (and not an organism which must first multiply and establish itself in the intestinal tract to produce reactions), onset of symptoms after ingestion is rapid and occurs usually within about 3 hours. Symptoms are acute and include nausea, vomiting, diarrhea, intestinal cramps, headache, and on occasion fever. In contrast to salmonellosis or botulism, the attack does not last more than 1 day and frequently terminates within 6 hours or less.

Trichinosis

Any discussion of food poisoning would be incomplete without a brief mention of trichinosis. This condition is the result of a generalized muscle infestation with the roundworm *Trichinella spiralis*. Encysted, dormant larvae of the worm are taken in through the consumption of infected pork which was insufficiently cooked to achieve destruction of the parasite.

Symptoms of the disease are fever and generalized muscular tenderness after an incubation period of about 1 to 2 weeks, followed by edema of the eyelids, gastrointestinal symptoms, headache, retinal hemorrhages, photophobia, and eosinophilia. The eosinophilia in conjunction with edema of the eyelids, headache, and muscular pains in the neck and muscles of respiration is almost pathognomonic. Eventually the invading larvae which remain outside of muscle tissue are destroyed and the survivors localize and encyst in muscles, particularly the diaphragm. At this point the infected individual becomes asymptomatic.

Many cases are mild enough to escape attention; others are quite severe, and a mortality of up to 5 percent has been reported in diagnosed cases. The incidence of human infection in the United States is very high and has been variously reported to be anywhere from 9 to 20 percent, depending on the locality. The condition can be prevented by the thorough cooking of all pork and pork products and avoidance of uncooked pork sausage meats. (Bear meat may also be infected but is statistically less significant.) The parasites can be destroyed by heating the meat harboring them to at least 160°F, by gamma irradiation at a dosage of 30,000 rads, or by freezing at 5°F for 20 days or more. Cooks and homemakers must be warned against preparing rare pork products; when cooking a pork roast, a thermometer inserted into the center of the thickest portion of the meat should indicate 185°F before roasting is terminated to ensure that temperatures lethal to the parasite are produced in all locations.

Trichinosis is very widespread among pigs, and the practice of feeding raw garbage to hogs serves to perpetuate and spread the condition since untreated garbage is usually contaminated with *T. spiralis* larvae. Today, in a number of communities special regulations force hog raisers to steam-sterilize all garbage before it is used for feeding purposes.

Heavy Metals

Metals which may be ingested in small quantities with foods and are toxic above certain levels include lead, arsenic, selenium, cadmium, and antimony. There are two major sources of lead ingestion: (1) lead contained in the paint covering objects which are chewed by young children, and (2) lead in the form of spray residues on edible crops. Fortunately, industrial practices and legal regulations effectively control this toxic contamination at present. Lead-containing enamels, glazes, and solders in cooking and food storage utensils constitute another potential source of lead contamination of foods and beverages. Lead toxicity is cumulative, and its onset almost unnoticeable.

The average arsenic content of most foods is less than 1 ppm. Marine crustaceans and shellfish may contain much more, but this is combined with organic matter in a form which is not absorbed. Arsenical insecticidal sprays are widely used for fruits and vegetables, but improved washing methods have rendered the risk from these negligible.

Cadmium is a powerful emetic. Acid fruits stored in cadmium-plated utensils may dissolve toxic amounts of this metal; cadmium plating should not be allowed to come in contact with foods.

Antimony is another emetic which has been used for glazes on enameled vessels and pottery. Several outbreaks have been traced to lemonade which has leached antimony from cheap gray enameled kettles.

Selenium may be found in excessive, toxic concentrations in cereals grown in certain areas in the United States. In commercial use, grain from such regions is mixed with selenium-free grain from other areas where the soil does not contain this element, before milling or before feeding to livestock.

Metallic mercury accidentally ingested (as from a broken thermometer bulb) is considered harmless. It is insoluble in water, dilute hydrochloric acid, and alkalies, and generally not subject to gastrointestinal absorption. Metallic mercury in industrial wastes, dumped into lakes and rivers, however, enters the food cycle (as mercury salts do) via microorganisms and plant life, usually in the form of methylated mercury ion which is concentrated via the food chain in fish.

Mussel Poisoning

A number of fish and shellfish found in tropical waters are poisonous; the nature of the poison is unknown in many cases and seems to vary with the species, geographical region, and season. In the United States mussel and clam poisoning is most common on the Pacific Coast, but is not restricted to this area. From June through October mussels and clams feed on a poisonous unicellular marine organism (*Gonyaulax*), which produces a toxic alkaloid resembling strychnine. Consumption of clams and mussels during these months may result in acute mussel poisoning. Symptoms may follow within 30 minutes; they include paresthesias around the mouth, followed by nausea, vomiting, abdominal cramps, dizziness, incoordination, and progressive paralysis; death may result from respiratory paralysis. The toxin has been isolated, and the empirical formula $C_{10}H_{17}N_7O_4$ has been worked out.

Poisonous Plants

A number of plants contain poisonous alkaloids which will cause toxic symptoms of varying severity depending on the amount ingested. Poisoning may occur particularly among children who are more apt to eat unknown but attractive leaves or berries. Examples of such plants are hemlock (coniine), Jimson weed (stramonium), foxglove (digitalis), monkshood (aconitine), and deadly nightshade (atropine).

Certain types of sweet peas (vetches) like *Lathyrus sativus* will cause lathyrism when eaten by man in large quantities. The condition is characterized in its earliest stages by a spastic paralysis, especially of the legs, with tremors and paresthesias, followed, in cases of prolonged consumption of the vetches or the active, toxic substances they contain—β-aminopropionitrile and amino-acetonitrile—by profound disorders in connective tissues, including bone deformities, hernias, and rupture of blood vessels. These plants survive periods of drought; consequently in countries like India and certain regions in Africa there is an increased incidence of lathyrism during famines when a significant percentage of the population is reduced to consuming vetches.

White snakeroot or richweed poisoning, characterized by vomiting, weakness, and prostration, may be caused by drinking the milk of cows that pasture where the noxious plant is plentiful. In commercial use milk is pooled from many sources, so that toxic concentrations of the etiologic trematol in processed milk are highly unlikely.

Fava bean poisoning (favism) is caused by the ingestion of fava beans (or even by exposure to the pollen of the blossoming plant) by individuals with an inborn deficiency of glucose-6-phosphate dehydrogenase. An as yet unknown toxic substance in fava beans produces a severe hemolysis in such individuals with vomiting, dizziness, prostration, and marked hemolytic anemia with icterus. In the Mediterranean basin, Asia, and Taiwan this sensitivity to broad (fava) beans affects a not inconsiderable proportion of the population.

In Guam, flour prepared from the seeds of the cycad plant is still sometimes used as human food. The toxic component in cycad nuts, cycasin, which has a chemical structure similar to that of the toxic industrial material dimethylnitrosamine, can have acute toxic and late carcinogenic effects on the consumer. Guamanians rid the cycad kernel of its toxic component by prolonged soaking in water followed by drying in the sun.

In the *raw* state, soy, kidney, navy, lima, and pinto beans contain natural toxic substances including trypsin inhibitors and hemaglutinins. These, however, are heat-labile and are inactivated by roasting or cooking.

Mycotoxins in Foods

Ergotism is probably the oldest known disease caused by toxic substances which are produced by fungi growing in food. Ergot poisoning is rare in the United States, but not uncommon in Europe, where the parasitic fungus of rye smut (*Claviceps purpurea*) is more widespread. Poisoning occurs because of ingestion of the powerful alkaloid ergot; this substance is found in the fruiting body of the fungus which is ground up and disseminated into the flour during milling. Ingestion of bread made from the unmixed, undiluted flour may result in severe and even fatal symptomatology referable to the circulatory or central nervous systems. Symptoms are due to the powerful vasoconstrictive action of the alkaloid and its induction of severe muscular contractions.

Molds are not uncommonly encountered on bread, fruit, or dairy products in the home. They usually belong to the genera *Aspergillus, Penicillium, Mucor,* and *Rhizopus.* None of the common fungi found in the food market or refrigerator in the United States has been implicated in *carcinogenesis,* but there have been reports of toxic reactions (usually vomiting and gastritis) after ingestion of foods *heavily* overgrown with common food molds. Some of these are known to be harmless, such as the fungus responsible for the flavor and texture of Camembert cheese.

In contrast, a grave and frequently fatal diathesis, alimentary toxic aleukia, is associated with the ingestion of grain on which cryophilic fungi have proliferated (or of foods prepared from such grain). *Fusarium sporotrichioides* and other fungi are implicated in this toxicosis, which is characterized by leucopenia, agranulocytosis, bone marrow depression, hemorrhages in a variety of tissues and organs, and, eventually, fatal secondary bacterial infections. The latest grave epidemic of this toxicosis, which caused tens of thousands of deaths, occurred in Russia toward the end of World War II when the hungry rural population consumed unharvested grain which had overwintered under snow and was heavily infested with the causative fungus.

In recent years significant attention has been focused on aflatoxin, a potent toxin elaborated by the ubiquitous fungus *Aspergillus flavus* in a variety of food crops when they are permitted to mold, particularly in peanuts, Aflatoxin has caused major epidemics of fatal hepatic necrosis in domestic fowl fed *Aspergillus*-contaminated peanuts; its chronic ingestion in lower dosages causes liver cancer in experimental animals. It is suspected to be the etiologic agent in "childhood cirrhosis" in India. The accidental ingestion of aflatoxin-contaminated peanut flour by a group of children in a hospital in Mysore, India, resulted in the prompt development of hepatomegaly followed by hepatic fibrosis and cirrhosis. The full significance of the aflatoxin problem has not yet been elucidated. In areas where agricultural and other practices permit extensive mold damage to food crops (as in the case of peanuts in India and Africa), the etiologic significance of chronic ingestion of traces of aflatoxin to endemic hepatic damage and oncogenicity cannot be dismissed.

Mushroom Poisoning

Poisonous mushrooms are distinguished from edible ones by specific botanical characteristics; persons unfamiliar with these morphologic criteria should not eat wild-growing mushrooms which they have gathered, since at times the risks of mushroom poisoning exceed the gastronomic rewards.

Two species of the genus *Amanita* are responsible for most cases of mushroom poisoning in the United States. The delicious but deadly *A.*

phalloides causes nearly 90 percent of fatalities, and *A. muscaria* is responsible for practically all other deaths from mycetismus.

In this country two types of poisoning are distinguished. The rapid type is caused by *A. muscaria,* which contains the alkaloid muscarine. In this type, symptoms will occur within 1 to 2 hours; they consist of vomiting, abdominal cramps, salivation, sweating, myosis, and collapse. Atropine is a specific antidote to which most persons respond well, and mortality is low.

The delayed type of poisoning is due to the ingestion of *A. phalloides,* which contains a number of yet-unidentified toxins. Here the symptoms occur after 6 to 16 hours; they consist of abdominal pain, extreme nausea, vomiting, and diarrhea. This is followed by extensive damage to the liver, kidney, and central nervous system. In this delayed type of mushroom poisoning the causative toxins have a chance to be well absorbed by the time countermeasures are taken, and the prognosis is correspondingly poor. The mortality is 50 percent or higher.

If the mushroom *Coprinus atramentarius* (inky cap) is eaten prior to the consumption of alcohol, the face of the drinker (and sometimes other parts of the body) turns a vivid purplish red. Apparently an antabuse-like reaction results from the interaction of some mushroom component and alcohol.

Miscellaneous Toxicity in Foods

In recent years the observation was made that patients who are receiving drugs which act as inhibitors of monoamine oxidase (MAO) as therapy for depression or hypertension will be subject to acute hypertensive crises and attacks of headache, palpitation, and flushing after the ingestion of certain foods. These very distressing attacks may have neurologic sequelae or may even lead to death. The foods involved—aged cheeses, Chianti wine, sherry, beer, broad beans, yeast extracts (more recently chocolate and pickled herring have also been implicated)—have in common the presence of the pressor amine tyramine, which is a potent blood pressure elevating agent. This pressor amine appears in the food as the result of decarboxylation of tyrosine by bacterial enzymes during aging and/or fermentation. Possibly tryptamine, histamine, and hydroxytyramine are also involved. Normally, monoamine oxidases in the gastrointestinal tract and other body tissues act as the first line of defense against ingested pressor amines. In patients who are treated with monoamine oxidase–inhibiting drugs, however, the food-derived pressor amines are not detoxified and the very distressing adverse effects ensue. Thus patients taking MAO-inhibitor drugs must be warned to avoid scrupulously consumption of the enumerated foods in any but the smallest quantities.

Certain predisposed individuals with an extremely low threshold to monosodium glutamate are subject to attacks of headache, temporary elevation of blood pressure, "facial pressure," a flushing or burning sensation, and chest pain after consumption of moderate to large quantities of this food flavoring agent. This disorder has been dubbed the Chinese restaurant syndrome since it appeared to be associated with Chinese dinners and is probably the sequel of the copious consumption of soy sauce, which contains a high concentration of monosodium glutamate. Fortunately for those addicted to Chinese cuisine, this dose-related syndrome appears to be limited to few individuals with a particularly low threshold of sensitivity to the substance.

Radioactive Contamination

Precautions associated with the use of foods suspected of radioactive contamination as a result of nuclear blasts are discussed in Chap. 40.

Prevention of Food Poisoning

Most instances of food poisoning occur through the mechanisms discussed in the early sections and involve, as the underlying cause, bacterial contamination. Such outbreaks can be avoided if the tenets of sanitary handling of foods are upheld at all times, preferably on a voluntary basis, but if necessary through strict enforcement of sanitary regulations promulgated by boards of health and similar agencies. This involves the elimination of chronic carriers from food-handling positions, the use of adequate refrigerated storage facilities in restaurants, a more effective separation of restaurant kitchens and rest rooms, the pasteurization of milk, thorough inspection of meats, pest control measures in food storage areas, insect control in food-handling establishments, and many others.

Most bacterial growth is inhibited in acid media; consequently, many fruits of low pH require a briefer or lower heat treatment than foods which are less acid in order to effect sterilization. Nevertheless, scrupulous care is necessary in handling all classes of foods because severe contamination may cause spoilage even in the lower ranges of hydrogen-ion concentration. Freezing cannot be relied on to sterilize food, and frozen foods, once thawed, should be regarded as particularly perishable products. The danger zone for bacterial reproduction in foods is between 50 and 120°F. Four hours may suffice to permit the growth of a sizable bacterial population, particularly in such favorable media as raw milk or ground meat. Whenever there is any reason to doubt the freshness or wholesomeness of a food product or dish, it should not be consumed and it should be disposed of in such a fashion that small children and domestic animals cannot reach and eat it. When a food is suspect, cowardice is the wisest course of action; the risks of casual testing by personal trial are disproportionate to the potential savings.

Chapter 42

Nutrition and Modern Food Technology

Since the dawn of history, man has been confronted with the problem of survival through alternate periods of glut and famine due to changes of season and the vagaries of climate. The solution evolved eventually, and man began to store the surplus of good years and seasons to nourish himself during the proverbial "seven lean years." The first documented, large-scale effort at preventive food storage was organized in biblical times by Joseph in Egypt, and this farsighted man may well be considered the prototype of the planner and entrepreneur in the fields of food and nutrition. Since then there have been many other milestones in man's efforts to prevent starvation and to assure an abundant diet at all times; yet the storage and preservation of foods remain a fundamental without which our civilization cannot exist.

Preservation of Foods

Since the conditions of present-day living demand that foods be transported over long distances and be stored for considerable periods, their limited natural keeping qualities must be improved. Some foods may be kept safely for years without the need for extensive processing. Thus cereals may be stored almost indefinitely, provided they are protected against spoilage through moisture and secured against infestation by insects and vermin. In the case of grains and seeds, natural dehydration serves as the protective process.

Dehydration

Man-made dehydration is one of the earliest methods of food preservation. Microbial spoilage depends on the presence of sufficient water, and drying of meat, fish, beans, fruits, and vegetables has been used since early days to effect the preservation of fresh foods. In recent years, aided particularly by the impetus of World War II, modern food technology has made immense strides in this particular field. Today's dried milk and dried eggs have a nutritive content practically identical with that of the fresh parent products. It is not as easy to make sweeping statements in the case of dehydrated or dried fruits and vegetables since results vary with each variety. In some instances vitamin losses are negligible; special processes, such as sulfuring in the case of fruits and steam blanching in the case of vegetables, tend to prevent losses of vitamin A and ascorbic acid. In general, about one-third to one-half of the thiamin in fruits and vegetables is lost during prolonged dehydration. Few data are available as yet concerning the preservation of riboflavin and niacin; theoretically both are more resistant to heating and oxidation than thiamin.

Canning

The salting and smoking of foods, though practiced for many centuries, is quantitatively less important today than in the past. Canning, freezing, and refrigeration have largely become the major modern methods of food preservation. The object in canning and bottling is the destruction of spoilage organisms. After suitable preparation the perishable raw materials are put into airtight, sealed containers, and a predetermined heat treatment serves to destroy the potential spoilage organisms which are capable of growing in the food. Once such approximate sterility is achieved, most canned foods remain edible for many years.

In modern commercial usage great care is taken to select specific varieties of raw material which lend themselves well to the canning process, to uphold sanitary conditions to the extreme in order to reduce to a practical minimum the number of bacteria in the yet-unsterilized food, and to shorten the time lag between harvest and process. Fruits and vegetables canned within 24 hours of picking often preserve a higher vitamin C content than similar foods bought "fresh" on the open market after prolonged shipping and storage and cooking in the home.

Retention of Nutrients in Canned Foods

Today, canning results in minimal nutritive losses. In general, it may be safely stated that there is no discernible loss in protein, fat, or carbohydrate. The vitamin content of canned foods reflects the variations in the nutrient values of the raw materials used, along with the methods employed in preparation and processing. Exposure to air (oxygen), contact with hot water, and heating—all conditions which are also at work in the home kitchen preparation of foods—are responsible for reductions in vitamin content which may occur during canning. However, with up-to-date equipment and methods, the vitamins contained in the raw foods are retained to a high degree in the canned product. The shortest blanching time at the highest temperatures consistent with the production of a high-quality product, and with a minimum exposure to oxygen, favors the greatest conservation of original vitamin content. Similarly, the use of new high-temperature, short-time processing techniques (used to sterilize semisolid products which traditionally were heat-sterilized through reliance on heat conduction only) permits the canning of products with retention of up to 90 percent of thiamin which, together with vitamin C, shares the distinction of being the most easily oxidized, heat-labile micronutrient subject to loss in the preparation of foods.

Exposure of a food to oxygen (air), particularly in the presence of enzymes and heavy metal ions like copper, may seriously affect the vitamin C content of the food product. Present-day methods permit the production of citrus juices which contain practically all the ascorbic acid found in the original fruit, and a similarly high retention is obtained in other products if the available information and advanced methods of processing are used.

The following data serve to give a general indication of vitamin retention in the canning of several representative fruits and vegetables.

Average Retention of Ascorbic Acid and Thiamin, Percent

	Ascorbic acid	Thiamin
Asparagus	92	67
Corn	...	34*
Green beans	55	71
Orange juice	98	
Peaches	71	76
Tomato juice	67	89

*New method of pressure cooking, up to 90 percent.

Nutritive losses during prolonged storage of canned foods are limited to the more vulnerable vitamins. In general, a 15 to 30 percent decrease in ascorbic acid may be expected during 1 year's storage at 80°F, whereas only 5

Average Retention of Carotene, Riboflavin, and Niacin, Percent

	Carotene	Riboflavin	Niacin
Asparagus	...	88	96
Corn	97	97	86
Green beans	87	96	92
Peaches	85	...	89
Tomatoes	67	100	98

to 15 percent is lost at 65°F, which is a more representative yearly average figure for most food warehouses in temperate climates. Depending on the pH of the food, thiamin losses are of a similar order of magnitude or somewhat larger. On the other hand, carotene, riboflavin, and niacin values decrease relatively slightly on storage.

Retention of Nutrients in Frozen Foods

Perhaps the most important development in food preservation in the last three decades is freezing. The nutritive loss which the food suffers during preparation for freezing (trimming, washing, blanching) is similar to that experienced in preparation for canning. Beyond this point, quick freezing prevents microbial spoilage. If the food is frozen quickly and maintained at 0°F, the subsequent losses in nutritive value are slight. Thus if the preparation for final freezing is efficient and well planned, the losses in nutrients may actually be smaller than those which take place during transportation, storage, and aging of "fresh" fruits and vegetables, followed by the preparatory steps which take place in the kitchen.

Ideally, frozen foods should be stored at 0°F. At that temperature, storage for 1 year does not result in significant vitamin losses. A rise in the storage temperature to 10°F may triple these small losses. At 30°F this rate increases about forty- or fiftyfold and microbial spoilage may accompany the attendant decrease in vitamin content.

Irradiation of Foods

The latest development in food preservation is sterilization by irradiation. Commercially produced irradiated foods are not yet available, and this aspect of food technology is still in its infant shoes. So far it has been amply demonstrated that foods may be sterilized by radiation if a sufficiently high dosage is used. Such foods are not dangerous since radioactivity is not induced by the dosages required for sterilization. However, undesirable changes in flavor, texture, color, and reduction in vitamin content still attend irradiation sterilization of a significant number of foods. In addition, high initial cost of installation and the slow rate of sterilization may make irradiation an uneconomical method of preserving foods. Thus several years may pass before irradiation will claim a significant proportion of the commercially processed foods consumed by the population.

Preparation of Foods in the Kitchen

The *processing* of fresh foods—trimming, washing, and cooking—in the home or institutional kitchen claims its share of nutrients. No matter how carefully washing and cooking are performed, loss of water-soluble and heat-labile or oxidation-prone constituents is inevitable. Similar to the situation in canning, losses in carotene, riboflavin, and niacin are not significant, though riboflavin may be destroyed by exposure to strong light. The final vitamin content of the finished food and the losses of thiamin and ascorbic acid due to oxidation and heating depend on the original freshness and vitamin content of the produce bought in the store and on the cooking habits of the cook. Suffice it to say that excessive losses of vulnerable vitamins and minerals can be prevented in the same fashion in which the industrial processes are improved, by avoiding prolonged exposure of hot foods to oxygen (air) and by minimizing the leaching of water-soluble constituents through the use of reasonable quantities of wash water and water used for boiling or cooking and by use of the cooking water (which contains water-soluble minerals and vitamins) in the food, instead of discarding it. Cooking in a covered pot and the briefer cooking period associated with pressure cooking tend to preserve thiamin and ascorbic acid.

Enrichment and Fortification

One of the most significant developments in food technology which serves to improve the nutritive value of refined or compounded and processed foods is enrichment with specific vitamins or minerals. It has been mentioned previously (Chap. 11) that the milling of low-extraction, fine white flour, cornmeal, and polished white rice results in unavoidable losses of some nutrients. In the last three decades the addition of thiamin, riboflavin, niacin, and iron to wheat flour, macaroni and noodle products, farina, rice, cornmeal, and corn grits has been gradually introduced as a legally required procedure in a large number of states and foreign countries.

The principle of *enrichment* connotes, by definition, the compensatory restoration, by addition of the pure vitamins and minerals, of the original natural levels of these elements in foods which routinely suffer nutritional loss during the process of milling or refining. On the other hand, *fortification* is a term applied to the addition of other than natural levels of vitamins or minerals to foods which are suitable vehicles of such nutrients, where such fortification may be sanctioned in view of specific, widespread nutritional deficiencies and when more natural routes of supplementation are not available.

Today, both enrichment and fortification have become accepted routine steps in the manufacture of certain staple foods, and they contribute considerably to the improvement of the nutritional welfare of the population. In practice, what may start as mere enrichment may become modified to a combination of enrichment and fortification. Enriched flour is a good example of how the enrichment was not limited to restoring previous natural values; in setting the legal requirements for enrichment, the human requirement and the general dietary situation with respect to the nutrients involved were also taken into consideration.

There exist a number of examples of nutritional fortification of popular food items which have now become accepted routine measures serving the interest of improved nutritional standards of the population. Most brands of margarine in this country are fortified to contain 15,000 IU of vitamin A per pound (the legal requirement calls for 9,000 units), and 2,000 IU of vitamin D. Practically all evaporated milk canned in this country is fortified to contain 400 units of vitamin D per quart of reconstituted milk. Similarly, vitamin D milk, which is pasteurized fresh milk, is fortified to contain 400 units of vitamin D per quart. By law, nonfat dry milk for aid shipments abroad must be fortified with 5,000 units of vitamin A and 500 units of vitamin D per 100 g of milk solids. For domestic use nonfat dry milk may be fortified under a standard which requires 500 units of vitamin A and 100 units of vitamin D per 8 fluid ounces of reconstituted fluid skim milk. This fortification of nonfat dry milk for domestic use should be mandatory. In Canada, where citrus fruits must be imported and where imported citrus juices are more expensive, legal standards—recognizing the need for a popularly available source of vitamin C—have created a fortified, standardized apple juice which contains a minimum of 35 mg of ascorbic acid per 100 ml of juice. Present-day precooked infant cereals are routinely enriched with iron, thiamin, and niacin; and iodized salt has become a household staple without which the goiter statistics in the United States (Chap. 12) would not appear as innocuous as they are today.

Nutrition Progress through Technology

Whenever modern methods of food manufacture are discussed in relation to the nutritive value of foods, it seems inevitable that a negative aspect—partial losses of a number of vulnerable nutrients during processing—will receive the glare of the limelight, while the large number of advantages are ignored or taken for granted. What is largely disregarded is that urbanization is an integral part of our civilization and the supply of food to an urbanized society entails food preservation and the manufacture of easily distributed and prepared food products. Furthermore, it is only because of the advances of modern food technology that the wide variety of foods, now taken for granted, exists at all and serves to balance the public nutritional intake. Advances in processing, preservation, and transportation of foods have been as important to the improvement of the nutritional standards of the population as advances in sanitation and pharmacology to its relative freedom from contagious diseases. There is no season of the year when an extensive variety of fresh and processed foods in liberal quantities is not available to the smallest community. Processed fish and seafoods are available where none were known, citrus fruits have become commonplace where sources of ascorbic acid had been scarce, and the sometimes monotonous diet of the farmhouse has become enriched and varied, all with the aid of advances in food technology.

Processed food products which in their advent were looked upon as expensive novelties soon came to occupy prominent places in the popular dietary and now serve to enrich the diet and to advance the cause of public health. The best example is, perhaps, the impact of modern processed foods on infant nutrition. There is no doubt today that infants are better nourished and enjoy a greatly reduced morbidity because of the production of sanitary, processed sources of milk and the addition of a wide variety of processed food products to their diet which contribute essential nutrients seldom supplied before when they were needed most. In brief, food processing has become an inseparable part of our civilization. It has innumerable advantages and some disadvantages. The former have raised our standards of nutrition, while the latter can, as enrichment has shown, be obviated with some enlightened thinking.

Chapter 43

Nutrition in Relation to Community Health

Nutrition may be defined as the science of foods and their relation to life and health. The preceding chapters have made the connection between nutrition and physiology abundantly clear, and further words are not needed to emphasize that a state of individual optimal health is not feasible without adequate nutrition. In the same vein, the general standards of health of a population are apt to be low wherever nutrition is inadequate. Thus nutrition and nutrition education are fundamental determinants, together with sanitation, preventive medicine, and others, of the overall concept of public health, and the nutritionist or dietitian is an indispensable member of the public health team.

Practical Aspects of Public Health Nutrition Work

The ramifications of public health nutrition work are seemingly endless. The objectives of public health nutrition efforts are to prevent disease and promote physical well-being through improvement of the nutritional status of the population. In furtherance of this aim the public health nutritionist works with official and voluntary health agencies, schools and colleges, social and welfare agencies, institutions, and individuals, in an advisory and educational capacity. Such work may take the form of food surveys or clinical and laboratory studies to ascertain and define local needs, or of home visits to ferret out nutritional problems and to suggest solutions; it may call for practical advice on such topics as nutrition in pregnancy, child feeding, family meal planning, proper cooking, weight control, geriatric nutrition, or special diets in disease. It may involve the organizing of educational campaigns complete with placards, exhibits, radio and television slogans, or the teaching of the basic tenets of good nutrition in local schools. Nutritionists or dietitians in public health work may have to extend consultation on food service and diet planning to institutions or homes for the chronically ill or aged who do not have the benefits of a house dietitian; they may have to develop teaching aids, good-breakfast projects, and animal nutrition demonstrations for schools or aid in the training of school-lunch personnel. The work may include consultation with social welfare agencies on foods, their nutritional values, and the wisest use in low-income family budgets. It may require participation in nutrition research projects or the conducting of diet interviews with patients in out-patient clinics, and it may on occasion call for educational talks to community groups.

Medical nutrition is an important and growing area of specialization for physicians engaged in practice, research, and teaching, especially in schools of medicine and public health.

Dietetics

Sir Robert Hutchinson defined dietetics as the science of applying the hitherto discovered facts about food and its use in the body to the feeding of the individual, the family, and the nation. One major aspect of the work of dietetics is to feed and maintain the sick; another just as important aspect is the education of the individual and the public in the best ways of nourishing themselves to prevent ill health.

In hospitals and sanatoria, the professional dietitian is in charge of diet planning and of the food service management. The hospital dietitian is also responsible for elicitation of diet histories from patients, for instruction of discharged patients in the planning of their maintenance diets, for the preparation of standard house diet manuals, and for teaching the principles of nutrition to student nurses. Here again, particularly in conjunction with dietary management of ill patients, the professional dietitian is an indispensable member of the health team, public or private.

The work of the professional dietitian is not limited to the therapeutic application of the knowledge of nutrition; increasing numbers of dietitians are active in preventive capacities, as it were, in charge of meal planning and food service administration in institutions other than hospitals, in large hotels and restaurants, and in school and industrial plant cafeterias. The latter two represent particularly fertile fields for the practice of preventive public health nutrition.

In-Plant Feeding in Industry

Ever since World War II increasing attention has been paid to the relationship between the efficiency and individual output of workers and their food intake. It has been shown in a number of studies that in the long run inadequate diets reflect on individual productivity. The poorly nourished worker, though outwardly healthy-appearing, may show more fatigue, may lose more time owing to illness, and may be less efficient and more accident-prone than the well-nourished worker. While in many industrial plants food supply is still considered a personal problem of the worker, an increasing number of industrial concerns and large offices have established systems of in-plant feeding at low cost for their employees as a matter of public spiritedness, convenience, and employee relations and morale, as well as of enlightened self-interest. Because of the tremendous number of people involved, providing this large segment of the population with well-planned, adequate nutrition for at least one meal per day makes industrial or office food service an important consideration in public health thinking. The office or plant cafeteria provides the opportunity for individual employees to obtain foods which will maintain them at a desired peak of physical efficiency throughout the greater portion of their working hours, and good food habits fostered by a well-planned meal pattern may influence the individuals' general health and thus, indirectly, their productive life span.

It would be futile to draw up detailed specifications as to what individual workers should eat in order to meet their nutritional requirements; persons eating in the office or plant cafeteria will select their own food largely according to their gastronomic preferences, long-standing food habits, and economic ability. It is important, however, that the cafeteria subtly influence this choice by providing desirable food items at low cost and that adequate nourishment be available at advantageous times to prevent excessive soft-drink-and-candy meal breaks and belated coffee-machine breakfasts. Direct education by leaflets and posters is also a good investment.

The nutritional needs of the industrial worker are largely the same as those of any other adult except for the intake of calories; the latter is determined by the physical exertion required by the individual job. (Since thiamin requirements are roughly proportional to the caloric intake, the thiamin intake must also increase in the case of jobs requiring unusual physical exertion. See Chap. 11.) Adequate breakfasts which provide more than just coffee and toast are needed to sustain physical activity and peak mental alertness throughout the entire morning and to prevent a late-morning slump. A morning meal which contains substantial amounts of protein, fat, and carbohydrate results in a less acute postprandial hyperglycemia than a meal which supplies primarily carbohydrates. The elevated postprandial blood glucose levels which follow the well-balanced type of meal return to depressive low fasting levels much more slowly, thus facilitating a sustained effort without an acute need to draw on reserves.

Experiments conducted at an industrial plant over a 2-year period have shown that among both men and women the work output was significantly greater when the dietary regimen included an adequate breakfast than when it was omitted. The addition of a midmorning break (consisting usually of coffee and rolls) when an adequate breakfast was eaten resulted in no advantage as far as maximum work output was concerned; where breakfast was omitted, a midmorning break showed a significant advantage, in maximum work output, for half the workers. Such data seem to indicate that it is in the interest of the employer to make breakfast service of the more desirable type available in the employees' cafeteria, especially in view of the fact that a large proportion of industrial and office workers limit themselves to a toast-and-coffee type of breakfast, taken hurriedly at home or at a quick-service fountain before entering the office or plant.

Meal service should be planned with the view to satisfying from one-third to two-thirds of the daily nutritional requirements in two meals, and it is essential that the main meal, lunch, provide at least one-third of the daily nutritive needs. Workers on swing and graveyard shifts should have the opportunity to obtain a satisfying, balanced meal since they are often nutritionally penalized because of their odd working hours. It is also highly desirable to have a "skeleton service" available outside of major meal times, particularly during minor breaks; such service should provide sandwiches (packaged, if necessary), milk or chocolate milk drinks, and citrus and tomato juices as an alternative to the usual vending-machine fare of coffee and candy.

School Lunch Program

The major points mentioned in connection with in-plant feeding apply equally well to school lunches. The principal difference, which is of utmost importance from the standpoint of fostering good nutrition, is that here children and adolescents are involved who require guidance in food choice even more than adults, and that the well-planned school lunch provides an excellent opportunity to establish desirable eating habits in young individuals who are still in their formative stages and whose food preferences have not yet become overly rigid.

In this country the Federal School Lunch Program has been established to encourage the feeding of nutritionally desirable meals at low cost to school children. A system of federal reimbursement of a portion of the cost of those meals which meet certain nutritional requirements serves as the inducement for compliance with desirable nutrition standards. In this program, a so-called type

A lunch is planned to provide one-third of the child's daily needs. Such a lunch must include at least the following: (1) $^1/_2$ pint of whole milk; (2) 2 ounces of lean meat, poultry, fish, or cheese (or one egg, or $^1/_2$ cup of cooked beans or peas, or 4 tablespoons of peanut butter); (3) a $^3/_4$-cup serving consisting of two or more vegetables or fruits or both; (4) one slice of whole-grain or enriched bread (or a serving of enriched biscuits, corn bread, rolls, or muffins); (5) 1 teaspoon of butter or fortified margarine. In the normal course of events, other components and food items are usually added to the school lunch to round off the meal gastronomically, to provide additional calories, and to add bulk and satiation value to the meal; the latter considerations are particularly important in the case of adolescents whose total requirements exceed those of children of grade school age.

Participation of schools in such a nutritionally desirable program is voluntary, just as the student's partaking of lunch meals at school is entirely voluntary. Thus not all students actually consume school lunches of laudable composition, but the majority have the opportunity to avail themselves of such meals, and the educational impact of desirable food choices fostered by well-planned school lunches is not to be dismissed lightly.

Nutrition Education

When the composition of the diet of different population groups is examined, it is usually observed that dietary adequacy increases as income rises. It is obvious that the chances for better diets increase with a higher per capita expenditure for food; however, once a certain minimum level of subsistence has been exceeded, the nutritional quality of the diet is no longer determined by cost alone and the factor of choice becomes paramount. Though ideally the selection of food should be determined primarily by nutritional considerations, gastronomic preferences, and family food habits acquired in childhood, regional or cultural food patterns as well as economic ability usually have the last word on the subject.

Since everyday application of nutrition knowledge lags behind scientific advances in the field, a significant proportion of the population does not enjoy the high level of health and mental and physical vigor which is potentially attainable. Nutrition education appears by far the most promising means to close this gap. Moreover, responsible nutrition education is just as essential for correcting misinformation as it is for conveying reliable information. Much the same happens in a new territory opened by science as in a newly discovered gold field; among others, adventurers rush in, and some of the ore mined lacks the true color of gold. Faddists and charlatans interested in quick profits are active in the popular realm of nutrition, and the attendant damage is best prevented through authoritative, trustworthy educational information.

The overall objective of nutrition education is to foster and establish nutritionally sound food practices. Changing the food habits of adults is particularly difficult since personal habits become rigid and ingrained with the passage of time. (Improved dietetic habits among the middle-aged and elderly will probably not be overly influential in the prevention of chronic, degenerative disease because of the damage well established in many individuals after a lifetime of faulty nutrition.) A strong motivation is usually required to make basic changes in faulty food habits, and even then the outcome is in doubt, as evidenced by the failure of most obese people to maintain a normal weight even after a temporary reduction which had been achieved by heroic means. Education toward desirable food habits is probably most successful in sick adults provided the special diet or changed food pattern is directly concerned with recovery and subsequent maintenance of health. It is doubtful, indeed, whether major and lasting voluntary changes in food habits can be wrought in many healthy adults unless very powerful motivation is provided. Nevertheless, a constant effort by physicians, medical societies, public health nutritionists, dietitians and nurses, community health councils, industry, informed parents, and the educational sections of mass media of communication and entertainment is beneficial in steadily shaping popular food habits.

Nutrition education has a particularly fertile field among the young, and the greatest promise lies in introducing desirable food attitudes where personality traits and personal habits have not yet fully solidified. Thus modern pediatric practice in infant feeding introduces the use of eggs, citrus juice, fruits, vegetables, and meat early in life and helps to accustom the infant to foods which should become part of his future meal pattern. The cooperation of parents is essential at this point, but it is usually obtained without great difficulty and considerably more readily than in the reverse case when the adult is the subject of the indoctrination.

Nutrition education in the classroom is of particular importance. Practical classroom projects are fruitful means of illustrating and bringing to life the more abstract teaching of elementary principles of good nutrition, especially in the lower levels. Teaching programs in schools tend to carry over into homes, and emphatic desires voiced by children often bring a food to the family table which otherwise would have little chance of appearing there. Practical indoctrination in the form of well-devised school lunches may also aid in changing food patterns in families of children who receive such meals in their schools.

Adolescents are particularly in need of nutrition information. On the one hand, this age group is noted for its poor food habits; on the other, its nutritive requirements are greater than those of most adults. Girls are particularly affected since many of them compound the demands made by growth with the physiologic stress and strain of early pregnancies. At the same time most adolescents, having a strong interest in personal physical improvement, represent a fertile field for the seeds of nutrition education. Perhaps the key figure in the battle for future longevity and optimal health is today's teen-age girl. It is she who will possibly soon bear children and who will influence by her dietetic practices the start which they get in life, and it is she—as the probable meal planner, cook, and food purchaser—who will determine the food pattern and shape the eating habits of her entire family.

Outlook

The science of nutrition has progressed a long way since the early days of James Lind, who, more than 200 years ago, cured scurvy with lemon juice in well-controlled experiments. In this country the nutritional level has risen tremendously as a result of a fortunate interplay of advances in the science of nutrition and the technology of foods and a rising standard of living. Because of this improvement of the national dietary, a new generation is growing up which is larger, healthier, and more resistant to disease than its predecessors. Nutrition education is gradually becoming part of the general program to improve communal health and contributes to the reduction of hidden and overt malnutrition. The once-prevalent classic malnutrition diseases—rickets, pellagra, goiter, and infantile scurvy—have all but disappeared. Overnutrition has become the national nutrition disease, and the attention of clinical nutrition research has shifted from deficiency diseases to the elucidation of the role of diet in the causation of chronic degenerative diseases.

Elsewhere, in the less developed areas of the world, the need for better nutrition, and particularly for economically available sources of protein, continues unabated. The elucidation of the etiology of the worldwide syndrome of kwashiorkor has done much to clarify specific nutritional needs in these areas. Local physicians, nutritionists, and government agencies, special teams of the World Health Organization, the Food and Agriculture Organization of the United Nations, and governmental and private institutions are endeavoring, within the limits imposed by the prevalent poverty, to raise the standards of nutrition and to teach the people to help themselves and to meet the human need for food and health.

The overall advances in the knowledge of human nutrition have been outstanding, and if some answers have so far eluded today's investigators, they will be found by the one who usually has the last word, the scientist of the future. The current incidence of cardiovascular diseases, renal diseases, and diabetes illustrates the opportunities that challenge nutrition scientists in their explorations. Just as the classic public health efforts devoted to sanitation and control of infection were instrumental in advancing yesterday's standards of health, we can expect that the science of nutrition will make crucial contributions to the future prevention of disease and to the continued advancement of human welfare.

Composition and Nutritive Value of Foods

Introduction to Tables

The Tables of Food Composition which follow are based largely on similar tables in *Handbook 8* of the U.S. Department of Agriculture and on the second, revised printing of the fourth edition of "Nutritional Data" (H. J. Heinz Company). Additional data have been included whenever available in reliable published literature. In the case of multiple values, representative averages were obtained and used.

The nutrient content of foods has been indicated by single figures, representing average values, rather than by ranges. Ranges, unless defined in terms of standard deviation and number of samples analyzed, with their sources, are unreliable. Most food analyses are not reported in such detail.

Furthermore, there is many a slip betwixt the crop and the lip. Harvesting, transporting, storing, processing, and final preparation for consumption are all stages at which nutrient losses can occur. "Fresh" foods may have been in storage for an unknown time when purchased. The nutritive value of canned foods and the effects of storage are well known and documented as the result of extensive studies carried out by the National Canners Association in collaboration with leading universities. Similar information is now available on frozen foods.

The following tables represent the best information available at the present time. Although they are adequate for preliminary calculation of diets and satisfactory for routine calculations of nutrient contents of diets, very precise work would seem to require laboratory analyses of the individual foods as consumed. This is particularly true of vitamins, which may vary considerably.

Notes Concerning Components

Proximate composition of food is the term which has come to be applied to the proportion of water, fat, carbohydrate, protein, and ash present in the food. Each component is made up of substances having some properties in common but may include smaller amounts of substances that are unrelated chemically.

Water content includes volatile substances in addition to free water. Most of the figures are based on loss of weight on drying to constant weight, either in a vacuum or air.

Protein values are calculated by multiplying the total nitrogen content by a suitable conversion factor. Foods also contain nonprotein nitrogen compounds, such as amino acids and the purine bases. Where the nonprotein nitrogen is fairly large, the figures for protein content have been adjusted to more nearly represent the sum of the true protein and amino acids present.

Fat refers in the main to ether-extractable materials. These include, in addition to the true fats, or glyceryl esters of fatty acids, various fatty acids, sterols, chlorophyll, and other pigments.

Carbohydrate is also called "total carbohydrate by difference." It is the difference between 100 percent and the sum of the percentages of protein, fat, ash, and water. It includes sugars and starches which the body uses entirely and also includes other forms of carbohydrate which the body uses to a smaller degree if at all, such as cellulose, lignin, pentosans, and some organic acids.

Fiber is that portion of the sample which resists solution when boiled in dilute acid and dilute alkali. It is usually composed of cellulose, hemicellulose, and lignin.

Calories are complicated. They are determined by multiplying the figures for percentage composition of protein, fat, and carbohydrate by factors dimensioned in calories per gram. For almost 50 years nutritionists got along very nicely with the factors of 4, 9, and 4, which were calculated by Atwater, who determined data on energy-yielding nutrients and coefficients of digestion for a large number of common foods. The physiologic energy value was derived from these by applying heats of combustion values to the digested nutrients and deducting a correction for loss in the urine. The Atwater factors were designed to facilitate the physiologic energy of average United States diets. They do not work so well when applied to diets of different types and to individual foods.

A committee of the Nutrition Division of the Food and Agriculture Organization of the United Nations has suggested the use of modified Atwater factors in computing the energy value of foods. These new values, published in the GAO pamphlet *Energy Yielding Components of Food and Computation of Calorie Values* (May 1947), were largely used in computing caloric values in the following tables. Their recommendations are summarized below.

This method of calculating caloric values has the disadvantage that it is difficult for the user of a table to check the compiler's arithmetic without knowing the specific factors used in the calculations.

Caloric Conversion Factors

Food group	Protein, kcal/g	Fat, kcal/g	Carbohydrate, kcal/g
Milk, etc.	4.27	8.79	3.87
Meat, fish	4.27	9.02	
Eggs	4.36	9.02	
Butterfat	. . .	8.79	
Animal fats	. . .	9.02	
Vegetable fats	. . .	8.84	
Cereals, 100% extraction	3.59	8.37	3.78
85–93% extraction	3.78	8.37	3.95
70–74% extraction	4.05	8.37	4.12
Other cereals	3.87	8.37	4.12
Dry beans, peas, and nuts	3.47	8.37	4.07
Potatoes	3.47	8.37	4.03
Vegetables	3.11	8.37	3.99
Fruits	3.36	8.37	3.60
Sugar	. . .	. . .	3.87

Calcium, phosphorus, and iron represent the total amounts of these elements present. The calcium in foods containing relatively large amounts of oxalic acid (such as spinach) is not all available. Data on the biologic availability of iron in different foods is limited, and short-cut chemical methods for estimating availability (such as the reaction with α- and ά-dipyridyl) are not entirely reliable. The phosphorus in phytates is relatively unavailable, and these salts of inositol hexaphosphoric acid may tie up some dietary calcium and iron in the intestinal tract.

Vitamin A values are expressed in international units. They have been based in part on biologic assay and in part on physical or chemical determinations of vitamin A itself or one of its precursors. For these tables, values expressed as micrograms of carotene were converted to international units of vitamin A on the basis that 0.6 μg of β-carotene and 1.2 μg of other carotenes had vitamin A activity equivalent to 1 IU of vitamin A.

B vitamins. Methods of extraction and assay for the three B vitamins included are still in the process of development. New procedures are giving greater sensitivity and precision, but these have not been applied to a great many foods. Consequently, many of the values in these tables are based on older methods. There is still considerable doubt concerning the adequacy of present methods for the release of bound forms of riboflavin. Niacin values in these tables were derived from data in the literature measuring niacin, niacinamide, and related active compounds; they do not include niacin potentially available through conversion of tryptophan present in the particular food item (Chap. 11).

Ascorbic acid values are based on determinations of reduced ascorbic acid, since this is the form in which nearly all this vitamin occurs in fresh products. Foods that have undergone processing or storage, however, may contain significant quantities of the oxidized form (dehydroascorbic acid). This would lead to underestimation of the vitamin C value of foods, except that some foods contain interfering substances (such as sulfhydryl compounds) which react chemically like the vitamin but do not have the same physiologic activity. These reductones are found especially in foods having a high carbohydrate content which have been subjected to heat or unfavorable storage conditions.

Average portions were a problem. The sizes and weights given are only approximations and have very little statistical significance. Dietetic scales should be used to weigh portions in any precise work.

Signs and Symbols Used

Dashes show that there is no value for a constituent reported in the literature, although it seems reasonable to assume that it should be present.

Trace (abbreviated Tr.) is used to indicate values that would round to zero with the number of decimal places carried in these tables. Zero means that, for all practical purposes, there is not enough of a constituent present to worry about.

CONVERSION EQUIVALENTS*

1 level standard teaspoon (tsp) = 5 ml, or $\frac{1}{6}$ fl oz
1 level standard tablespoon (tbsp) = 15 ml, or $\frac{1}{2}$ fl oz
1 fluid ounce (fl oz) = 29.6 ml
1 measuring cup = 237 ml, or 8 fl oz
1 quart (2 pints, 4 cups) = 947 ml
1 pound (lb) = 454 g
1 ounce (avoirdupois) = 28.3 g
1 kilogram (kg) = 2.2 lb
1 liter = 1.057 qt
100 milliliters (ml) = $3\frac{1}{3}$ fl oz

*Values are slightly rounded off to yield practical, workable figures.

Tables of Food Composition

TABLES OF FOOD
CONSTITUENTS OF 100 g

Name		PROXIMATE COMPOSITION						MINERALS	
Name	Cal-ories	Water, g	Pro-tein, g	Fat, g	Ash, g	Total carbohy-drates, g	Crude fiber, g	Calcium, mg	Phos-phorus, mg
DAIRY PRODUCTS									
Butter	716	15.5	.6	81	2.5	.4	0	20	16
Buttermilk	36	90.5	3.5	.1	.8	5.1	0	118	93
Cheese									
Blue mold	368	40	21.5	30.5	6.0	2.0	0	315	339
Cheddar	3 3	37	25.0	32.2	3.7	2.1	0	725	495
Cheddar, processed	370	40	23.2	29.9	4.9	2.0	0	673	787
Cottage	95	76.5	19.5	.5	1.5	2.0	0	96	189
Cream	371	51	9.0	37.0	1.0	2.0	0	68	97
Swiss	370	39	27.5	28.0	3.8	1.7	0	925	563
Swiss, processed	355	40	26.4	26.9	5.1	1.6	0	887	867
Cream, light	204	72.5	2.9	20.0	.6	4.0	0	97	77
Cream, whipping	330	59	2.3	35.0	.5	3.2	0	78	61
Ice cream, plain	207	62.1	4.0	12.5	.8	20.6	0	123	99
Milk, cow's									
Fluid, whole	68	87.0	3.5	3.9	.7	4.9	0	118	93
Fluid, nonfat	36	90.5	3.5	.1	.8	5.1	0	123	97
Evaporated, cnd.	138	73.7	7.0	7.9	1.5	9.9	0	243	195
Nonfat solids, dry	362	3.5	35.6	1.0	7.9	52.0	0	1,300	1,030
Malted, beverage	104	78.2	4.6	4.4	1.0	11.8	0	135	123
Chocolate-flavored	74	83.0	3.2	2.2	.8	10.6	0	109	91
Milk, goat's, fluid	67	87.4	3.3	4.0	.7	4.6	0	129	106
Sherbet	123	68.1	1.5	.0	.4	30.0	—	50	40
Whey, dried	344	6.2	12.5	1.2	7.7	72.4	0	679	576
FATS, OILS, AND SHORTENINGS									
Butter	716	15.5	.6	81	2.5	.4	0	20	16
Fats, cooking, vegetable	884	0	0	100	0	0	0	0	0
Lard	902	0	0	100	0	0	0	0	0
Margarine	720	15.5	.6	81	2.5	.4	0	20	16
Mayonnaise	708	16	1.5	78	1.5	3.0	0	19	60
Oils, salad or cooking	884	0	0	100	0	0	0	0	0
Salad dressing, French	394	39.6	.6	35.5	4.0	20.3	.3	0	0
Salt pork, fat	783	8.0	3.9	85	3.5	0	0	Tr.	Tr.
FRUITS									
Berries									
Blackberries, raw	57	84.8	1.2	1.0	.5	12.5	4.2	32	32
Blueberries, raw	61	83.4	.6	.6	.3	15.1	1.2	16	13
Blueberries, cnd., sweet	98	73	.4	.4	.2	26	1.0	41	6

COMPOSITION
OF EDIBLE PORTION

MINERALS			VITAMINS					AVERAGE PORTION		
Iron, mg	Sodium, mg	Potassium, mg	A, IU	B₁, mg	B₂, mg	Nicotinic acid, mg	C, mg	Total calories	Measure	Weight in grams
.0	980	23	3,300	Tr.	.01	.1	0	100	1 tbsp	14
.1	130	140	Tr.	.04	.18	.1	1	86	1 cup	244
.5	—	—	1,240	.03	.61	.4	0	104	1 oz	28
1.0	700	92	1,400	.02	.42	Tr.	0	113	1 oz (1″ cube)	28
.9	1,500	80	1,300	.02	.41	Tr.	0	105	1 oz	28
.3	290	72	20	.02	.31	.1	0	27	1 oz	28
.2	250	74	1,450	.01	.22	.1	0	106	1 oz	28
.9	710	100	1,450	.01	.40	.1	0	105	1 oz	28
0.9	—	—	1,390	.01	.40	.1	0	101	1 oz	28
.1	50	91	830	.03	.14	.1	1	30	1 tbsp	15
0	40	56	1,440	.02	.11	.1	1	50	1 tbsp	15
.1	100	90	520	.04	.19	.1	1	167	1 slice	81
.1	50	140	160	.04	.17	.1	1	166	1 cup	244
.1	52	150	Tr.	.04	.18	.1	1	87	1 cup	246
.2	100	270	400	.05	.36	.2	1	346	1 cup	252
.6	528	1,130	40	.35	1.96	1.1	7	28	1 tbsp	8
.3	—	—	250	.07	.21	—	1	281	1 cup	270
.1	4	33	90	.03	.16	.1	1	185	1 cup	250
.1	34	180	160	.04	0.11	0.3	1	164	1 cup	244
0	174	218	0	.02	.08	Tr.	0	118	½ cup	96
—	—	—	50	.49	2.5	.8	—	—	—	—
0	980	23	3,300	Tr.	.01	.1	0	100	1 tbsp	14
0	4	0	0	0	0	0	0	1768	1 cup	200
0	.3	.2	0	0	0	0	0	126	1 tbsp	14
0	1,100	58	3,300	0	0	0	0	100	1 tbsp	14
1.0	590	25	210	.04	.04	0	0	92	1 tbsp	13
0	.2	.1	0	0	0	0	0	124	1 tbsp	14
0	—	—	0	0	0	0	0	60	1 tbsp	15
0.6	1,800	27	0	.18	.04	.9	0	470	2 oz	60
.9	.2	150	200	.04	.04	.4	21	82	1 cup	144
.8	.6	89	280	.02	.02	.3	16	85	1 cup	140
.5	—	—	40	0.01	0.01	0.2	13	245	1 cup	249

TABLES OF FOOD
CONSTITUENTS OF 100 g

Name	Calories	Water, g	Protein, g	Fat, g	Ash, g	Total carbohydrates, g	Crude fiber, g	Calcium, mg	Phosphorus, mg
PROXIMATE COMPOSITION								**MINERALS**	
FRUITS—Continued									
Cranberries, raw	48	87.4	.4	.7	.2	11.3	1.4	14	11
Cranberry sauce, cnd., sweet	198	48.1	.1	.3	.1	51.4	.4	8	7
Currants, red, raw	55	84.4	1.2	.2	.6	13.6	4.0	36	33
Gooseberries	39	88.9	.8	.2	.4	9.7	1.9	22	28
Loganberries, raw	62	82.9	1.0	.6	.5	15.0	1.4	35	19
Raspberries, black, raw	74	80.6	1.5	1.6	.6	15.7	6.8	40	37
Raspberries, red, raw	57	84.1	1.2	.4	.5	13.8	4.7	40	37
Raspberries, red, frz.	98	74.3	.7	.2	.2	24.7	2.1	12	17
Strawberries, raw	37	89.9	.8	.5	.5	8.3	1.4	28	27
Strawberries, frozen	95	74.8	.5	.2	.2	24.4	.6	13	16
Citrus fruit									
Grapefruit, raw	40	88.8	.5	.2	.4	10.1	.3	22	18
Grapefruit, cnd., sw.	72	79.8	.6	.2	.4	19.1	.2	13	14
Lemons	32	89.3	.9	.6	.5	8.7	.9	40	22
Limes	37	86.0	.8	.1	.8	12.3	.9	40	22
Oranges	45	87.2	.9	.2	.5	11.2	.6	33	23
Tangerines	44	87.3	.8	.3	.7	10.9	1.0	33	23
Melons									
Cantaloupes	20	94.0	.6	.2	.6	4.6	.6	17	16
Honeydew	32	90.5	.5	.0	.5	8.5	.4	17	16
Watermelon	28	92.1	.5	.2	.3	6.9	.6	7	12
Tree, vine, and other fruits									
Apples, raw	58	84.1	.3	.4	.3	14.9	1.0	6	10
Apples, dry, unckd.	277	23	1.4	1.0	1.4	73.2	3.9	19	48
Apricots, raw	51	85.4	1.0	.1	.6	12.9	.6	16	23
Apricots, cnd., sw.	80	77.3	.6	.1	.6	21.4	.4	10	15
Apricots, dry	262	24	5.2	.4	3.5	66.9	3.2	86	119
Avocado	245	65.4	1.7	26.4	1.4	5.1	1.8	10	38
Bananas	88	74.8	1.2	.2	.8	23	.6	8	28
Cherries, all, raw	61	83.0	1.1	.5	.6	14.8	.3	18	20
Cherries, red, sour, canned	48	86.6	.8	.3	.4	11.9	.1	11	12
Dates, dried	284	20	2.2	.6	1.8	75.4	2.4	72	60
Figs, cnd., sw.	113	68.5	.8	.3	.4	30.0	.9	35	21
Figs, dried	270	24	4.0	1.2	2.4	68.4	5.8	186	111

COMPOSITION
OF EDIBLE PORTION

MINERALS			VITAMINS					AVERAGE PORTION		
Iron, mg	Sodium, mg	Potas- sium, mg	A, IU	B₁, mg	B₂, mg	Nico- tinic acid, mg	C, mg	Total calories	Measure	Weight in grams
.6	1	65	40	.03	.02	.1	12	54	1 cup	113
.3	1	17	30	.02	.02	.1	2	550	1 cup	277
.9	2	160	120	.04	—	—	36	30	¹/₂ cup	55
.5	.7	87	290	—	—	—	33	59	1 cup	150
1.2	—	—	200	.03	.07	.3	24	90	1 cup	144
.9	.3	190	0	.02	.07	.3	24	100	1 cup	134
.9	.5	130	130	.02	.07	.3	24	70	1 cup	123
.6	.7	97	80	.02	.07	.6	21	84	3 oz	86
.8	.8	180	60	.03	.07	.3	60	54	1 cup	149
.6	1.5	107	33	.02	.06	.5	43	82	3 oz	86
.2	.5	200	Tr.	.04	.02	.2	40	77	1 cup sections	194
.3	—	—	Tr.	.03	.02	.2	30	181	1 cup	249
.6	.7	130	0	.04	Tr.	.1	50	20	1, 2″ diam.	100
.6	1	100	—	.04	Tr.	.1	27	19	1, 1¹/₂″ long	68
.4	.3	170	190	.08	.03	.2	49	70	1 med., 3″ diam.	215
.4	2	110	420	.07	.03	.2	31	35	1 med., 2¹/₂″ diam.	114
.4	12	230	3,420	.05	.04	.5	33	37	¹/₂, 5″ diam.	385
.4	—	—	40	.05	.03	.2	23	49	1, 2 × 7″ wedge	150
.2	.3	110	590	.05	.05	.2	6	97	¹/₂ sl., ³/₄×10″	345
.3	.2	74	90	.04	.03	.2	5	87	1 med. (2¹/₂″ diam.)	150
1.4	—	—	0	.10	.10	1.0	12	315	1 cup	114
.5	.6	440	2,790	.03	.05	.8	7	54	3	114
.3	2	65	1,350	.02	.02	.3	4	97	4 med. halves, 2 tbsp	122
4.9	11	1,700	7,430	.01	.16	3.3	12	280	40 halves	150
.6	3	340	290	.06	.13	1.1	16	280	¹/₂, 3¹/₂ × 3¹/₄″	114
.6	.5	420	430	.04	.05	.7	10	132	1 med., 6×1¹/₂″	150
.4	1	260	620	.05	.06	.4	8	94	1 cup pitted	154
.3	3	55	720	.03	.02	.2	6	122	1 cup pitted	254
2.1	1	790	60	.09	.10	2.2	0	505	1 cup pitted	177
.4	1	105	50	.03	.03	.4	Tr.	130	3, 2 tbsp syrup	115
3.0	34	780	80	.16	.12	1.7	0	57	1 large, 1×2″	21

TABLES OF FOOD
CONSTITUENTS OF 100 g

Name	PROXIMATE COMPOSITION							MINERALS	
	Cal-ories	Water, g	Pro-tein, g	Fat, g	Ash, g	Total carbohy-drates, g	Crude fiber, g	Calcium, mg	Phos-phorus, mg
FRUITS—Continued									
Grapes, raw									
American (slip skin)	70	81.9	1.4	1.4	.4	14.9	.5	17	21
European									
(adherent skin)	66	81.6	.8	.4	.5	16.7	.5	17	21
Guavas, raw	70	80.6	1.0	.6	.7	17.1	5.5	30	29
Papaya, raw	43	88.3	.6	.1	—	10.0	—	19	13
Peaches, raw	46	86.9	.5	.1	.5	12.0	.6	8	22
Peaches, cnd., sw.	68	80.9	.4	.1	.4	18.2	.4	5	14
Peaches, frz., sw.	88	76.3	.5	.1	.8	22.8	.4	4	12
Peaches, dry, unckd.	265	24	3.0	.6	3.0	69.4	3.5	44	126
Pears, raw	63	82.7	.7	.4	.4	15.8	1.4	13	16
Pears, cnd., sw.	68	81.1	.2	.1	.2	18.4	.8	8	10
Plums, raw	50	85.7	.7	.2	.5	12.9	.5	17	20
Plums, cnd., sw.	76	78.6	.4	.1	.5	20.4	.3	8	12
Prunes, dry	268	24	2.3	.6	2.1	71.0	1.6	54	85
Raisins, dry	268	24	2.3	.5	2.0	71.2	—	78	129
Rhubarb, frz.	74	80.2	.6	.2	.6	19.2	.9	99	14
FRUIT JUICES AND OTHER FRUIT PRODUCTS									
Apple juice, frozen									
or canned	50	85.9	.1	0	.3	13.8	—	6	10
Apple sauce, frz.									
or cnd., sw.	72	79.8	.2	.1	.2	19.7	.6	4	8
Apricot nectar	52	86.1	.3	.1	.5	12.4	.2	9	13
Fruit cocktail,									
canned, sweet	70	80.6	.4	.2	.3	18.6	.4	9	12
Grape juice, cnd., sw.	67	81	.4	0	.4	18.2	—	10	10
Grapefruit juice,									
canned, sweet	52	85.3	.5	.1	.4	13.7	.1	8	13
Lemon juice, cnd.	24	91.4	.4	.2	.3	7.7	0	14	11
Lime juice, fresh	24	91.0	.4	0	.3	8.3	0	14	11
Olives, green	132	75.2	1.5	13.5	5.8	4.0	1.2	87	17
Olives, ripe, Mission	191	71.8	1.8	21.0	2.8	2.6	1.5	87	17
Orange juice, fresh	44	87.5	.8	.2	.4	11.0	.1	19	16
Orange juice, cnd.	44	87.5	.8	.2	.4	11.1	.1	10	18
Orange and grapefruit									
juice, cnd., sw.	52	85.1	.5	.1	.4	13.9	.1	9	15
Pineapple juice, cnd.	49	86.2	.3	.1	.4	13.0	.1	15	8
Prune juice, cnd.	71	80	.4	0	.3	19.3	—	25	40
Tangerine juice, cnd.	39	89.2	.9	.3	.4	9.2	—	19	16
Tomato juice, cnd.	21	93.5	1.0	.2	1.0	4.3	.2	7	15

COMPOSITION
OF EDIBLE PORTION

MINERALS			VITAMINS					AVERAGE PORTION		
Iron, mg	Sodium, mg	Potassium, mg	A, IU	B_1, mg	B_2, mg	Nicotinic acid, mg	C, mg	Total calories	Measure	Weight in grams
.6	3	84	80	.06	.04	.2	4	84	1 cup	153
.6	4	180	80	.06	.04	.2	4	102	1 cup, 40 grapes	160
.7	—	—	250	.07	.04	1.2	302	49	1 small	80
.3	—	—	2,400	.05	.13	—	36	73	1, 2½×7" wedge	170
.6	.5	160	880	.02	.05	.9	8	45	1 med., 2½×2" diam.	114
.4	5	31	450	.01	.02	.7	4	175	1 cup	258
.7	3	124	133	.01	.04	.7	13	99	4 oz	112
6.9	12	1,100	3,250	.01	.20	5.4	19	424	1 cup	160
.3	2	100	20	.02	.04	.1	4	95	1, 3×2½" diam.	182
.2	8	52	Tr.	.01	.02	.1	2	80	2 halves, 2 tbsp syrup	117
.5	.6	170	350	.06	.04	.5	5	30	1, 2" diam.	60
1.1	18	110	230	.03	.03	.4	1	186	1 cup	256
3.9	6	600	1,890	.10	.16	1.7	3	94	4 large	40
3.3	21	720	50	.15	.08	.5	Tr.	430	1 cup	160
.8	6	212	83	.02	.06	.2	7	202	1 cup	273
.5	4	100	40	.02	.03	Tr.	1	124	1 cup	249
.4	.3	55	30	.02	.01	Tr.	1	185	1 cup	254
.3	2.9	98	1,090	Tr.	.01	Tr.	1	170	1 cup	254
.4	9	160	160	.01	.01	.4	2	180	1 cup	257
.3	1	120	—	.04	.05	.2	Tr.	120	6 oz	180
.3	.4	150	Tr.	.03	.02	.2	35	131	1 cup	251
.1	1.1	—	0	.04	Tr.	.1	42	4	1 tbsp	15
.1	—	175	0	.04	Tr.	.1	27	57	1 cup	246
1.6	2,400	55	300	Tr.	—	—	—	72	10 "mammoth"	65
1.6	980	23	60	Tr.	Tr.	—	—	106	10 "mammoth"	65
.2	3.6	182	190	.08	.03	.2	49	108	1 cup	246
.3	.5	190	100	.07	.02	.2	42	135	1 cup	251
.3	.4	170	40	.05	.02	.2	38	132	1 cup	251
.5	.5	140	80	.05	.02	.2	9	121	1 cup	249
1.8	2	260	—	.03	.08	.4	1	170	1 cup	240
.2	.6	170	420	.06	.03	.2	26	95	1 cup	246
.4	230	230	1,050	.05	.03	.8	16	50	1 cup	242

TABLES OF FOOD
CONSTITUENTS OF 100 g

	PROXIMATE COMPOSITION							MINERALS	
Name	Cal- ories	Water, g	Pro- tein, g	Fat, g	Ash, g	Total carbohy- drates, g	Crude fiber, g	Calcium, mg	Phos- phorus, mg
GRAINS AND GRAIN PRODUCTS									
Breakfast									
cereals									
Bran flakes	292	3.6	10.8	1.9	4.9	78.8	3.9	61	622
Corn flakes*	385	3.6	8.1	.4	2.9	85.0	.6	11	58
Farina, ckd.*	44	89.2	1.3	.1	.3	9.1	0	3	13
Oat breakfast cereal*	396	4.0	14.5	7.0	4.3	70.2	2.0	160	350
Oatmeal, ckd.	63	84.8	2.3	1.2	.7	11.0	.2	9	67
Puffed rice*	392	3.5	5.9	.6	2.3	87.7	.5	21	116
Puffed wheat*	355	3.8	10.8	1.6	3.6	80.2	1.7	46	329
Rice flakes*	392	3.5	5.9	.6	2.3	87.7	.5	21	116
Wheat flakes*	355	3.8	10.8	1.6	3.6	80.2	1.7	46	329
Wheat, whole meal*	344	8.2	12.7	1.7	2.1	75.3	2.2	46	392
FLOURS, MEALS, AND OTHER FARINACEOUS MATERIALS									
Barley, pearled, light	349	11.1	8.2	1.0	.9	78.8	.5	16	189
Buckwheat flour, light	348	12	6.4	1.2	.9	79.5	.5	11	88
Corn grits*, ckd.	51	87.1	1.2	.1	.6	11.0	.1	1	10
Cornmeal, whole	362	12	9.0	3.4	1.1	74.5	1.0	6	178
Cornmeal, degermed*	363	12	7.9	1.2	.5	78.4	.6	6	99
Farina*	370	10.5	10.9	.8	.4	77.4	.4	28	112
Flour, rye, dark	318	11	16.3	2.6	2.0	68.1	2.4	54	536
Flour, wheat, 80% extn.	365	12	12.0	1.3	.7	74.1	.5	24	191
Flour, wheat, self-rising*	350	12	9.2	1.0	4.0	73.8	.4	272	484
Flour, wheat, all-purpose*	364	12	10.5	1.0	.4	76.1	.3	16	87
Flour, wheat, cake	364	12	7.5	.8	.3	79.4	.2	17	73
Rice, brown	360	12	7.5	1.7	1.1	77.7	.6	39	303
Rice, converted	362	12	7.6	.3	.4	79.4	.2	24	136
Rice, white	362	12.3	7.6	.3	.4	79.4	.2	24	136
Soybean flour, defatted	228	11.0	44.7	1.1	5.5	37.7	2.3	265	623
Starch, pure	362	12	.5	.2	.3	87	.1	0	0
Tapioca, dry	360	12.6	.6	.2	.2	86.4	.1	12	12
Wheat germ	361	11.0	25.2	10.0	4.3	49.5	2.5	84	1,096
Wild rice	364	8.5	14.1	.7	1.4	75.3	1.0	19	339
BAKED AND COOKED PRODUCTS									
Breads									
Boston brown*	219	44.5	4.8	2.1	2.6	46.0	.3	185	158
Cracked wheat*	259	36.0	8.5	2.2	1.9	51.4	.5	83	126
French or Vienna*	270	35.5	8.1	2.7	1.7	52.0	.2	24	71
Raisin*	284	30.2	7.1	3.1	1.8	57.8	.2	80	104

*Enriched, fortified, or restored to legal standard when one exists.

COMPOSITION
OF EDIBLE PORTION

MINERALS			VITAMINS					AVERAGE PORTION		
Iron, mg	Sodium, mg	Potassium, mg	A, IU	B₁, mg	B₂, mg	Nicotinic acid, mg	C, mg	Total calories	Measure	Weight in grams
5.1	1,400	1,200	0	.46	.23	8.7	0	117	1 cup	40
2.2	660	160	0	.41	.10	2.2	0	96	1 cup	25
.2	11	10	0	.04	.03	.2	0	105	1 cup	238
4.1	—	—	0	.82	.19	1.9	0	100	1 cup	25
.7	.3	55	0	.10	.02	.2	0	150	1 cup	238
1.8	.9	100	0	.46	.08	5.5	0	55	1 cup	14
4.2	4	340	0	.56	.18	6.4	0	43	1 cup	12
1.8	720	180	0	.46	.08	5.5	0	117	1 cup	30
4.2	1,300	320	0	.56	.18	6.4	0	125	1 cup	35
3.4	2	380	0	.55	.15	4.4	0	103	¼ cup	30
2.0	3	160	0	.12	.08	3.1	0	710	1 cup	204
1.0	—	—	0	.08	.04	.4	0	342	1 cup	98
.3	—	—	40	.04	.03	.4	0	122	1 cup	242
1.8	—	—	440	.30	.08	1.9	0	459	1 cup	127
2.9	.7	120	300	.44	.26	3.5	0	527	1 cup	145
1.3	2	86	0	.37	.26	1.3	0	625	1 cup	169
4.5	1	860	0	.61	.22	2.7	0	285	1 cup	80
1.3	1	120	0	.26	.07	2.0	0	400	1 cup, stirred	110
2.9	1,500	90	0	.44	.26	3.5	0	384	1 cup, stirred	110
2.9	1	86	0	.44	.26	3.5	0	400	1 cup, stirred	110
.5	—	—	0	.03	.03	.7	0	364	1 cup, stirred	100
2.0	9	150	0	.32	.05	4.6	0	748	1 cup	208
.8	4	170	0	.20	.03	3.8	0	677	1 cup	187
.8	2	130	0	.07	.03	1.6	0	692	1 cup	191
13.0	—	—	70	1.10	.35	2.9	0			
0	4	4	0	0	0	0	0	29	1 tbsp	8
1.0	5	19	0	0	0	0	0	547	1 cup	152
8.1	2	780	0	2.05	.80	4.6	0	246	1 cup	68
—	7	220	0	.45	.63	6.2	0	593	1 cup	163
2.9	280	360	140	.13	.17	1.9	0	105	1, ¾″ slice	48
2.0	620	250	0	.25	.19	2.5	0	60	1, ½″ slice	23
1.8	—	—	0	.24	.15	2.2	0	1225	1 lb	453
1.8	—	—	10	.24	.15	2.2	0	65	1, ½″ slice	23

TABLES OF FOOD
CONSTITUENTS OF 100 g

| | | | | | | Total | | | |
Name	Cal-ories	Water, g	Pro-tein, g	Fat, g	Ash, g	carbohy-drates, g	Crude fiber, g	Calcium, mg	Phos-phorus, mg
PROXIMATE COMPOSITION								**MINERALS**	
BAKED AND COOKED PRODUCTS—Continued									
Rye (¹/₃ rye flour)	244	35.3	9.1	1.2	2.0	52.4	.4	72	147
White, 4% nonfat milk solids*	275	34.7	8.5	3.2	1.8	51.8	.2	79	92
Whole wheat	240	36.6	9.3	2.6	2.5	49.0	1.5	96	263
Bread crumbs, dry	385	8.5	11.9	4.5	2.6	72.5	.2	111	129
Cakes									
Angel food	270	31.6	8.4	.3	1.0	58.7	0	6	24
Foundation	350	25.1	5.9	11.7	1.4	55.9	.1	126	120
Fruit, dark	354	22.9	5.2	13.8	2.2	55.9	1.2	97	126
Plain	327	26.8	6.4	8.2	1.6	57.0	.1	155	137
Sponge	291	31.8	7.9	5.0	.9	54.4		28	110
Corn bread*	219	49.2	6.7	4.7	2.8	36.6	.2	139	155
Crackers, graham	393	5.5	8.0	10.0	2.2	74.3	.8	20	203
Crackers, saltines	431	4.6	9.2	11.8	3.3	71.1	.4	19	92
Custard, baked	114	77.3	5.3	5.4	.8	11.2	0	114	119
Doughnuts	425	18.7	6.6	21.0	1.0	52.7	.2	73	286
Fig bars	350	13.8	4.2	4.8	1.4	75.8	1.7	69	69
Gingerbread	327	30.4	3.9	12.0	2.1	51.6	.1	114	71
Macaroni,* dry	377	8.6	12.8	1.4	.7	76.5	.4	22	165
Macaroni and cheese, ckd.	211	58.1	8.1	11.0	3.1	19.7	.1	191	169
Muffins*	280	37.4	8.0	8.4	2.2	42.1	.1	206	191
Noodles (egg), ckd.	67	83.8	2.2	.6	.6	12.8	.1	4	35
Pancakes, wheat*	218	55.4	6.8	9.2	2.0	26.6	.1	158	154
Pancakes, buckwheat	176	62.0	6.1	8.4	2.6	20.9	.5	249	362
Pies									
Apple	246	47.8	2.1	9.5	1.1	39.5	.7	7	24
Mince	252	43.0	2.5	6.9	2.0	45.6	.5	16	40
Pumpkin	202	58.9	4.2	9.6	1.5	25.8	.6	54	81
Pretzels	369	8.0	8.8	3.2	5.5	74.5	.3	12	71
Rolls, plain*	309	28.5	9.0	5.5	1.9	55.1	.2	55	96
Rolls, sweet	323	28.4	8.5	7.8	1.5	53.8	.2	63	104
Rye wafers	324	6.5	12.4	1.2	4.6	75.3	2.1	50	400
Spaghetti,* cooked	149	60.6	5.1	.6	3.5	30.2	.2	9	65
Waffles*	287	40	9.3	10.6	2.3	37.8	.1	192	204
NUTS AND NUT PRODUCTS									
Almonds, dry	597	4.7	18.6	54.1	3.0	19.6	2.7	254	475
Brazil nuts, shelled	646	5.3	14.4	65.9	3.4	11.0	2.1	186	693
Cashews, roasted	578	3.6	18.5	48.2	2.7	27.0	1.3	46	428

*Enriched, fortified, or restored to legal standard when one exists.

COMPOSITION
OF EDIBLE PORTION

MINERALS			VITAMINS					AVERAGE PORTION		
Iron, mg	Sodium, mg	Potassium, mg	A, IU	B₁, mg	B₂, mg	Nicotinic acid, mg	C, mg	Total calories	Measure	Weight in grams
1.6	590	160	0	.18	.08	1.5	0	57	1, ½" slice	23
1.8	640	180	0	.24	.15	2.2	0	63	1, ½" slice	23
2.2	930	230	0	.30	.13	3.0	0	55	1, ½" slice	23
2.6	—	—	0	.27	.22	3.1	0	339	1 cup	88
.3	—	—	0	.01	.14	.2	0	110	2" sec. of 8" cake	41
.5	—	—	160	.03	.08	.2	0	230	1 sq., 3×2×1¾"	66
2.8	—	—	160	.14	.14	1.1	0	106	2×2×½"	30
.4	—	—	120	.03	.08	.3	0	161	1, 2¾" cupcake	50
1.4	—	—	520	.05	.15	.2	0	117	2" sec. of 8" cake	40
1.9	—	—	130	.17	.23	1.3	0	103	1, 2¾" muffin	48
1.9	710	330	0	.30	.12	1.5	0	55	2 medium	14
1.0	1,100	120	0	.06	.04	1.0	0	34	2, 2" square	8
.5	—	—	340	.05	.20	.1	Tr.	283	1 custard cup	248
.7	—	—	140	.16	.13	1.2	0	136	1	32
1.3	—	—	0	.02	.06	.9	0	87	1 large bar	25
2.5	—	—	100	.04	.08	1.0	0	180	1, 2" cube	55
2.9	1	160	0	.88	.37	6.0	0	463	1 cup dry	123
.5	—	—	450	.03	.16	.4	Tr.	464	1 cup	220
1.6	—	—	100	.18	.21	1.5	0	135	1, 2¾" muffin	48
.5	—	—	30	.14	.06	1.0	0	107	1 cup	60
1.3	—	—	200	.18	.21	1.3	Tr.	60	1, 4" diam.	27
1.2	—	—	110	.16	.16	.9	Tr.	48	1, 4" diam.	27
.4	—	—	160	.03	.02	.2	1	330	4" sec. of 9" pie	220
2.2	—	—	10	.07	.04	.4	1	340	4" sec. of 9" pie	135
.8	—	—	1,910	.03	.12	.3	0	265	4" sec. of 9" pie	131
.7	1,700	130	0	.01	.04	.7	0	18	5 small sticks	5
1.8	—	—	0	.24	.15	2.2	0	120	1 (¹⁄₁₂ lb)	39
1.8	—	—	0	.24	.15	2.2	0	178	1	55
4.4	1,500	600	0	.32	.20	1.2	0	43	2	13
1.1	—	—	0	.17	.10	1.4	0	220	1 cup	148
1.8	—	—	360	.18	.27	1.3	0	216	1, 4½×5⅝×½"	75
4.4	160*	710*	0	.25	.67	4.6	Tr.	850	1 cup	140
3.4-	1	670	Tr.	.86	—	—	—	905	1 cup	140
5.0	200*	560*	—	.63	.19	2.1	—	810	1 cup	140

*When roasted and salted.

TABLES OF FOOD
CONSTITUENTS OF 100 g

	PROXIMATE COMPOSITION							MINERALS	
Name	Cal-ories	Water, g	Pro-tein, g	Fat, g	Ash, g	Total carbohy-drates, g	Crude fiber, g	Calcium, mg	Phos-phorus, mg
NUTS AND NUT PRODUCTS—Continued									
Chestnuts, fresh	191	53.2	2.8	1.5	1.0	41.5	1.1	48	48
Coconut, dry, sw.	556	3.3	3.6	39.1	.8	53.2	4.1	43	191
Peanuts, roasted	559	2.6	26.9	44.2	2.7	23.6	2.4	74	393
Peanut butter	576	1.7	26.1	47.8	3.4	21.0	2.0	74	393
Pecans, raw	696	3.0	9.4	73.0	1.6	13.0	2.2	74	324
Walnuts, Eng., raw	654	3.3	15.0	64.4	1.7	15.6	2.1	83	380
MEAT									
Beef									
Chuck, ckd.	309	51	26	22	.7	0	0	11	117
Hamburger, ckd.	364	47	22	30	1.1	0	0	9	158
Porterhouse, ckd.	342	49	23	27	1.1	0	0	11	170
Rib roast, ckd.	319	51	24	24	1.2	0	0	10	185
Round, ckd.	233	59	27	13	1.3	0	0	11	224
Corned beef, cnd.	216	59.3	25.3	12	3.4	0	0	20	106
Corned beef hash, cnd.	141	70.4	13.7	6.1	2.6	7.2	.2	26	146
Dried or chipped beef	203	47.7	34.3	6.3	11.6	0	0	20	404
Roast beef, cnd.	224	60	25	13	2	0	0	16	116
Lamb									
Med. fat, raw	317	55.8	15.7	27.7	.8	0	0	9	157
Rib chop, raw	356	51.9	14.9	32.4	.8	0	0	9	138
Rib chop, ckd.	418	40	24	35	1.2	0	0	11	200
Leg roast, raw	235	63.7	18.0	17.5	.9	0	0	10	213
Leg roast, ckd.	274	56	24	19	1.1	0	0	10	257
Pork									
Bacon, fried	607	13	25	55	6	1	0	25	255
Bacon, Canadian, raw	231	56	22.1	15	6.2	.3	0	13	210
Ham, fresh, raw	344	53	15.2	31	.8	0	0	9	168
Ham, cured, ckd.	397	39	23	33	5.4	.4	0	10	166
Pork luncheon meat, cnd.	289	55.2	14.9	24.3	4.1	1.5	.2	9	161
Veal									
Veal, med. fat	190	68	19.1	12	1.0	0	0	11	193
Veal cutlet, ckd.	219	60	28	11	1.4	0	0	12	258
Stew meat, ckd.	296	53	25	21	.8	0	0	11	124
VARIETY MEATS AND MIXTURES									
Brains	125	78.9	10.4	8.6	1.4	.8	0	16	330
Chili con carne	200	66.9	10.3	14.8	2.2	5.8	.2	38	152
Heart, beef, raw	108	77.6	16.9	3.7	1.1	.7	0	9	203

COMPOSITION
OF EDIBLE PORTION

MINERALS			VITAMINS					AVERAGE PORTION		
Iron, mg	Sodium, mg	Potas- sium, mg	A, IU	B$_1$, mg	B$_2$, mg	Nico- tinic acid, mg	C, mg	Total calories	Measure	Weight in grams
4.1	2	410	0	.08	.24	1.0	0	95	20	250
3.6	16	770	0	Tr.	Tr.	Tr.	0	344	1 cup shreds	62
1.9	460*	700*	0	.30	.13	16.2	0	805	1 cup	144
1.9	120	820	0	.12	.13	16.2	0	92	1 tbsp	16
2.4	.3	420	50	.72	.11	.9	2	752	1 cup of halves	108
2.1	2	450	30	.48	.13	1.2	3	654	1 cup of halves	100
3.1	51	360	0	.05	.20	4.1	0	265	3 oz	86
2.8	107	345	0	.08	.19	4.8	0	316	3 oz	86
3.0	69	334	0	.06	.18	4.7	0	293	3 oz	86
3.0	107	345	0	.06	.18	4.3	0	266	3 oz	86
3.4	68	400	0	.08	.22	5.5	0	197	3 oz	86
4.3	1,300	60	0	.02	.24	3.4	0	180	3 oz	86
1.3	540	200	Tr.	.03	.14	2.9	0	120	3 oz	86
5.1	4,300	200	0	.07	.32	3.8	0	115	2 oz	56
2.4	—	—	0	.02	.23	4.2	0	189	3 oz	86
2.4	—	—	0	.14	.20	4.5	0	273	3 oz	86
2.2	98	340	0	.13	.18	4.3	0	409	4 oz	115
3.0	—	—	0	.14	.26	5.6	0	480	4 oz	115
2.7	78	380	0	.16	.22	5.2	0	202	3 oz	86
3.1	—	—	0	.14	.25	5.1	0	314	3 oz	86
3.3	2,400	390	0	.48	.31	4.8	0	97	2 slices	16
3.3	—	—	0	.91	.25	5.2	0	262	4 oz	115
2.3	—	—	0	.74	.18	4.0	0	296	3 oz	86
2.9	1,100	340	0	.54	.21	4.2	0	340	3 oz	86
2.2	—	—	0	.32	.22	2.8	0	165	2 oz	57
2.9	48	330	0	.14	.25	6.4	0	219	4 oz	115
3.5	—	—	0	.08	.28	6.1	0	184	3 oz	86
3.0	—	—	0	.05	.24	4.6	0	252	3 oz	86
3.6	150	340	0	.23	.26	4.4	18	106	3 oz	86
1.4	—	—	150	.02	.12	2.2	—	170	1/3 cup	85
4.6	90	160	30	.58	.89	7.8	6	92	3 oz	86

*When roasted and salted.

TABLES OF FOOD
CONSTITUENTS OF 100 g

| | | | | | | PROXIMATE COMPOSITION | | MINERALS | |
NAME	Cal-ories g	Water, g	Pro-tein, g	Fat, g	Ash, g	Total carbohy-drates, g	Crude fiber, g	Calcium, mg	Phos-phorus, mg
VARIETY MEATS AND MIXTURES—Continued									
Kidneys, beef, raw	141	74.9	15.0	8.1	1.1	.9	0	9	221
Liver, beef, raw	136	69.7	19.7	3.2	1.4	6.0	0	7	358
Liver, beef, fried	208	57.2	23.6	7.7	1.8	9.7	0	8	486
Liver, calf, raw	141	70.8	19.0	4.9	1.3	4.0	0	6	343
Liver, pork, raw	134	72.3	19.7	4.8	1.5	1.7	0	10	362
Sausage, bologna	221	62.4	14.8	15.9	3.3	3.6	—	9	112
Sausage, frankfurter, cooked	248	62	14	20	2	2	—	6	49
Sausage, liverwurst	263	59.0	16.7	20.6	2.2	1.5	—	9	238
Sausage, pork, raw	450	41.9	10.8	44.8	2.1	0	0	6	100
Sweetbreads, cooked	178	67.2	22.7	9.1	—	0	0	14	596
Tongue, beef	207	68	16.4	15	.9	.4	0	9	187
FISH AND SEAFOODS									
Bluefish, baked	155	69.2	27.4	4.2	1.9	0	0	23	293
Caviar, sturgeon	243	57.0	26.9	15.0	—	—	0	30	300
Clams, raw	81	80.3	12.8	1.4	2.1	3.4	0	96	139
Cod, raw	74	82.6	16.5	.4	1.2	0	0	10	194
Cod, dried	375	12.3	81.8	2.8	7.0	0	0	50	891
Crabs, cnd. or ckd.	104	77.2	16.9	2.9	1.7	1.3	0	45	182
Flounder, raw	68	82.7	14.9	.5	1.3	0	0	61	195
Frog legs, raw	73	81.9	16.4	.3	1.1	0	0	18	147
Haddock, ckd.	158	66.9	18.7	5.5	1.9	7.0	0	18	182
Halibut, raw	126	75.4	18.6	5.2	1.0	0	0	13	211
Halibut, ckd.	182	64.2	26.2	7.8	1.9	0	0	14	267
Herring, raw	191	67.2	18.3	12.5	2.7	0	0	10	256
Herring, kippered	211	61.0	22.2	12.9	4.0	0	0	66	254
Lobster, raw	88	79.2	16.2	1.9	2.2	.5	0	61	184
Lobster, cnd.	92	77.2	18.4	1.3	2.7	.4	0	65	192
Mackerel, cnd.	182	66.0	19.3	11.1	3.2	0	0	185	274
Oysters, raw	84	80.5	9.8	2.1	2.0	5.6	0	94	143
Oyster stew	91	82.6	5.3	5.4	1.4	5.3	0	117	110
Salmon, raw	223	63.4	17.4	16.5	1.0	0	0	—	289
Salmon, cnd.	203	64.7	19.7	13.2	2.4	0	0	154	289
Sardines, cnd.	214	57.4	25.7	11.0	4.7	1.2	0	386	586
Pilchards, cnd.	200	65.2	17.7	13.5	2.9	.7	0	381	168
Scallops, raw	78	80.3	14.8	.1	1.4	3.4	0	26	208
Shad, raw	168	70.2	18.7	9.8	1.4	0	0	—	260
Shrimp, cnd.	127	66.2	26.8	1.4	5.8	—	0	115	263
Swordfish, ckd.	178	64.8	27.4	6.8	1.7	0	0	20	251
Tuna fish, cnd.	198	60.0	29.0	8.2	2.7	0	0	8	351

COMPOSITION
OF EDIBLE PORTION

MINERALS			VITAMINS					AVERAGE PORTION		
Iron, mg	Sodium, mg	Potas- sium, mg	A, IU	B₁, mg	B₂, mg	Nico- tinic acid, mg	C, mg	Total calories	Measure	Weight in grams
7.9	210	310	1,150	.37	2.55	6.4	13	120	3 oz	86
6.6	110	380	43,900	.26	3.33	13.7	31	117	3 oz	86
7.8	—	—	53,500	.26	3.96	14.8	31	118	2 oz	57
10.6	110	380	22,500	.21	3.12	16.1	36	121	3 oz	86
18.0	77	350	14,200	.40	2.98	16.7	23	115	3 oz	86
2.2	1,300	230	0	.18	.19	2.7	0	117	2 slices, ⅛×4″	211
1.2	1,100	220	0	.16	.18	2.5	0	124	1, 7×¾″	51
5.4	892	149	5,750	.17	1.12	4.6	0	150	2 oz	57
1.6	740	140	0	.43	.17	2.3	0	158	2, 3½″ long	35
1.6	69	243	—	.08				204	4 oz	115
2.8	100	260	0	.12	.29	5.0	0	235	4 oz	115
.7	—	—	—	.12	.11	2.2	—	178	4 oz	115
1.4	—	—	—	—	—	—	—	208	3 oz	86
7.0	180	240	110	.10	.18	1.6	—	92	4 oz	115
.4	60	360	0	.06	.09	2.2	2	85	4 oz	115
3.6	8,100	160	0	.08	.45	10.9	0	106	1 oz	28
.9	1,000	110	—	.05	.06	2.5	—	90	3 oz	86
.8	—	—	—	.06	.05	1.7	—	78	4 oz	115
1.1	—	—	0	.14	.25	1.2	—	82	4 oz	115
.6	—	—	—	.04	.09	2.6	—	158	1 fillet, 4×3×½″	100
.7	56	540	440	.07	.06	9.2	—	145	4 oz	115
.8	—	—	—	.06	.07	10.5	—	230	1 fillet, 4×3×½″	126
1.1	—	—	110	.02	.15	3.4	—	191	1 small	100
1.4	—	—	0	Tr.	.28	2.9	—	211	1 small	100
.6	210	180	—	.13	.06	1.9	—	88	½ average	100
.8	—	—	—	.03	.07	2.2	—	78	3 oz	86
2.1	—	—	430	.06	.21	5.8	—	155	3 oz	86
5.6	73	110	320	.15	.20	1.2	—	200	13–19 med., 1 cup	238
1.5	—	—	280	.06	.18	.4	—	244	1 cup, 6–8 oysters	240
.9	48	410	310	.10	.23	7.2	9	192	3 oz	86
.9	540	300	230	.03	.14	7.3	0	120	3 oz	86
2.7	510	560	220	.02	.17	4.8	0	182	3 oz, drained	86
4.1	760	260	30	.01	.30	7.4	0	171	3 oz	86
1.8	150	420	0	.04	.10	1.4	—	90	4 oz	115
.5	—	—	—	.15	.24	8.4	—	191	4 oz	115
3.1	140	220	60	.01	.03	2.2	0	110	3 oz	86
1.1	—	—	2,300	.05	.06	10.3	0	223	1 steak, 3×3×½″	125
1.4	800	240	80	.05	.12	12.8	0	170	3 oz, drained solids	86

TABLES OF FOOD
CONSTITUENTS OF 100 g

						PROXIMATE COMPOSITION		MINERALS	
Name	Cal-ories	Water, g	Pro-tein, g	Fat, g	Ash, g	Total carbohy-drates, g	Crude fiber, g	Calcium, mg	Phos-phorus, mg
POULTRY AND EGGS									
Chicken, fryers, raw	112	74.5	20.5	2.7	1.1	0	0	15	188
Chicken, roasters, raw	200	66.0	20.2	12.6	1.0	0	0	14	200
Chicken, cnd.	199	61.9	29.8	8.0	2.4	0	0	14	148
Chicken liver	141	69.6	22.1	4.0	1.7	2.6	0	16	240
Duck	322	54.3	16.1	28.6	1.0	0	—	9	172
Goose	366	49.7	15.9	33.6	.9	0	0	9	176
Turkey	268	58.3	20.1	20.2	1.0	0	0	23	320
Eggs, raw									
White	50	87.8	10.8	0	.6	.8	0	6	17
Yolk	361	49.4	16.3	31.9	1.7	.7	0	147	586
Whole	162	74.0	12.8	11.5	1.0	.7	0	54	210
Eggs, dried									
White	398	3	85.9	0	4.8	6.3	0	48	135
Yolk	693	3	31.2	61.2	3.3	1.3	0	282	1,123
Whole	592	5	46.8	42.0	3.6	2.5	0	190	767
SUGARS AND SWEETS									
Candied peel									
Citron	314	18.0	.2	.3	1.3	80.2	1.4	83	24
Ginger root	340	12	.3	.2	.4	87.1	.7	—	—
Lemon, orange, or									
grapefruit	316	17.4	.4	.3	1.3	80.6	2.3	—	—
Butterscotch	410	5.0	0	8.9	.5	85.6	0	20	7
Caramels	415	7.0	2.9	11.6	1	77.5	0	126	90
Chocolate, sweetened,									
milk	503	1.1	6	33.5	1.7	55.7	.5	216	283
Chocolate, with almonds	532	.6	8	38.6	1.8	50.0	.6	206	249
Chocolate creams	394	9	4	14	1	72	—	—	—
Fondant	352	8	0	0	1	91	0	0	0
Fudge, plain	411	5	1.7	11.3	.7	81.3	.3	48	67
Hard candy	383	1	0	0	0	99	0	0	0
Marshmallows	325	15	3	0	1	81	—	0	0
Peanut brittle	441	2	8.3	15.5	1.3	72.8	.8	38	124
Chocolate, bitter	501	2.3	5.5	52.9	3.2	29.2	2.6	98	446
Chocolate, plain, sw.	471	1.4	2	29.8	1.4	62.7	1.4	63	287
Chocolate syrup	209	39.0	1.2	1.1	.6	56.6	.6	15	86
Cocoa, breakfast	293	3.9	8	23.8	5.0	48.9	4.6	125	712
Cocoa beverage, all									
milk	95	79.0	3.8	4.6	.9	10.9	.1	119	114
Honey	294	20	.3	0	.2	79.5	—	5	16

COMPOSITION
OF EDIBLE PORTION

MINERALS			VITAMINS					AVERAGE PORTION		
Iron, mg	Sodium, mg	Potas- sium, mg	A, IU	B$_1$, mg	B$_2$, mg	Nico- tinic acid, mg	C, mg	Total calories	Measure	Weight in grams
1.8	78	320	0	.10	.24	5.6	0	210	1 breast	224
1.5	110	250	0	.08	.16	8.0	0	227	4 oz	115
1.8	—	—	0	.04	.16	6.4	0	169	3 oz	86
7.4	51	160	32,200	.20	2.46	11.8	20	106	2 med. livers	75
2.4	—	—	—	.12	.40	7.9	8	370	4 oz	115
2.4	—	—	—	.14	—	—	13	420	4 oz	115
3.8	40–92	310–320	Tr.	.09	.14	8.0	0	304	4 oz	115
.2	110	100	0	0	.26	.1	0	15	1 white	31
7.2	26	100	3,210	.27	.35	Tr.	0	61	1 yolk	17
2.7	81	100	1,140	.10	.29	.1	0	77	1 medium egg	54
1.6	—	—	0	0	2.05	.7	0	223	1 cup whites	56
13.8	—	—	5,540	.50	.66	.1	0	666	1 cup yolks	96
8.8	—	—	3,740	.34	1.06	.2	0	640	1 cup	108
.8	290	120	—	—	—	—	—	89	1 oz	28
—	—	—	—	—	—	—	—	85	1 small piece	25
—	50	12	—	—	—	—	—	32	1 small piece	10
1.8	—	—	0	0	Tr.	Tr.	0	20	$^3/_4$" sq. × $^3/_8$"	5
2.3	—	—	170	.02	.14	.1	Tr.	42	$^7/_8$" sq. × $^1/_2$"	10
4.0	86	420	150	.10	.38	.8	0	30	$^3/_4$×1$^1/_2$×$^1/_4$"	6
2.9	—	—	140	.13	.51	1.1	0	32	$^3/_4$×1$^1/_2$×$^1/_4$"	6
—	10	110	—	—	—	—	0	55	1$^1/_4$" diam. × $^3/_4$"	14
0	—	—	0	0	0	0	0	28	1" sq. × $^5/_8$"	8
.3	—	—	220	.01	.07	.1	Tr.	185	2" sq. × $^5/_8$"	45
0	—	—	0	0	0	0	0	31	3, $^3/_4$" diam.	8
0	41	6	0	0	0	0	0	98	5, 1$^1/_4$" diam.	30
2.0	—	—	30	.09	.05	4.9	0	66	1$^1/_2$×3"	15
4.4	4	830	60	.05	.24	1.1	0	30	$^3/_4$×1$^1/_2$×$^1/_4$"	6
2.8	35	230	30	.03	.15	.6	0	28	$^3/_4$×1$^1/_2$×$^1/_4$"	6
1.4	60	130	—	—	—	—	—	40	1 tbsp	19
11.6	57	1,400	30	.12	.38	2.3	0	15	2 tsp	5
.4	—	—	160	.04	.19	.2	1	236	1 cup	250
.9	7	10	0	Tr.	.04	.2	4	62	1 tbsp	21

TABLES OF FOOD
CONSTITUENTS OF 100 g

Name	Cal-ories	Water, g	Pro-tein, g	Fat, g	Ash, g	Total carbohy-drates, g	Crude fiber, g	Calcium, mg	Phos-phorus, mg
PROXIMATE COMPOSITION								**MINERALS**	
SUGARS AND SWEETS—Continued									
Jams, marmalades, etc.	278	28	.5	.3	.4	70.8	.6	12	12
Jellies	252	34.5	.2	0	.3	65.0	0	12	12
Molasses, cane, light	252	24	—	—	6.3	65	—	165	45
Molasses, cane blackstrap	213	24	—	—	.5	55	—	579	85
Syrup, table blends	286	25	0	0	.6	74	—	46	16
Sugars, cane or beet	385	.5	0	0	0	99.5	0	—	—
Sugar, brown	370	3	0	0	1.2	95.5	—	76	37
Corn sugar	348	7.5	—	—	.3	90	—	—	—
Maple sugar	348	7.5	—	—	.9	90	—	—	—
ROOT AND TUBER VEGETABLES									
Beets, red, raw	42	87.6	1.6	.1	1.1	9.6	.9	27	43
Beets, cooked	41	88.3	1.0	.1	.8	9.8	.8	21	31
Beets, canned	34	90.3	.9	.1	.8	7.9	.5	15	29
Carrots, raw	42	88.2	1.2	.3	1.0	9.3	1.1	39	37
Carrots, canned	30	91.5	.6	.5	1.0	6.4	.8	26	26
Parsnips, raw	78	78.6	1.5	.5	1.2	18.2	2.2	57	80
Parsnips, cooked	60	83.5	1.0	.5	1.1	13.9	2.1	57	80
Potatoes, sweet, raw	123	68.5	1.8	.7	1.1	27.9	1.0	30	49
Potatoes, sweet, boiled	123	68.5	1.8	.7	1.1	27.9	1.0	30	49
Potatoes, sweet, candied	179	57.4	1.5	3.6	1.3	36.2	.8	36	45
Potatoes, white, raw	83	77.8	2.0	.1	1.0	19.1	.4	11	56
Potatoes, white, baked	98	73.8	2.4	.1	1.2	22.5	.5	13	66
Potatoes, white, boiled	83	77.8	2.0	.1	1.0	19.1	.4	11	56
Radishes, raw	20	93.6	1.2	.1	1.0	4.2	.7	37	31
Rutabagas, raw	38	89.1	1.1	.1	.8	8.9	1.3	55	41
Rutabagas, cooked	32	90.8	.8	.1	.8	7.5	1.4	55	41
Turnips, raw	32	90.9	1.1	.2	.7	7.1	1.1	40	34
Turnips, cooked	27	92.3	.8	.2	.7	6.0	1.2	40	34
LEAF AND STEM VEGETABLES									
Asparagus, raw	21	93.0	2.2	.2	.7	3.9	.7	21	62
Asparagus, ckd.	20	92.5	2.4	.2	1.3	3.6	.8	19	53
Asparagus, cnd.	18	93.6	1.9	.3	1.3	2.9	.5	18	43

COMPOSITION
OF EDIBLE PORTION

MINERALS			VITAMINS					AVERAGE PORTION		
Iron, mg	Sodium, mg	Potassium, mg	A, IU	B₁, mg	B₂, mg	Nicotinic acid, mg	C, mg	Total calories	Measure	Weight in grams
.3	7–13	8–78	10	.02	.02	.2	6	55	1 tbsp	20
.3	—	—	10	.02	.02	.2	4	50	1 tbsp	20
4.3	80	1,500	—	.07	.06	.2	→	50	1 tbsp	20
11.3	—	—	—	.28	.25	2.1	—	43	1 tbsp	20
4.1	68	4	0	0	.01	.1	0	57	1 tbsp	20
—	.3	0.5	—	—	—	—	—	48	1 tbsp	12
2.6	24	230	0	0	0	0	0	51	1 tbsp	14
—	1	0.4	0	0	0	0	0	45	1 tbsp	13
—	—	—	—	—	—	—	—	104	Piece 1¾×1¼×½"	30
1.0	54	350	20	.02	.05	.4	10	56	1 cup, diced	134
.7	—	—	20	.02	.04	.3	7	68	1 cup, ckd., diced	165
.6	36	120	20	.01	.02	.1	5	82	Canned, 1 cup	246
.8	51	410	12,000	.06	.06	.5	4	45	Grated, 1 cup	110
.6	280	110	17,500	.02	.02	.3	3	44	Diced, 1 cup	145
.7	7	740	0	.08	.12	.2	18	94	⅔ cup, diced	120
.7	—	—	0	.06	.10	.2	12	94	Diced, 1 cup	155
.7	4	530	7,700	.09	.05	.6	22	185	1, 6×1¾"	150
.7	—	—	7,700	.09	.05	.6	20	252	1, 5×2.5"	205
.9	—	—	6,250	.04	.04	.5	9	270	1, 6×1¾", candied	150
.7	.8	410	20	.11	.04	1.2	17	83	1 med., 2½" diam.	100
.8	—	—	20	.11	.05	1.4	17	97	1 med., 2½" diam.	100
.7	—	—	20	.10	.04	1.2	15ɩ	120	1 med.	142
1.0	9	260	30	.03	.02	.3	24	4	4 small	40
.4	5	260	330	.07	.08	.9	36	45	Diced, ¾ cup	120
.4	—	—	350	.05	.07	.7	21	50	Ckd., diced, 1 cup	155
.5	58	230	Tr.	.05	.07	.5	28	43	1 cup, diced	134
.5	58	—	Tr.	.04	.06	.4	18	42	1 cup, diced	155
.9	2	240	1,000	.16	.19	1.4	33	16	6, 6" stalks	75
1.0	—	—	1,040	.13	.17	1.2	23	36	1 cup cut spears	175
1.7	410	130	600	.07	.10	.9	15	22	6 med. spears	126

TABLES OF FOOD
CONSTITUENTS OF 100 g

Name		PROXIMATE COMPOSITION						MINERALS	
	Cal-ories	Water, g	Pro-tein, g	Fat, g	Ash, g	Total carbohy-drates, g	Crude fiber, g	Calcium, mg	Phos-phorus, mg
LEAF AND STEM VEGETABLES—Continued									
Beet greens, raw	27	90.4	2.0	.3	1.7	5.6	1.4	118	45
Beet greens, ckd.	27	90.4	2.0	.3	1.7	5.6	1.4	118	45
Brussels sprouts, raw	47	84.9	4.4	.5	1.3	8.9	1.3	34	78
Brussels sprouts, ckd.	47	84.9	4.4	.5	1.3	8.9	1.3	34	78
Brussels sprouts, frz.	36	88.4	3.3	.2	.9	7.3	1.3	31	64
Cabbage, raw	24	92.4	1.4	.2	.8	5.3	1.0	46	31
Cabbage, ckd.	24	92.4	1.4	.2	.8	5.3	1.0	46	31
Celery, raw	18	93.7	1.3	.2	1.1	3.7	.7	50	40
Chard, leaves, raw	27	91	2.6	.4	1.2	4.8	.8	105	36
Chard, leaves and stalks, ckd.	21	91.8	1.4	.2	2.2	4.4	.9	105	36
Chicory, French endive	21	94.2	1.6	.3	1.0	2.9	.8	18	21
Chives	52	86.0	3.8	.6	1.8	7.8	2.0	48	57
Dandelion greens, ckd.	44	85.8	2.7	.7	2.0	8.8	1.8	187	70
Endive, raw	20	93.3	1.6	.2	.9	4.0	.8	79	56
Kale, raw	40	86.6	3.9	.6	1.7	7.2	1.2	225	62
Kale, frz.	32	89.8	3.2	.5	.9	5.6	.9	132	52
Kohlrabi, raw	30	90.1	2.1	.1	1.0	6.7	1.1	46	50
Lettuce, headed	15	94.8	1.2	.2	.9	2.9	.6	22	25
Mustard greens, ckd.	22	92.2	2.3	.3	1.2	4.0	.8	220	38
Onions, mature, raw	45	87.5	1.4	.2	.6	10.3	.1	32	44
Onions, mature, ckd.	38	89.5	1.0	.2	.6	8.7	.8	32	44
Onions, young green	45	87.6	1.0	.2	.6	10.6	1.8	135	24
Parsley	50	83.9	3.7	1.0	2.4	9.0	1.8	193	84
Sauerkraut, cnd.	22	91.2	1.4	.3	2.7	4.4	.9	36	18
Spinach, raw	20	92.7	2.3	.3	1.5	3.2	.6	81	55
Spinach, ckd.	26	90.8	3.1	.6	1.9	3.6	1.0	124	33
Spinach, cnd.	20	92.3	2.3	.4	1.8	3.0	.7	90	33
Turnip greens, raw	30	89.5	2.9	.4	1.8	5.4	1.2	259	50
Turnip greens, ckd.	30	89.5	2.9	.4	1.8	5.4	1.2	259	50
Watercress	18	93.6	1.7	.3	1.1	3.3	.5	195	46
FLOWER, FRUIT, AND SEED VEGETABLES									
Artichoke	63	83.7	2.9	.4	1.1	11.9	3.2	47	94
Beans Red kidney, raw, dry	336	12.2	23.1	1.7	3.6	59.4	3.5	163	437

COMPOSITION
OF EDIBLE PORTION

MINERALS			VITAMINS					AVERAGE PORTION		
Iron, mg	Sodium, mg	Potassium, mg	A, IU	B₁, mg	B₂, mg	Nicotinic acid, mg	C, mg	Total calories	Measure	Weight in grams
3.2	130	570	6,700	.08	.18	.4	34	27	1 cup	100
3.2	—	—	7,440	.05	.16	.4	15	39	1 cup	145
1.3	11	450	400	.08	.16	.7	94	47	1 cup	100
1.3	—	—	400	.04	.12	.5	47	60	1 cup, cooked	130
1.2	11	300	550	.10	.12	.6	83	36	1 cup	100
.5	5	230	80	.06	.05	.3	50	24	Shredded, 1 cup	100
.5	—	—	90	.05	.05	.3	31	40	Ckd., diced, 1 cup	170
.5	110	300	0	.05	.04	.4	7	18	Raw, diced, 1 cup	100
2.5	84	380	8,720	.06	.18	.4	38	27	Leaves, 1½ cups	100
2.5	—	—	3,110	.04	.06	.4	17	30	1 cup	145
.7	—	—	10,000	.05	.20	—	15	3	¼ sm. head	15
8.4	—	—	500	.12	—	—	70	4	1 tbsp, chopped	7
3.1	76	430	15,170	.13	.12	.7	16	80	1 cup greens, ckd.	180
1.7	18	400	3,000	.07	.12	.4	11	90	1 lb, raw	460
2.2	110	410	7,540	.10	.26	2.0	115	70	1¾ cup	175
1.2	29	254	8,000	.07	.17	.8	60	56	1¾ cup	175
.6	—	—	Tr.	.06	.05	.2	61	41	1 cup	138
.5	12	140	540	.04	.08	.2	8	7	2 lg. or 4 sm. leaves	50
2.9	48	450	7,180	.06	.18	.7	45	31	1 cup greens	140
.5	1	130	50	.03	.04	.2	9	50	1, 2½″ diam.	110
.5	—	—	50	.02	.03	.2	6	79	1 cup	210
.9	—	—	50	.03	.04	.2	24	23	6 small, less tops	50
4.3	8	880	8,230	.11	.28	1.4	193	1	1 tbsp	3.5
.5	630	140	40	.03	.06	.1	16	32	Cnd., drained, 1 cup	150
3.0	82	780	9,420	.11	.20	.6	59	22	Raw, 4 oz	115
2.0	—	—	11,780	.08	.20	.6	30	46	Cooked, 1 cup	80
1.6	320	260	6,790	.02	.10	.3	14	45	Canned, 1 cup	232
2.4	10	440	9,540	.09	.46	.8	136	15	Raw, ½ cup	50
2.4	—	—	10,600	.06	.41	.7	60	43	Cooked, 1 cup	145
2.0	—	—	4,720	.08	.16	.8	77	5	½ cup	20
1.9	43	430	390	.15	.03	—	11	33	1, 3″ diam.	50
6.9	—	—	0	.57	.22	2.5	2	638	1 cup	190

TABLES OF FOOD
CONSTITUENTS OF 100 g

		PROXIMATE COMPOSITION						MINERALS	
Name	Cal-ories	Water, g	Pro-tein, g	Fat, g	Ash, g	Total carbohy-drates, g	Crude fiber, g	Calcium, mg	Phos-phorus, mg
FLOWER, FRUIT AND SEED VEGETABLES—Continued									
Beans, Continued									
Red kidney, cnd.									
or ckd.	90	76.0	5.7	.4	1.5	16.4	.9	40	124
Others, raw, dry	338	11.5	21.4	1.6	3.9	61.6	4.0	163	437
Others, bkd., pork									
and molasses	125	70.0	5.8	3.0	2.0	19.2	.9	56	113
Others, bkd., pork									
and tomato sauce	113	71.7	5.8	2.1	2.0	18.4	1.0	41	113
Lima, green, raw	128	66.5	7.5	.8	1.7	23.5	1.5	63	158
Lima, green, ckd.	95	74.9	5.0	.4	1.4	18.3	2.0	29	77
Lima, green, cnd.	71	80.9	3.8	.3	1.5	13.5	1.3	27	73
Lima, green, frz.	100	73.2	6.1	.2	1.5	19.0	1.7	23	102
Lima, dry	333	12.6	20.7	1.3	3.8	61.6	4.3	68	381
Snap, green, raw	35	88.9	2.4	.2	.8	7.7	1.4	65	44
Snap, green, ckd.	22	92.5	1.4	.2	1.2	4.7	.5	36	23
Snap, green, cnd.	18	93.5	1.0	.1	1.2	4.2	.6	27	19
Snap, green, frz.	27	91.6	1.7	.1	.5	6.2	1.1	45	33
Broccoli, raw	29	89.9	3.3	.2	1.1	5.5	1.3	130	76
Broccoli, ckd.	29	89.9	3.3	.2	1.1	5.5	1.3	130	76
Broccoli, frz.	30	90.2	3.4	.3	.8	5.3	1.1	61	63
Cauliflower, raw	25	91.7	2.4	.2	.8	4.9	.9	22	72
Cauliflower, ckd.	25	91.7	2.4	.2	.8	4.9	.9	22	72
Cauliflower, frz.	22	92.7	2.1	.2	.6	4.3	.9	18	45
Corn, sweet, raw	92	73.9	3.7	1.2	.7	20.5	.8	9	120
Corn, sweet, ckd.	85	75.5	2.7	.7	.9	20.2	—	5	52
Corn, sweet, cnd.	67	80.5	2.0	.5	.9	16.1	.8	4	51
Cucumbers, raw	12	96.1	.7	.1	.4	2.7	.5	10	21
Eggplant, raw	24	92.7	1.1	.2	.5	5.5	.9	15	37
Lentils, dry split	339	12.2	24.0	1.2	2.2	60.4	1.7	34	292
Mushrooms, raw	16	91.1	2.4	.3	1.1	4.0	.9	9	115
Mushrooms, canned	11	93.0	1.4	.2	1.0	3.7	—	7	90
Okra, cooked	32	89.8	1.8	.2	.8	7.4	1.0	82	62
Peas, green, raw	98	74.3	6.7	.4	.9	17.7	2.2	22	122
Peas, green, cooked	70	81.7	4.9	.4	.9	12.1	2.2	22	122
Peas, green, cnd.	68	82.3	3.4	.4	1.0	12.9	1.4	25	67
Peas, green, frz.	83	80.3	5.7	.4	.8	12.9	1.8	24	92
Peas, dry, split	344	10.0	24.5	1.0	2.8	61.7	1.2	33	268
Peppers, green, raw	25	92.4	1.2	.2	.5	5.7	1.4	11	25
Pumpkin, raw	31	90.5	1.2	.2	.8	7.3	1.3	21	44

COMPOSITION
OF EDIBLE PORTION

| MINERALS | | | VITAMINS | | | | | AVERAGE PORTION | | |
Iron, mg	Sodium, mg	Potassium, mg	A, IU	B₁, mg	B₂, mg	Nicotinic acid, mg	C, mg	Total calories	Measure	Weight in grams
1.9	—	—	0	.05	.05	.8	0	230	Cnd., or ckd., 1 cup	255
6.9	1	1,300	0	.67	.23	2.2	2	642	1 cup	190
2.1	480	210	30	.05	.04	.5	2	325	Baked, 1 cup	260
1.8	400	140	80	.05	.04	.5	2	295	Baked, 1 cup	260
2.3	1	680	280	.21	.11	1.4	32	96	Green, raw, 1/2 cup	75
1.7	—	—	290	.14	.09	1.1	15	152	Cooked, 1 cup	160
1.7	310	210	130	.04	.04	.5	8	176	Cnd., 1 cup	249
2.3	181	489	220	.11	.06	1.14	21	75	Frozen, 1/2 cup	75
7.5	22.5	1,758	0	.48	.18	2.0	2	610	Dry, 1 cup	183
1.1	.9	300	630	.08	.11	.5	19	26	Raw, 1/4 cup	75
.7	—	—	660	.05	.09	.4	10	27	Cooked, 1 cup	125
1.4	410	120	410	.03	.04	.3	4	27	Canned, 1 cup	125
.8	2	204	570	.07	.11	.4	7	20	Frozen, 1/4 cup	75
1.3	16	400	3,500	.10	.21	1.1	118	25	Raw, 1 cup	120
1.3	—	—	3,400	.07	.15	.8	74	44	Cooked, 1 cup	150
.8	16	244	2,850	.07	.13	.6	62	36	Frozen, 1 cup	120
1.1	24	400	90	.11	.10	.6	69	31	Raw, 1 1/4 cups	125
1.1	—	—	90	.06	.08	.5	28	30	Cooked, 1 cup	120
.6	11	234	33	.06	.06	.4	55	27	Frz., 1 1/4 cups	125
.5	.3–.4	240–370	390	.15	.12	1.7	12	92	1 ear, 8" long	100
.6	—	—	390	.11	.10	1.4	8	85	Ckd., 1 ear, 5"	140
.5	205	200	200	.03	.05	.9	5	140	Cnd., 1 cup	116
.3	.9	230	0	.03	.04	.2	8	6	6, 1/8" slices	50
.4	.9	190	30	.04	.05	.6	5	60	2 slices	250
7.4	3	1,200	570	.56	.24	2.2	5	204	1/4 cup	60
1.0	5	520	0	.10	.44	4.9	5	8	1/2 cup, diced	50
.8	400	150	0	.02	.25	2.0	—	28	Canned, 1 cup	244
.7	1	220	740	.06	.06	.8	20	28	Cooked, 8 pods	85
1.9	1	370	680	.34	.16	2.7	26	74	1/2 cup	75
1.9	—	—	720	.25	.14	2.3	15	111	Cooked, 1 cup	60
1.8	270	96	540	.11	.06	1.0	8	145	Canned, 1 cup	60
2.2	160	153	670	.33	.10	1.9	17	124	Frozen, 1 cup	150
5.1	42	880	370	.77	.28	3.1	2	689	Dry, split, 1 cup	200
.4	.6	170	630	.04	.07	.4	120	16	1 medium	76
.8	.6	480	3,400	.05	.08	.6	8	37	Raw, 3/4 cup	120

TABLES OF FOOD
CONSTITUENTS OF 100 g

	PROXIMATE COMPOSITION							MINERALS	
Name	Cal-ories	Water, g	Pro-tein, g	Fat, g	Ash, g	Total carbohy-drates, g	Crude fiber, g	Calcium, mg	Phos-phorus, mg
FLOWER, FRUIT AND SEED VEGETABLES—Continued									
Pumpkin, cnd.	33	90.2	1.0	.3	.6	7.9	1.2	20	36
Soybeans, dry	331	7.5	34.9	18.1	4.7	34.8	5.0	227	586
Soybean flour, med. fat	264	9	42.5	6.5	4.8	37.2	2.6	244	610
Soybean sprouts, raw	46	86.3	6.2	1.4	.8	5.3	.8	48	67
Squash, summer, raw	16	95.0	.6	.1	.4	3.9	.5	15	15
Squash, summer, frz.	21	93.4	1.4	.1	.4	4.7	.6	14	32
Squash, winter, raw	38	88.6	1.5	.3	.8	8.8	1.4	19	28
Squash, winter, ckd.	47	85.7	1.9	.4	1.0	11.0	1.8	24	35
Squash, winter, frz.	33	89.2	1.2	.4	.51	8.8	1.2	27	33
Succotash, frz.	97	66.3	4.5	.4	.8	21.4	.9	15	90
Tomatoes, raw	20	94.1	1.0	.3	.6	4.0	.6	11	27
Tomatoes, canned	19	94.2	1.0	.2	.7	3.9	.4	11	27
Tomato ketchup	98	69.5	2.0	.4	3.6	24.5	.4	12	18
Tomato puree, cnd.	36	89.2	1.8	.5	1.3	7.2	.4	11	37
MISCELLANEOUS									
Beer (4% alcohol)	20–48	90.2	.6	0	.2	4.4	—	4	26
Coffee, black	4	99	.2	0	—	.7	0	4	4
Cola beverages	46	88	—	—	—	12	—	—	—
Ginger ale	35	91	—	—	—	9	—	—	—
Popcorn	386	4.0	12.7	5.0	1.6	76.7	2.2	11	281
Potato chips	544	3.1	6.7	37.1	4.0	49.1	1.1	30	152
Yeast, bakers', compressed	86	70.9	10.6	.4	2.4	13.0	.3	25	605
Yeast, brewers', dry	273	7.0	36.9	1.6	7.9	37.4	.8	106	1,893

COMPOSITION
OF EDIBLE PORTION

MINERALS			VITAMINS					AVERAGE PORTION		
Iron, mg	Sodium, mg	Potassium, mg	A, IU	B₁, mg	B₂, mg	Nicotinic Acid, mg	C, mg	Total calories	Measure	Weight in grams
.7	2	240	3,400	.02	.06	.5	—	76	Canned, 1 cup	228
8.0	4	1,900	110	1.07	.31	2.3	Tr.	695	Dry, 1 cup	210
13.0	1	1,700	110	.82	.34	2.6	0	232	1 cup	88
1.0	—	—	180	.23	.20	.8	13	50	Raw, 1 cup	107
.4	.2	150	260	.05	.09	.8	17	40	1 3/4 cups, diced	250
.6	4	169	150	.07	.04	.4	6	44	Ckd., diced, 1 cup	210
.6	.3	240	4,950	.05	.12	.5	8	95	1 3/4 cups, diced	250
.8	—	—	6,190	.05	.15	.6	7	97	Mashed, 1 cup	205
1.3	.2	209	4,280	.03	.07	.5	7	82	1 3/4 cups, diced	250
1.2	73	279	167	.11	.06	1.5	7	205	3/4 cup, ckd.	210
.6	3	230	1,100	.06	.04	.5	23	30	1 med., 2×2 1/2"	150
.6	18	130	1,050	.06	.03	.7	16	46	Canned, 1 cup	242
.8	1,300	800	1,880	.09	.07	2.2	11	17	1 tbsp	17
1.1	—	—	1,880	.09	.07	1.8	28	90	1 cup	249
0	8	46	0	Tr.	.03	.2	0	72–173	12 oz	360
.5	.03	16.2	—	—	—	—	0	9	1 cup	230
—	1	52	—	—	—	—	—	83	6 oz	180
—	8	.6	—	—	—	—	—	63	6 oz	180
2.7	2,000	240	0	.39	.12	2.2	0	54	1 cup, popped	14
1.9	340	880	50	.18	.11	3.2	11	108	10 medium, 2"	20
4.9	4	360	0	.45	2.07	28.2	0	24	1 oz	28
18.2	150	1,700	0	9.69	5.45	36.2	0	22	1 tbsp	8

Index